SECOND EDITION

SECTIONAL ANATOMY BY MRI

SECOND EDITION

SECTIONAL ANATOMY BY MRI

GEORGES Y. EL-KHOURY, M.D.
Professor
Departments of Radiology and Orthopaedic Surgery
University of Iowa College of Medicine
Iowa City, Iowa

RONALD A. BERGMAN, Ph.D.
Professor
Department of Anatomy
University of Iowa College of Medicine
Iowa City, Iowa

WILLIAM J. MONTGOMERY, M.D.
Associate Professor
Department of Radiology
University of Florida College of Medicine
Gainesville, Florida

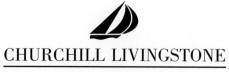

CHURCHILL LIVINGSTONE

An Imprint of Elsevier Science
New York, Edinburgh, London, Philadelphia

CHURCHILL LIVINGSTONE
An Imprint of Elsevier Science

The Curtis Center
Independence Square West
Philadelphia, Pennsylvania 19106

Library of Congress Cataloging-in-Publishing Data

EI-Khoury, Georges Y.
    Sectional anatomy by MRI / Georges Y. EI-Khoury, Ronald A.
Bergman, William J. Montgomery.—2nd ed.
        p. cm.
    Rev. ed. of: Sectional anatomy by MRI/CT / Georges Y. EI-Khoury,
Ronald A. Bergman, William J, Montgomery. 1990.
    Includes bibliographical references and index.
    ISBN 0-443-08890-X
    1. Human anatomy—Atlases. 2. Magnetic resonance imaging-
-Atlases. 3. Tomography—Atlases. I. Bergman, Ronald A. (Ronald
Arly). II. Montgomery, William J. III. EI-Khoury,
Georges J. Sectional anatomy by MRI. IV. Title.
    [DNLM: 1. Anatomy, Regional—atlases. 2. Magnetic Resonance
Imaging—atlases. QS 17 E44sa 1995]
    QM25.E38 1995
    611.9 0222—dc20
    DNLM/DLC   94-32581

Second Edition © Churchill Livingstone Inc. 1995
First Edition © Churchill Livingstone Inc. 1990

Permissions may be sought directly from Elsevier's Health Sciences Rights Department in Philadelphia, USA:
phone: (+1)215-238-7869, fax: (+1)215-238-2239, email: healthpermissions@elsevier.com. You may also
complete your request on-line via the Elsevier Science homepage (http://www.elsevier.com), by selecting
'Customer Support' and then 'Obtaining Permissions'.

Churchill Livingstone and the Sail Boat Design are trademarks of Elsevier Science.

Distributed in the United Kingdom by Churchill Livingstone, Robert Stevenson House, 1–3 Baxter's Place, Leith
Walk, Edinburgh EH1 3AF, and by associated companies, branches, and representatives throughout the world.

The cover illustrations are by Leonardo da Vinci and were made available by the Windsor Castle, Royal Library.
They are used by the gracious permission of Her Majesty, Queen Elizabeth II.

Printed in China

Last digit is the print number   7

To our wives, Salam, Phyllis, and Nancy.
Without their love and support
this work
would not have been possible.

CONTRIBUTORS

Thomas J. Gilbert, M.D.

Assistant Professor, Department of Radiology, University of Minnesota Medical School; Orthopedic Radiologist, Suburban Radiologic Consultants, Minneapolis, Minnesota

Hiroshi Honda, M.D.

Assistant Professor, Department of Radiology, Kyushu University Faculty of Medicine, Fukuoka, Japan

Daniel J. Loes, M.D.

Assistant Clinical Professor, Department of Radiology, University of Minnesota Medical School; Director of Neuroradiology and Magnetic Resonance Imaging, Suburban Radiologic Consultants, Minneapolis, Minnesota

Christopher F. Pope, M.D.

Associate Clinical Professor, Department of Medicine, University of Vermont College of Medicine, Burlington, Vermont; Director, Section of Magnetic Resonance Imaging, Department of Radiology, Maine Medical Center, Portland, Maine

William Stanford, M.D.

Professor, Department of Radiology, University of Iowa College of Medicine; Chief, Division of Cardiovascular Radiology, Department of Radiology, University of Iowa Hospitals and Clinics, Iowa City, Iowa

Saara M.S. Totterman, M.D.

Associate Professor, Department of Radiology, University of Rochester School of Medicine and Dentistry; Director, Magnetic Resonance Center, Department of Radiology, University of Rochester Medical Center, Rochester, New York

Craig W. Walker, M.D.

Assistant Professor, Department of Radiology, University of Nebraska College of Medicine, Omaha, Nebraska

Camelia G. Whitten, M.D.

Musculoskeletal Radiologist, Department of Radiology, St. Cloud Hospital, St. Cloud, Minnesota

PREFACE TO THE SECOND EDITION

Traditionally, neuroradiologists have been expected to be experts in the anatomy of the central nervous system and encasing structures. Other radiologists investigating different organ systems are currently held to similar standards. Young physicians who have chosen diagnostic imaging as a career need to realize early in their studies the importance of mastering anatomy. In medicine, anatomy commands a status analogous to that of currency or money in commerce; there is no commerce without money. Anatomy is the currency or language of medicine. Communication among health professionals can be severely hampered without the accurate use of anatomy.

Advances and refinements in pulse sequences and surface coils have enhanced the ability of radiologists to identify a wide variety of soft-tissue structures. These advances have affected all subspecialties but the impact has been most pronounced in musculoskeletal radiology. There is little doubt that the survival of musculoskeletal radiology as a subspecialty has been enhanced by the advent of magnetic resonance imaging (MRI). MR evaluation of ligaments, tendons, muscles, vessels, and nerves is now commonplace.

Sectional Anatomy by MRI is intended for radiologists and other clinicians interested in sectional anatomy. In this edition, the computed tomographic (CT) images have been eliminated to avoid redundancy. We have recruited the help of several experts who contributed images and other material for this atlas.

In our daily practice, we saw the need for a detailed reference for anatomic relationships and names of structures. The first edition served this purpose well. Since the first edition was published, the technology has matured, and progress in MR has plateaued somewhat. We are again hopeful that this atlas will fulfill the needs of practicing radiologists.

Georges Y. El-Khoury, M.D.
Ronald A. Bergman, Ph.D.
William J. Mongtomery, M.D.

PREFACE TO THE FIRST EDITION

In recent years, as a response to giant strides in imaging technology, there has been a surge of interest in anatomy by radiologists. The most acute need has been in the area of the musculoskeletal system. However, most of the current books and atlases that we have consulted in our clinical practice have failed to provide necessary information and to satisfy our curiosity. Yet, detailed anatomic reviews with our anatomist colleagues resulted in a deeper understanding of our imaging studies, improved our insight into disease processes, and enhanced our ability to communicate with the referring physicians.

As work in sectional anatomy proceeded, this new excitement and enthusiasm grew and, in some instances, became contagious. Our residents demanded more instruction in clinical anatomy, and we established courses to teach sectional anatomy to fourth year medical students and to introduce sectional anatomy at the freshman level. The desire to share our new mode of providing information led us to contact Toni M. Tracy, President of Churchill Livingstone Inc., who encouraged us to prepare a detailed sectional anatomy atlas.

This atlas, *Sectional Anatomy by MRI/CT*, is intended to be used by radiologists and other clinicians interested in sectional anatomy, and by anatomists, principally as an anatomic reference for the body sectioned in all three standard planes.

There are some areas of necessary duplication within the atlas. For instance, the coronal and sagittal sections of the pelvis include the proximal thigh. Similarly, in the thigh, there are images of the adjacent pelvic region. We think this is of value, as visualization of adjacent structures beyond the traditional compartments are frequently necessary in clinical practice. We also believe that the systematic study of anatomy in multiple planes leads to a greater understanding of the spatial relationships between structures.

The book is divided into anatomic regions. These regions are then imaged in the three standard planes. The more familiar axial plane is portrayed first, followed by the coronal and sagittal planes. All images are from normal volunteers; no cadaveric studies are included. This accounts for some of the variability in muscle mass and body fat between different subjects.

Computed tomography (CT) has been used in conjunction with magnetic resonance imaging (MRI) in the abdomen and thorax. CT is used to demonstrate the axial anatomy of the upper abdomen, because respiratory motion degrades MRI quality. Images from a ciné-CT (ultrafast) scanner have been used to augment the MRI of the thorax.

In this atlas, axial sections start proximally or cephalad and advance distally or caudally. Coronal sections start posteriorly or dorsally and advance anteriorly or ventrally, and sagittal sections, in most regions, start medially and advance laterally. Through figure labelling, the anatomic make-up of the image is identified, and the atlas uses the following abbreviations: *m.*, muscle; *mm.*, muscles; *a.*, artery; *aa.*, arteries; *v.*, vein; *vv.*, veins.

Subjects were scanned lying in the anatomic position, i.e., the subject lying straight with the feet together and the toes directed upward, arms by the side, and palms of the hands facing upward. In sections of the foot, the definition of axial and coronal is strictly based on the position of the feet of the recumbent subject in the anatomic position.

For us, the creation of this book has fulfilled a need that started with the early days of CT and became acute with the advent of MRI. We are hopeful that *Sectional Anatomy by MRI/CT* will also fulfill this need for others.

Georges Y. El-Khoury, M.D.
Ronald A. Bergman, Ph.D.
William J. Montgomery, M.D.

ACKNOWLEDGMENTS

We are indebted to Phyllis S. Bergman for her expert editorial help and to Mary McBride and Marna Getting for their diligent secretarial assistance. We are also grateful to Heidi Berns and Sally Hofdahl, who took meticulous care in preparing many of the images for the book. During the past fifteen years, Dr. E.A. Franken, Jr., established and nurtured a healthy academic environment within which to work and create. We will be ever thankful for his support.

Georges Y. El-Khoury, M.D.
Ronald A. Bergman, Ph.D.
William J. Montgomery, M.D.

CONTENTS

Chapter 1

NECK

Soft Tissue Neck

The soft tissue neck is usually considered to extend from the hard palate to the clavicles. It can be subdivided by the hyoid bone into suprahyoid and infrahyoid regions. The suprahyoid neck extends above the hard palate and includes the extracranial soft tissue structures of the face excluding the orbits and paranasal sinuses. The caudal extent of the infrahyoid neck also lacks a distinct boundary as contents of this region normally extend into the superior mediastinum and axillary regions.

The suprahyoid neck is divided into eight main spaces: parapharyngeal, masticator, parotid, carotid, pharyngeal mucosa, retropharyngeal, prevertebral, and posterior cervical spaces. The oral cavity, which is frequently imaged with the suprahyoid neck, contains two compartments: the sublingual and submandibular spaces. The parapharyngeal space is a nonfascially enclosed area containing mainly fat. Its central position in the suprahyoid neck helps to outline anatomy and pathology in the remaining suprahyoid neck spaces. The masticator space contains the muscles of mastication and the posterior body and ramus of the mandible. The parotid space contains the parotid gland, the intraparotid branches of the facial nerve, the retromandibular vein, and intraparotid lymph nodes. The carotid space contains the internal carotid artery; internal jugular vein; sympathetic plexus; and glossopharyngeal, vagus, and spinal accessory nerves (cranial nerves IX through XI) as they exit the jugular foramen; and lymph nodes. The pharyngeal mucosa space contains primarily mucosa and the lymphoid tissue of Waldeyer's ring. The retropharyngeal space is primarily a potential space, although it normally contains small medial and lateral retropharyngeal lymph nodes. The prevertebral space contains prevertebral musculature, posterior paraspinal musculature, and the bony vertebral column. The posterior cervical space contains spinal accessory lymph nodes, the spinal accessory nerve (cranial nerve XI), and fat.

The infrahyoid neck contains five main spaces: visceral, carotid, retropharyngeal, prevertebral, and posterior cervical spaces. The visceral space, unique to the infrahyoid neck, contains the thyroid gland, parathyroid glands, larynx, trachea, esophagus, and recurrent laryngeal nerve. The remaining infrahyoid spaces are shared with the suprahyoid neck. The carotid space in the infrahyoid neck contains the common carotid artery, vagus nerve (cranial nerve X), internal jugular vein, and deep cervical lymph nodes. The prevertebral space in the infrahyoid neck contains the phrenic nerve and brachial plexus, as well as the prevertebral and paraspinal musculature.

Neck anatomy may also be delineated by surgical and gross anatomic triangles created by muscle attachments and the hyoid bone. The sternocleidomastoid muscle divides the neck into anterior and posterior triangles. The hyoid bone and the anterior bellies of the digastric muscles subdivide the suprahyoid anterior triangle into a medial submental triangle and the lateral submandibular triangles. The superior belly of the omohyoid muscle divides the infrahyoid anterior triangle into medial muscular and more lateral carotid triangles. The inferior belly of the omohyoid muscle divides the posterior triangle into the more superior occipital triangle and an inferior subclavian triangle.

2

1. These sagittal images begin in the midline and progress laterally.

2. The level of the true vocal cord on sagittal images can be located by identifying either the superior margin of the cricoid cartilage or the inferior margin of the arytenoid cartilages.

3. The spinous processes are interconnected via interspinous muscles and ligaments.

4. Portions of the sphenoid and occipital bones unite to form the clivus.

Figure 1.1.1

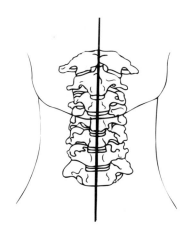

Clivus

Nasopharynx

C1 anterior arch

Genioglossus m.

Oropharynx

Epiglottis

Mylohyoid and geniohyoid mm.

Hypopharynx

Cricoid cartilage

Trachea

Manubrium

Basion

Opisthion

C1 posterior arch

Semispinalis capitis m.

Mylohyoid m

Transverse arytenoid m.

Level of true vocal cords

Trapezius m.

Figure 1.1.2

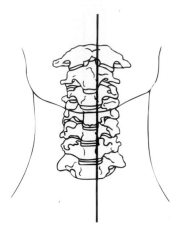

1. The ligamentum nuchae, the cervical portion of the supraspinous ligament, attaches inferiorly to the C7 spinous process and superiorly to the external occipital protuberance.

2. The laryngeal ventricle is located between the false and true vocal cords.

3. The hyoid bone divides the neck into suprahyoid and infrahyoid regions.

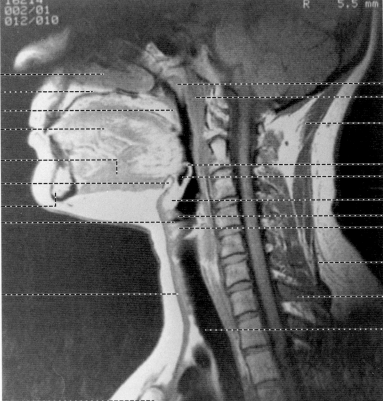

Inferior conchae
Hard palate
Palatopharyngeus m.
Genioglossus m.
Mylohyoid and geniohyoid mm.
Hyoid bone
Mandible, body
Laryngeal vestibule
Infrahyoid mm.
Manubrium

Adenoids
Longus capitis m.
Semispinalis capitis m.
Epiglottis
Vallecula
Preepiglottic space
False vocal cords
True vocal cords
Ligamentum nuchae
C7 spinous process
Trachea

1. The sternohyoid and sternothyroid muscles originate from the posterior margin of the sternal manubrium.

2. The sternal head of the sternocleidomastoid muscle arises from the anterior margin of the sternal manubrium.

Figure 1.1.3

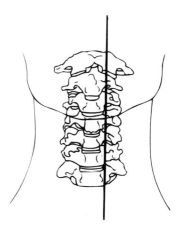

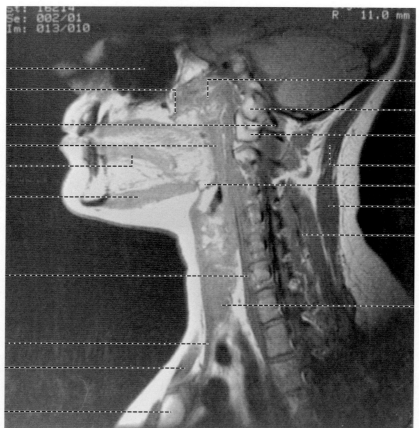

Maxillary antrum

Tensor veli palatini m.

Vertebral a.

Superior constrictor m.

Genioglossus m.

Mylohyoid and geniohyoid mm.

Longus colli m.

Sternohyoid and sternothyroid mm.

Sternocleidomastoid m., sternal head

Manubrium

Levator veli palatini m.

Occipital condyle

C1 lateral mass

Semispinalis capitis m.

Hyoid bone

Trapezius m.

Multifidus M.

Thyroid gland

Figure 1.1.4

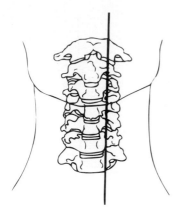

1. The suboccipital muscles consist of the rectus capitis posterior major and minor and the oblique capitus superior and inferior.

2. The suboccipital triangle is delineated by the oblique capitis superior and inferior muscles and the rectus capitis posterior muscle.

3. The suboccipital triangle contains the vertebral artery as it pierces the dura of the posterior atlanto-occipital membrane to gain entrance to the subarachnoid space.

4. The first spinal nerve also transverses the suboccipital triangle.

5. The thyroid gland is covered anteriorly by strap muscles.

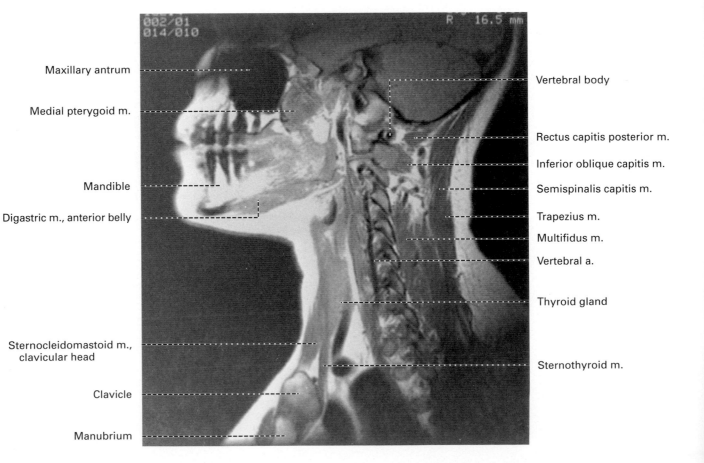

1. A communicating vein between the anterior jugular veins crosses through the suprasternal space of Burn anterior to the infrahyoid strap muscles.

Figure 1.1.5

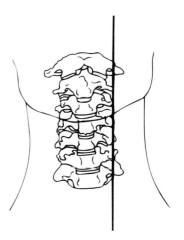

Maxillary antrum

Lateral pterygoid m.

Medial pterygoid m.

Mandible

Longus colli m.

Common carotid a.

Sternocleidomastoid m., clavicular head

Sternothyroid m.

Communicating v.

Clavicle, head

Rectus capitis posterior m.

Inferior oblique capitis m.

Semispinalis capitis m.

Trapezius m.

Suprasternal space of Burn

Figure 1.1.6

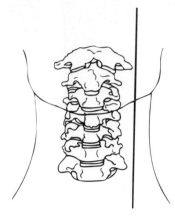

1. In addition to being more lateral, the lateral pterygoid muscle is also located superior to its neighbor the medial pterygoid muscle.

2. The superior and inferior relationships of the pterygoid muscles are determined by the insertion of the lateral pterygoid muscle onto the mandibular condyle and meniscus and the insertion of the medial pterygoid muscle onto the posterior mandibular ramus.

3. The submandibular gland is located inferior to the medial pterygoid muscle and the angle of the mandible.

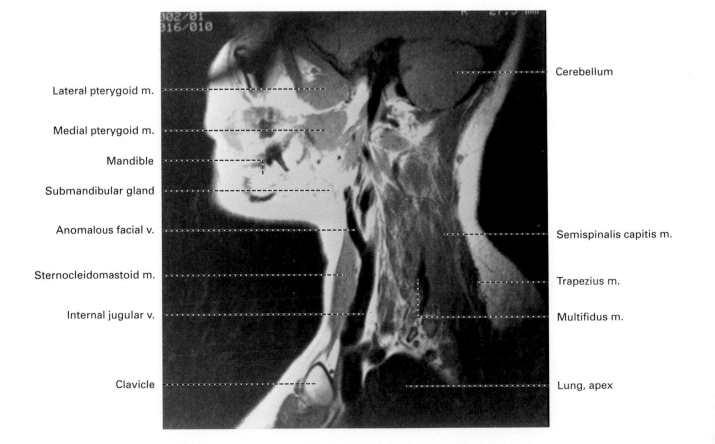

1. The clavicular head of the sternocleidomastoid muscle can be identified on this section.

2. The middle and posterior scalene, levator scapulae, and splenius capitis muscles, respectively, form the "floor" of the posterior cervical space (posterior triangle) in an anteroinferior to posterosuperior direction.

Figure 1.1.7

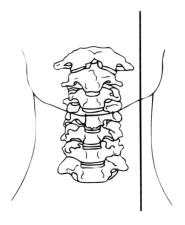

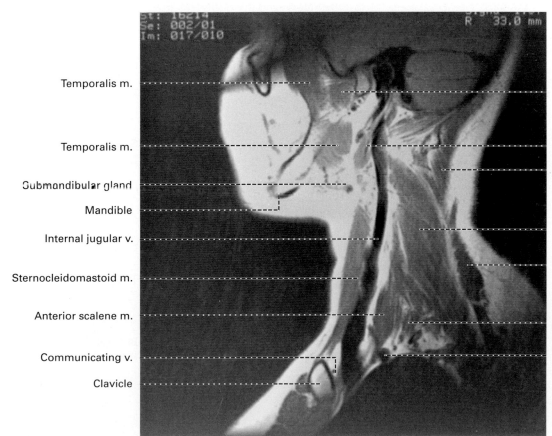

Figure 1.1.8

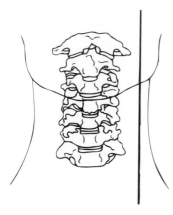

1. The anterior scalene muscle is positioned between the anteriorly located subclavian vein and the posteriorly located subclavian artery.

2. The brachial plexus and subclavian artery pass between the anterior and middle scalene muscles.

3. The sternocleidomastoid and trapezius muscles delineate the posterior triangle (posterior cervical space).

4. The posterior cervical space contains the spinal accessory nerve (cranial nerve XI) and the spinal accessory lymph node chain.

5. Both the sternocleidomastoid and trapezius muscles are innervated by the spinal accessory nerve.

6. The posterior belly of the digastric muscle innervated by the facial nerve (cranial nerve VII) extends from the mastoid process to the hyoid bone.

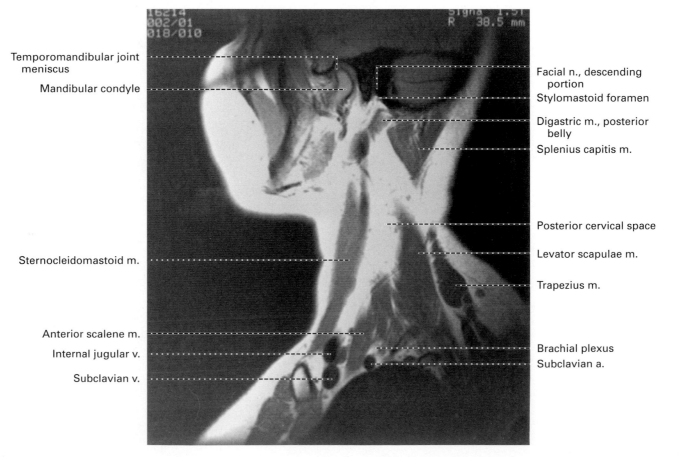

Temporomandibular joint meniscus
Mandibular condyle
Sternocleidomastoid m.
Anterior scalene m.
Internal jugular v.
Subclavian v.

Facial n., descending portion
Stylomastoid foramen
Digastric m., posterior belly
Splenius capitis m.
Posterior cervical space
Levator scapulae m.
Trapezius m.
Brachial plexus
Subclavian a.

1. The mastoid process is a traction epiphysis that grows until skeletal maturity under the pull of primarily the sternocleidomastoid muscle.

2. The masseter muscle originates from the zygomatic arch.

3. The retromandibular vein courses through the parotid gland and empties into the external jugular vein, which lies on the superficial surface to the sternocleidomastoid muscle.

4. The sternocleidomastoid muscle has two heads originating from the sternum and the clavicle and one insertion on the mastoid process of the temporal bone.

Figure 1.1.9

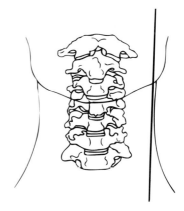

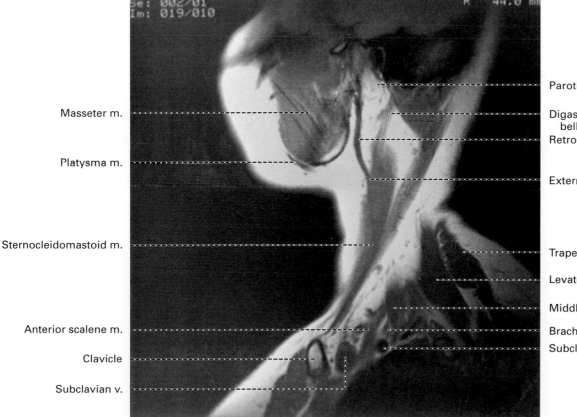

Figure 1.2.1

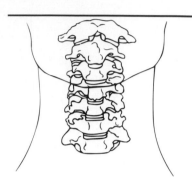

1. This axial image is at the level of the hard palate.

2. The lower nasopharynx can be identified by three landmarks: the fossa of Rosenmüller, the torus tubarius, and the eustachian tube orifice.

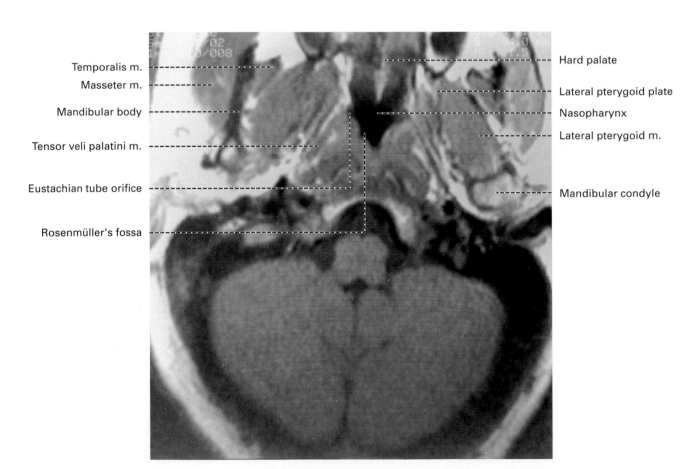

Temporalis m. — Hard palate

Masseter m. — Lateral pterygoid plate

Mandibular body — Nasopharynx

Tensor veli palatini m. — Lateral pterygoid m.

Eustachian tube orifice — Mandibular condyle

Rosenmüller's fossa

1. The parotid duct (Stensen's duct) courses lateral to the masseter muscle before piercing the buccinator muscle to enter the oral cavity at the level of the second upper molar tooth.

2. The lower head of the lateral pterygoid muscle originates from the lateral surface of the lateral pterygoid plate whereas the medial pterygoid muscle arises primarily from the medial surface of the lateral pterygoid plate.

3. The muscles of mastication, which include the masseter, temporalis, lateral pterygoid, and medial pterygoid muscles, are innervated by the mandibular division (V3) of the trigeminal nerve (cranial nerve V).

Figure 1.2.2

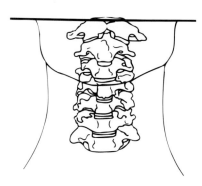

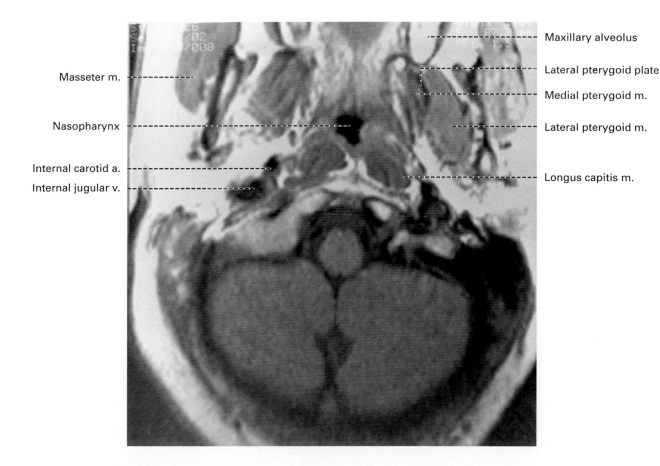

Maxillary alveolus

Lateral pterygoid plate

Medial pterygoid m.

Masseter m.

Lateral pterygoid m.

Nasopharynx

Internal carotid a.

Longus capitis m.

Internal jugular v.

Figure 1.2.3

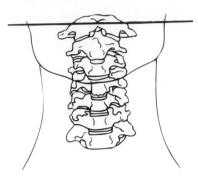

1. The buccinator muscle acts as a sphincter for Stenson's duct; it prevents air from entering the parotid gland.

2. The lingual septum divides the free tongue into right and left halves.

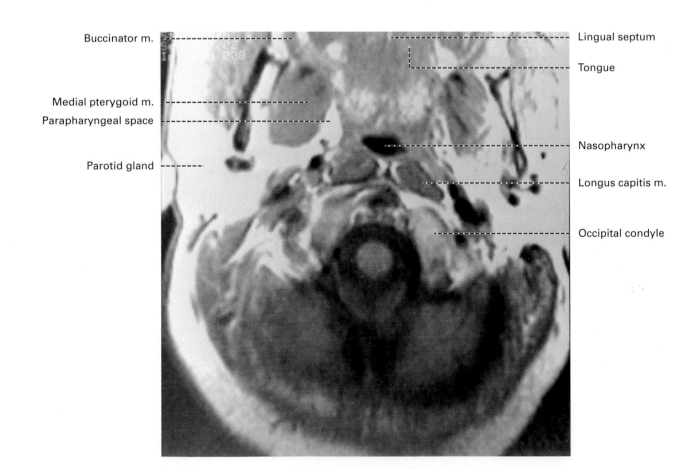

Buccinator m.

Medial pterygoid m.

Parapharyngeal space

Parotid gland

Lingual septum

Tongue

Nasopharynx

Longus capitis m.

Occipital condyle

1. The parapharyngeal space, a nonfascially enclosed space that contains little more than fat and a few small vessels, is a key anatomic space in the suprahyoid neck owing to its central position between the masticator space, parotid space, carotid space, and pharyngeal muscosal space.

2. Within the parotid gland, the retromandibular veins are situated lateral to the external carotid artery (facial branch).

3. The intraparotid facial nerve, which divides the parotid gland into the surgically important superficial and deep lobes, courses immediately lateral to the retromandibular vein.

4. At the C1 level, the vertebral arteries course laterally to the ring of C1 before turning medially and cephalad to enter the subarachnoid space over the posterior arch of C1.

Figure 1.2.4

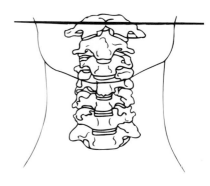

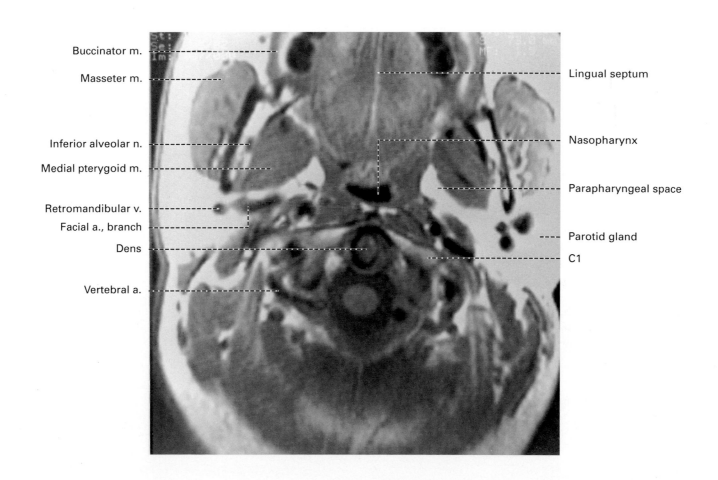

Figure 1.2.5

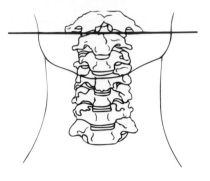

1. The uvula, a midline inferior extension of the soft palate, projects into the oropharynx.

2. The semispinalis capitis and the rectus capitis posterior muscles are the largest muscle groups immediately inferior to the occipital bone.

3. The superior constrictor muscle forms the bed of tonsils, enclosing the palatine tonsils, the palatoglossus muscles, which form the anterior tonsillar pillars, and the palatopharyngeus muscles, which form the posterior tonsillar pillars.

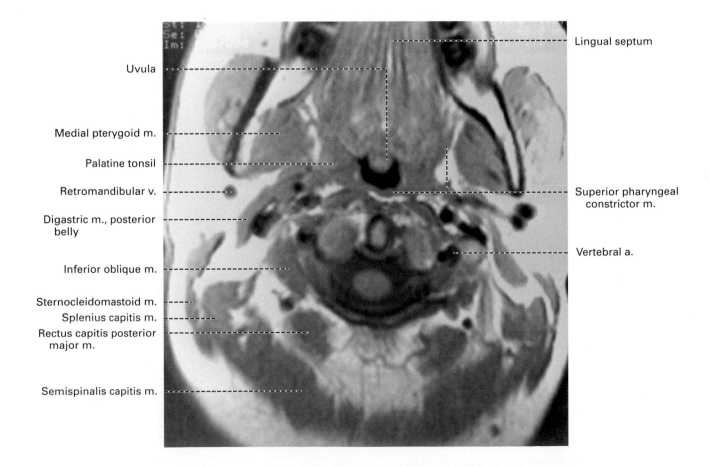

1. The internal jugular vein follows the oblique course of the sternocleidomastoid muscle; it lies posterolateral to the internal carotid artery near the skull base and anterolateral to the common carotid artery in the lower neck.

2. The vagus nerve travels between the internal carotid artery and internal jugular vein.

3. The carotid sheath contains the internal jugular vein, vagus nerve, and the common and internal carotid arteries.

4. The cervical sympathetic chain is embedded within the posteromedial aspect of the carotid sheath.

5. The lateral retropharyngeal lymph nodes, which are normally prominent in children, are located anteromedial to the internal carotid artery at the level of the skull base.

Figure 1.2.6

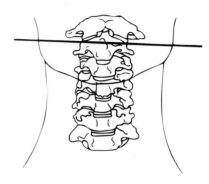

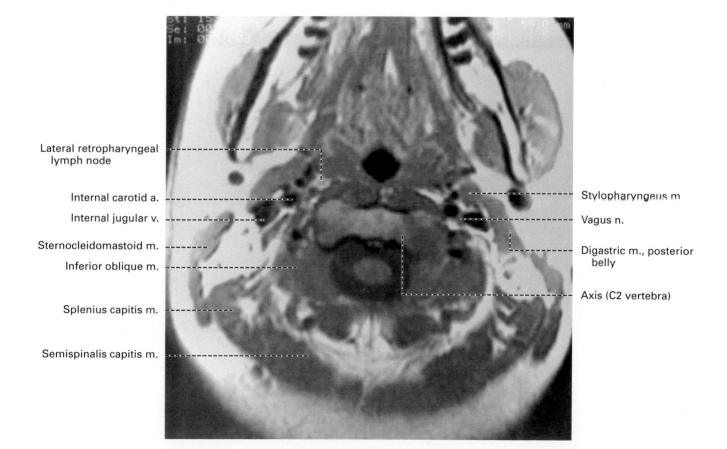

Lateral retropharyngeal lymph node

Internal carotid a.

Internal jugular v.

Sternocleidomastoid m.

Inferior oblique m.

Splenius capitis m.

Semispinalis capitis m.

Stylopharyngeus m

Vagus n.

Digastric m., posterior belly

Axis (C2 vertebra)

Figure 1.2.7

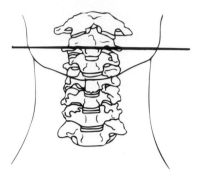

1. The mylohyoid muscle separates the deeper sublingual space from the more superficially located submandibular space.

2. The sublingual and submandibular spaces are in direct communication posteriorly along the free edge of the mylohyoid.

3. The hyoglossus muscle is a useful landmark; Wharton's duct (submandibular duct) and the hypoglossal nerve (cranial nerve XII) travel superficially and the lingual artery passes deep with respect to this muscle.

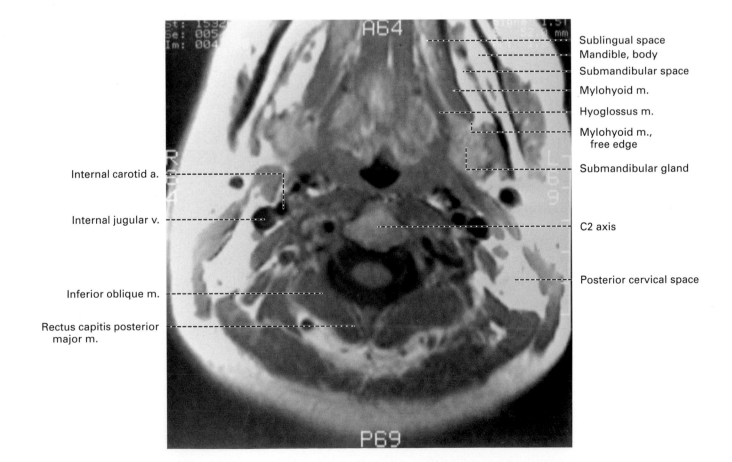

1. The suprahyoid muscles, composed of the digastric, mylohyoid, stylohyoid, and geniohyoid muscles, are responsible for elevating the hyoid bone during swallowing.

2. In the suprahyoid neck, the floor of the posterior cervical space (posterior triangle) is formed by the levator scapulae and splenius capitus muscles.

Figure 1.2.8

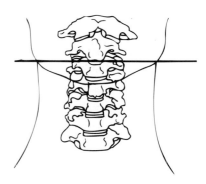

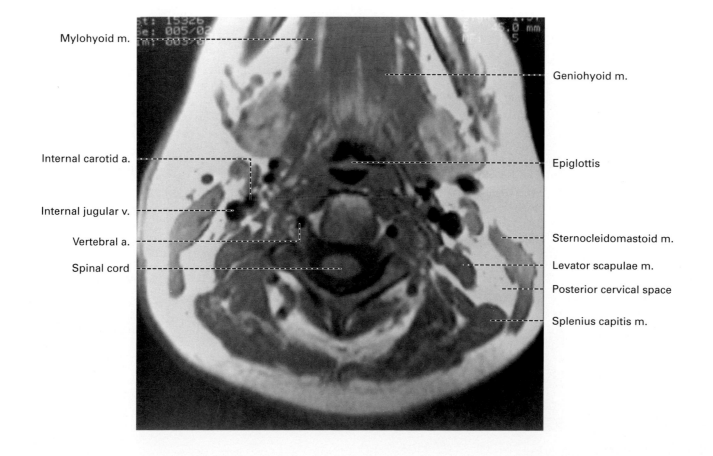

Figure 1.2.9

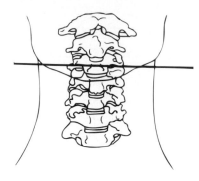

1. The hyoid bone marks the level of the third cervical vertebra.

2. Due to its fascial and muscular attachments, the hyoid bone divides the neck into two main compartments: the suprahyoid neck and the infrahyoid neck.

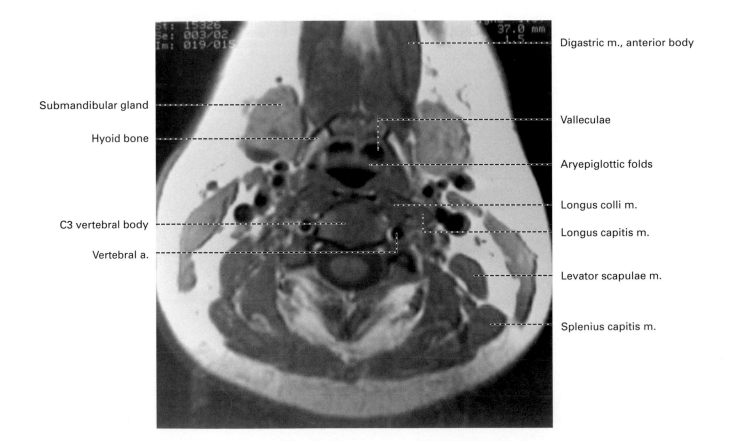

1. The carotid artery bifurcation is usually located immediately below the level of the hyoid bone.

2. The internal carotid artery most often is posterolateral to the external carotid artery at its point of origin.

Figure 1.2.10

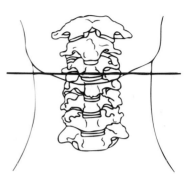

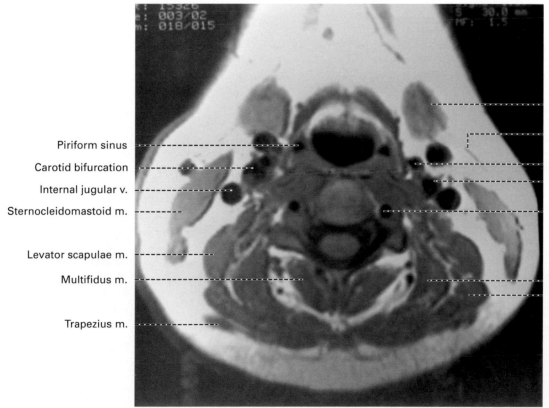

Piriform sinus

Carotid bifurcation

Internal jugular v.

Sternocleidomastoid m.

Levator scapulae m.

Multifidus m.

Trapezius m.

Submandibular gland

Platysma m.

External carotid a.

Internal carotid a.

Vertebral a.

Semispinalis capitis m.
Splenius capitis m.

Figure 1.2.11

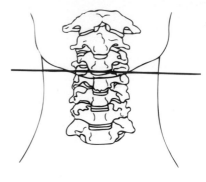

1. The infrahyoid muscles, also known as the strap muscles, consist of the sternohyoid, thyrohyoid, omohyoid, and sternothyroid muscles.

2. The infrahyoid muscles aid tongue movements by stabilizing the hyoid bone and assist phonation by moving the larynx.

3. The aryepiglottic folds form the medial margins of the pyriform sinuses.

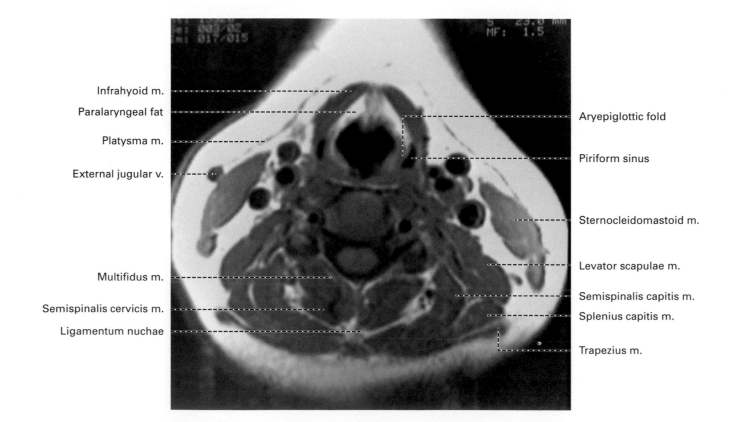

1. The platysma muscle, which lies in the superficial fascia, extends from the mandible to the upper thoracic region.

2. Known as the cervical equivalent of the facial muscle, the platysma as well as the other facial muscles are innervated by the facial nerve (cranial nerve VII).

Figure 1.2.12

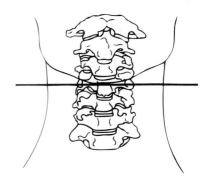

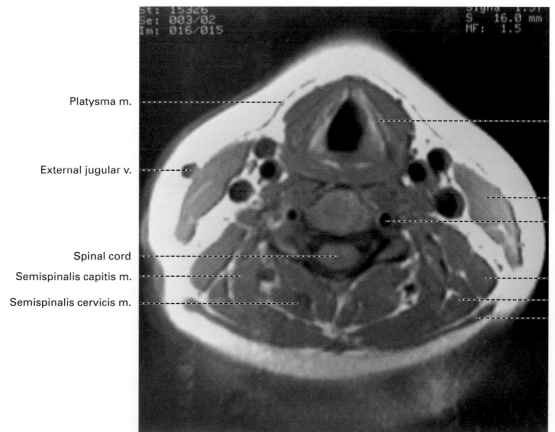

Platysma m.

External jugular v.

Spinal cord
Semispinalis capitis m.
Semispinalis cervicis m.

Thyroid cartilage

Sternocleidomastoid m.
Vertebral a.

Levator scapulae m.
Splenius capitis m.
Trapezius m.

Figure 1.2.13

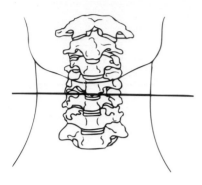

1. This axial image is at the level of the true vocal cords.

2. The true vocal cords are attached posteriorly to the arytenoid cartilages and are connected to each other via the anterior commissure.

3. The striated muscle fibers of the inferior constrictor muscle blend with the smooth muscle fibers of the esophagus at the level of the cricoid cartilage.

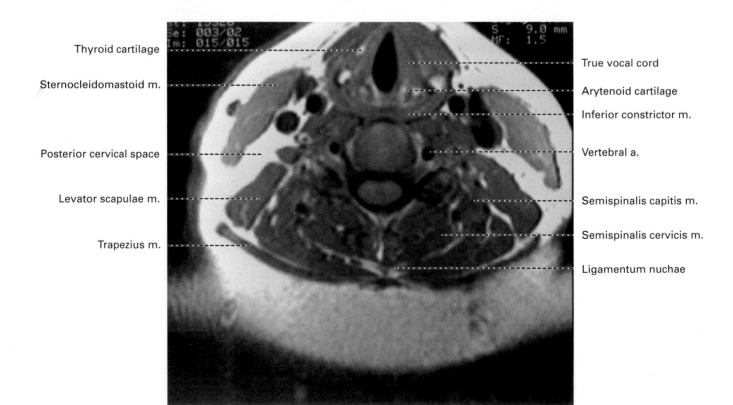

Thyroid cartilage

Sternocleidomastoid m.

Posterior cervical space

Levator scapulae m.

Trapezius m.

True vocal cord

Arytenoid cartilage

Inferior constrictor m.

Vertebral a.

Semispinalis capitis m.

Semispinalis cervicis m.

Ligamentum nuchae

1. The cricothyroid membrane is the safest place to perform an emergent tracheostomy as numerous vessels and the thyroid gland are potential hazards below the cricoid cartilage.

2. The external jugular vein is located superficial to the sternocleidomastoid muscle and deep to the platysma muscle.

Figure 1.2.14

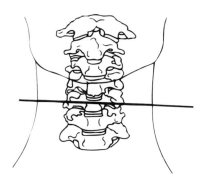

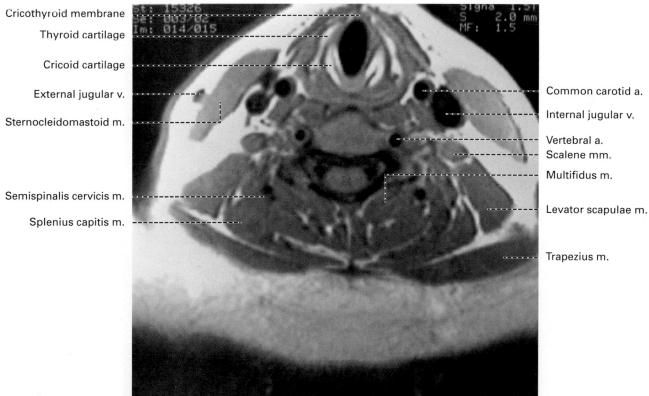

Cricothyroid membrane
Thyroid cartilage
Cricoid cartilage
External jugular v.
Sternocleidomastoid m.
Semispinalis cervicis m.
Splenius capitis m.

Common carotid a.
Internal jugular v.
Vertebral a.
Scalene mm.
Multifidus m.
Levator scapulae m.
Trapezius m.

Figure 1.2.15

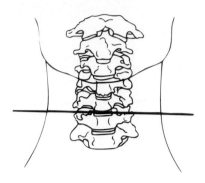

1. This axial image is located at the level of the cricoid cartilage.

2. The thyroid gland, located between the infrahyoid muscles and the airway, usually extends from the base of the thyroid cartilage to the level of the fifth or sixth tracheal ring.

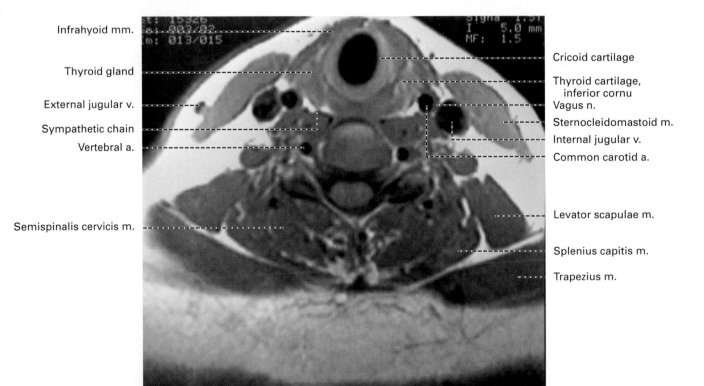

Infrahyoid mm.

Thyroid gland

External jugular v.

Sympathetic chain

Vertebral a.

Semispinalis cervicis m.

Cricoid cartilage

Thyroid cartilage, inferior cornu

Vagus n.

Sternocleidomastoid m.

Internal jugular v.

Common carotid a.

Levator scapulae m.

Splenius capitis m.

Trapezius m.

1. The thyrohyoid muscle is the only strap muscle that does not cover the thyroid gland.

2. The esophagus arises from the pharynx just below the level of the cricoid cartilage.

3. The vertebral arteries usually enter the spinal column via the foramen transversarium at the level of C6.

Figure 1.2.16

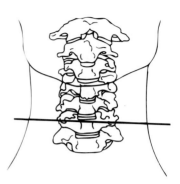

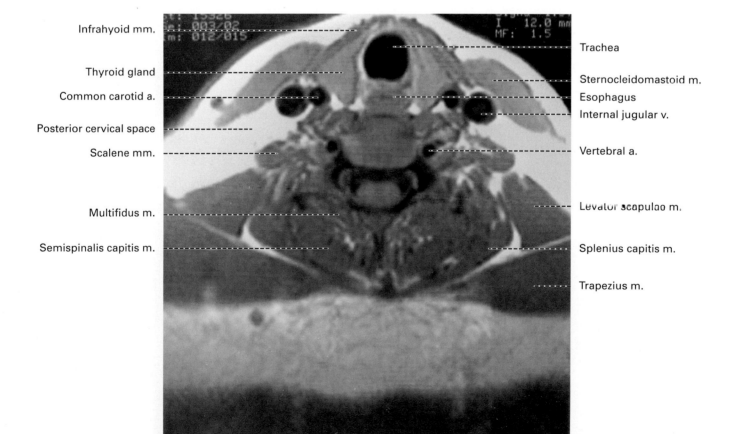

Infrahyoid mm.

Thyroid gland

Common carotid a.

Posterior cervical space

Scalene mm.

Multifidus m.

Semispinalis capitis m.

Trachea

Sternocleidomastoid m.

Esophagus

Internal jugular v.

Vertebral a.

Levator scapulae m.

Splenius capitis m.

Trapezius m.

Figure 1.2.17

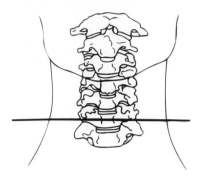

1. Through much of the infrahyoid neck, the levator scapulae muscle can be readily identified by its triangular shape.

2. The posterior cervical space in the infrahyoid neck is bordered by the sternocleidomastoid muscle anteriorly, the levator scapulae and scalene muscles medially, and the trapezius muscle posteriorly.

3. The omohyoid has superior and inferior muscle bellies that are connected via a tendon attached to the sternocleidomastoid muscle.

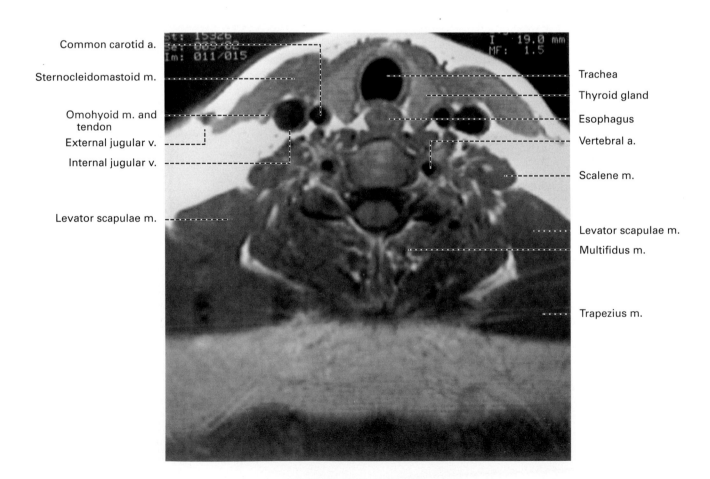

Common carotid a.

Sternocleidomastoid m.

Omohyoid m. and tendon

External jugular v.

Internal jugular v.

Levator scapulae m.

Trachea

Thyroid gland

Esophagus

Vertebral a.

Scalene m.

Levator scapulae m.

Multifidus m.

Trapezius m.

1. The parathyroid glands, which are located on the posterior surface of the thyroid gland, are normally too small to visualize.

Figure 1.2.18

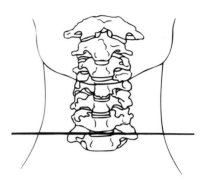

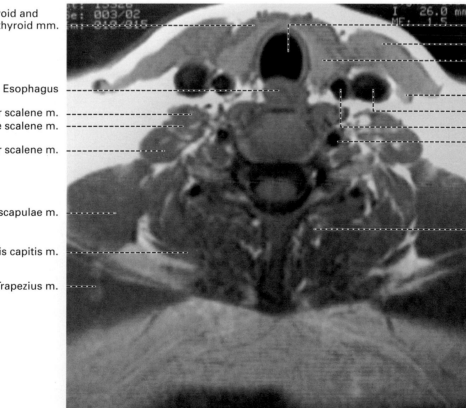

Sternohyoid and
sternothyroid mm.

Esophagus

Anterior scalene m.
Middle scalene m.

Posterior scalene m.

Levator scapulae m.

Semispinalis capitis m.

Trapezius m.

Trachea
Sternocleidomastoid m.
Thyroid gland

Omohyoid tendon
Internal jugular v.
Common carotid a.
Vertebral a.

Multifidus m.

Figure 1.2.19

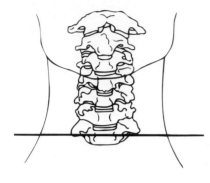

1. The recurrent laryngeal nerve can be found in the tracheal esophageal groove.

2. Although the carotid sheath (and its fascial components) cannot be visualized, the sympathetic trunk, located within the posteromedial portion of the carotid sheath, occasionally can be identified.

3. At this level the vagus nerve (cranial nerve X) is located between and posterior to the internal jugular vein and common carotid artery.

4. The phrenic nerve descends along the anterior surface of the anterior scalene muscle.

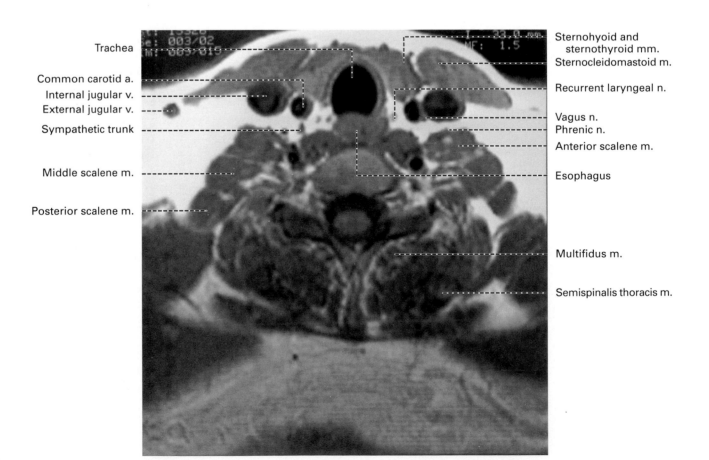

Trachea

Common carotid a.
Internal jugular v.
External jugular v.
Sympathetic trunk

Middle scalene m.

Posterior scalene m.

Sternohyoid and
sternothyroid mm.
Sternocleidomastoid m.

Recurrent laryngeal n.

Vagus n.
Phrenic n.
Anterior scalene m.

Esophagus

Multifidus m.

Semispinalis thoracis m.

1. The scalene muscles originate from the transverse processes of C2 to C6. (Only the posterior scalene muscles have attachment to C2.)

2. The anterior and middle scalene muscles insert on the first rib; the posterior scalene muscle inserts on the second rib.

3. Although the jugular veins are approximately equal in size in this individual, the right internal jugular vein is often larger than the left jugular vein because the superior sagittal venous sinus frequently drains unilaterally through the right transverse sinus.

Figure 1.2.20

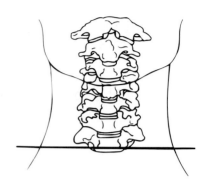

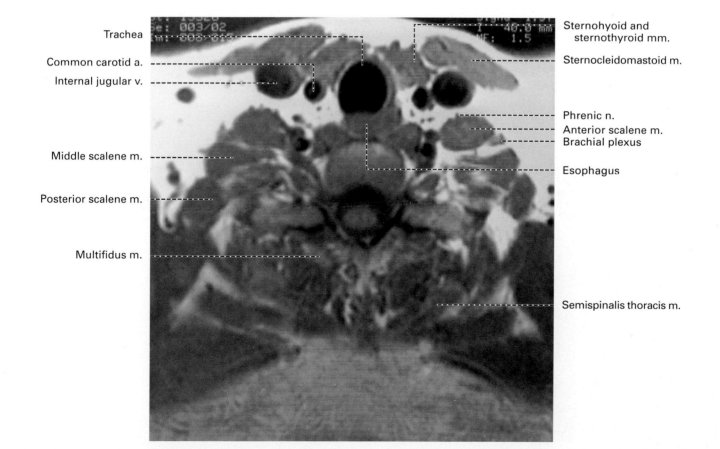

Trachea

Common carotid a.

Internal jugular v.

Middle scalene m.

Posterior scalene m.

Multifidus m.

Sternohyoid and sternothyroid mm.

Sternocleidomastoid m.

Phrenic n.

Anterior scalene m.

Brachial plexus

Esophagus

Semispinalis thoracis m.

Figure 1.2.21

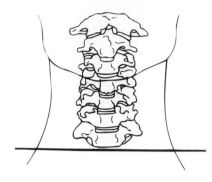

1. The nerve roots of the brachial plexus travel between the anterior and middle scalene muscles.

2. The phrenic nerve descends on the anterior surface of the anterior scalene muscle.

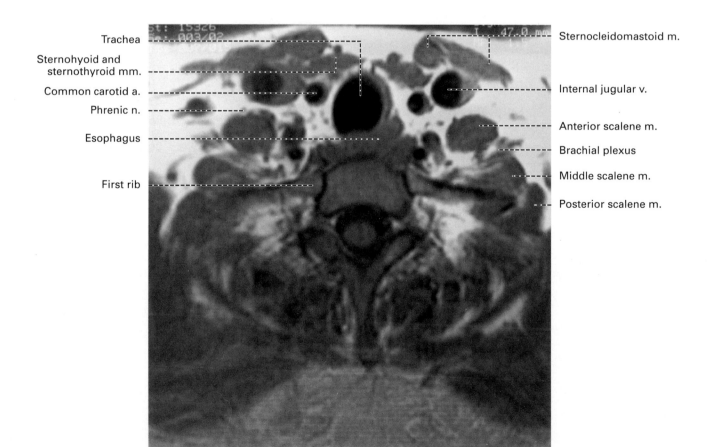

Trachea

Sternohyoid and
sternothyroid mm.

Common carotid a.

Phrenic n.

Esophagus

First rib

Sternocleidomastoid m.

Internal jugular v.

Anterior scalene m.

Brachial plexus

Middle scalene m.

Posterior scalene m.

1. The sternohyoid muscle is located more superficially than the sternothyroid muscle.

Figure 1.2.22

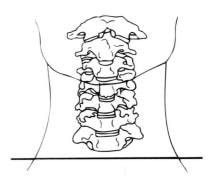

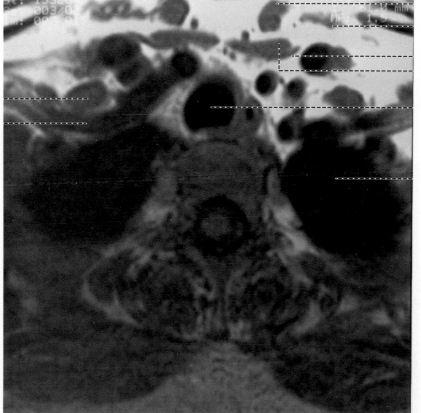

Sternocleidomastoid m., sternal head

Sternocleidomastoid m., clavicular head

Sternothyroid m.

Sternohyoid m.

Anterior scalene m.

Subclavian a.

Trachea

Lung, apex

Figure 1.3.1

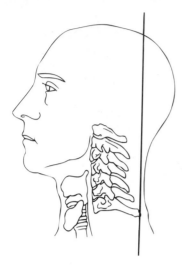

1. Coronal images through the neck progress from posterior to anterior.

2. The spinal accessory nerve (cranial nerve XI) innervates the trapezius muscle after innervating the sternocleidomastoid muscle.

3. The semispinalis capitis muscle is a member of the transversospinalis muscle group. The main members of this group are the multifidus and rotatores muscles; these muscles are also present in the thoracic and lumbar regions.

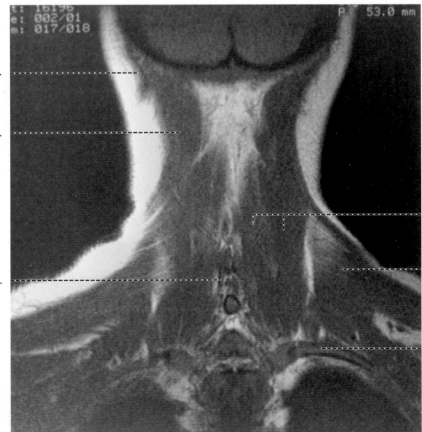

Splenius capitis m.

Semispinalis capitis m.

Interspinalis m.

Semispinalis cervicis and semispinalis capitis mm.

Trapezius m.

First rib

1. The semispinalis cervicis muscles are also part of the cervical transversospinalis muscle group. These muscles, along with the erector spinae muscle group, help to extend, laterally flex, and rotate the vertebral column.

2. The interspinalis muscles are short muscular fascicles connecting adjacent spinous processes.

Figure 1.3.2

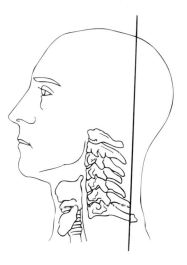

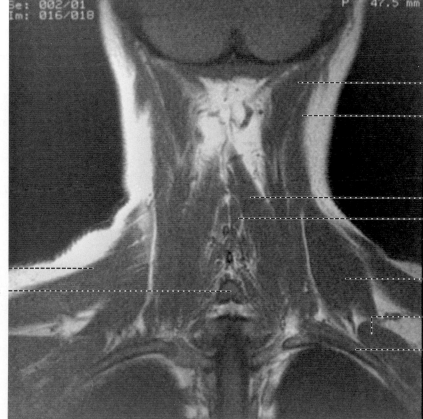

Semispinalis capitis m.

Splenius capitis m.

Semispinalis cervicis m.

Interspinous m.

Trapezius m.

Levator scapulae m.

C7 spinous process

Serratus anterior m.

First rib

Figure 1.3.3

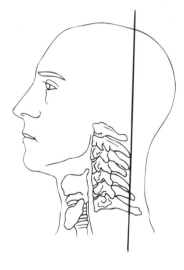

1. The occipital artery travels between the splenius capitis and semispinalis capitis muscles.

2. The multifidus muscles originate from the articular processes of the lower four cervical vertebral bodies and insert into the spine of the vertebra above the vertebra of origin.

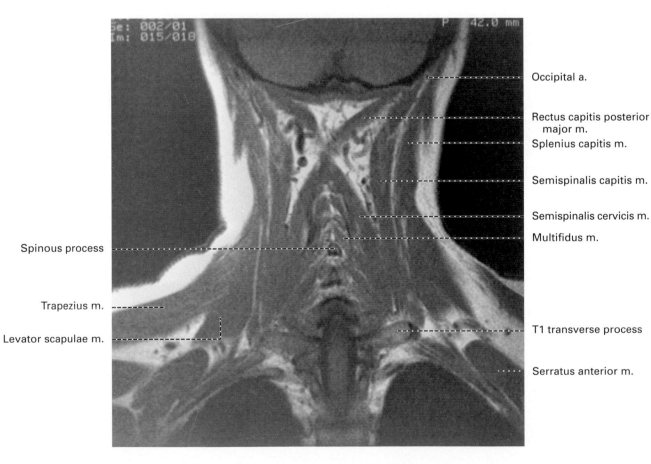

Spinous process

Trapezius m.

Levator scapulae m.

Occipital a.

Rectus capitis posterior major m.

Splenius capitis m.

Semispinalis capitis m.

Semispinalis cervicis m.

Multifidus m.

T1 transverse process

Serratus anterior m.

1. The splenius capitis muscle lies superficial to the semispinalis capitis muscle.

2. The splenius muscle originates from the midline ligamentum nuchae. Its fibers travel upward and laterally like a bandage around the posterior neck.

3. The rectus capitis posterior major muscles originate from the spinous process of the axis and insert laterally on the occiput.

Figure 1.3.4

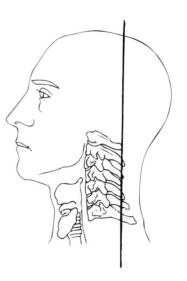

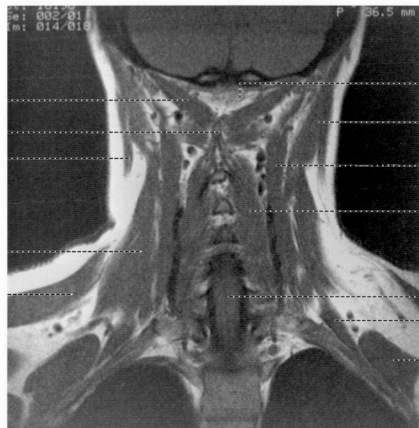

Rectus capitis major m.

C2 spinous process

Sternocleidomastoid m.

Levator scapulae m.

Trapezius m.

Rectus capitis posterior minor m.

Splenius capitis m.

Semispinalis capitis m.

Semispinalis cervicis m.

Cervical cord

Posterior scalene m.

Serratus anterior m.

Figure 1.3.5

1. The suboccipital muscle group consists of the superior and inferior oblique capitis muscles and the rectus capitis posterior major and minor muscles.

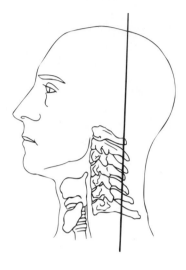

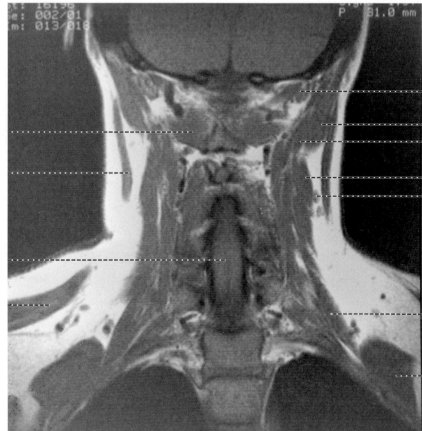

Inferior oblique m.

Sternocleidomastoid m.

Cervical cord

Trapezius m.

Superior oblique m.

Splenius capitis m.

Longissimus capitis m.

Levator scapulae

Posterior cervical space lymph node

Posterior scalene m.

Serratus anterior m.

1. The splenius, levator scapulae, and the middle and posterior scalenes form the floor of the posterior space.

2. The roof of the posterior cervical space (posterior triangle) is formed by the sternocleidomastoid muscle.

Figure 1.3.6

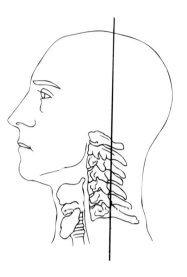

Superior oblique m.
C1 posterior arch
Inferior oblique m.
Posterior cervical space

Splenius capitis m.

Sternocleidomastoid m.

Levator scapulae m.

Cervical cord

Middle and posterior scalene mm.

Brachial plexus elements

Serratus anterior m.

Figure 1.3.7

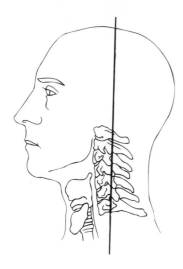

1. The brachial plexus travels between the anterior and middle scalene muscles on its course to the upper limb.

2. The brachial plexus is formed from nerve roots C4 to T1.

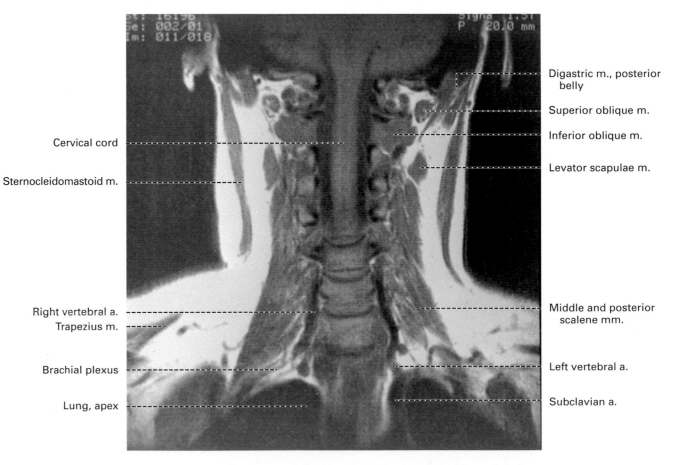

1. The vertebral arteries travel in the spinal column within the foramen transversarium, usually from C6 to C1.

2. The vertebral artery gains entrance to the subarachnoid space by piercing the posterior atlanto-occipital membrane above the arch of C1.

3. The oblique capitis inferior muscle is located between the atlas and the axis.

Figure 1.3.8

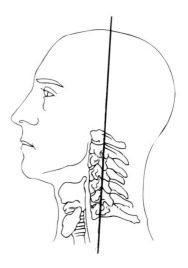

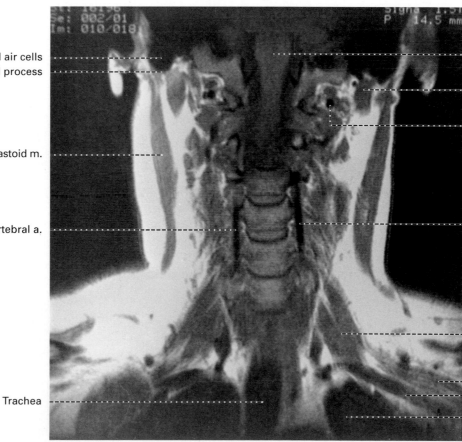

Mastoid air cells

Mastoid process

Sternocleidomastoid m.

Right vertebral a.

Trachea

Medulla oblongata

Digastric m., posterior belly

Vertebral a.

Left vertebral a.

Anterior scalene m.

Brachial plexus

Subclavian a.

Lung, apex

Figure 1.3.9

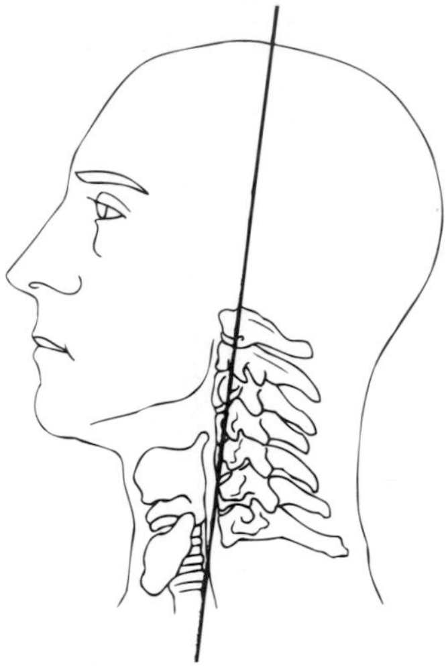

1. The anterior scalene muscle arises from the anterior tubercles of the transverse processes of C3 to C6 and inserts on the first rib.
2. Oblique coronal images would be required to see optimally the scalene muscles.
3. The brachial plexus usually travels superiorly with respect to the subclavian artery as it enters the upper limb.

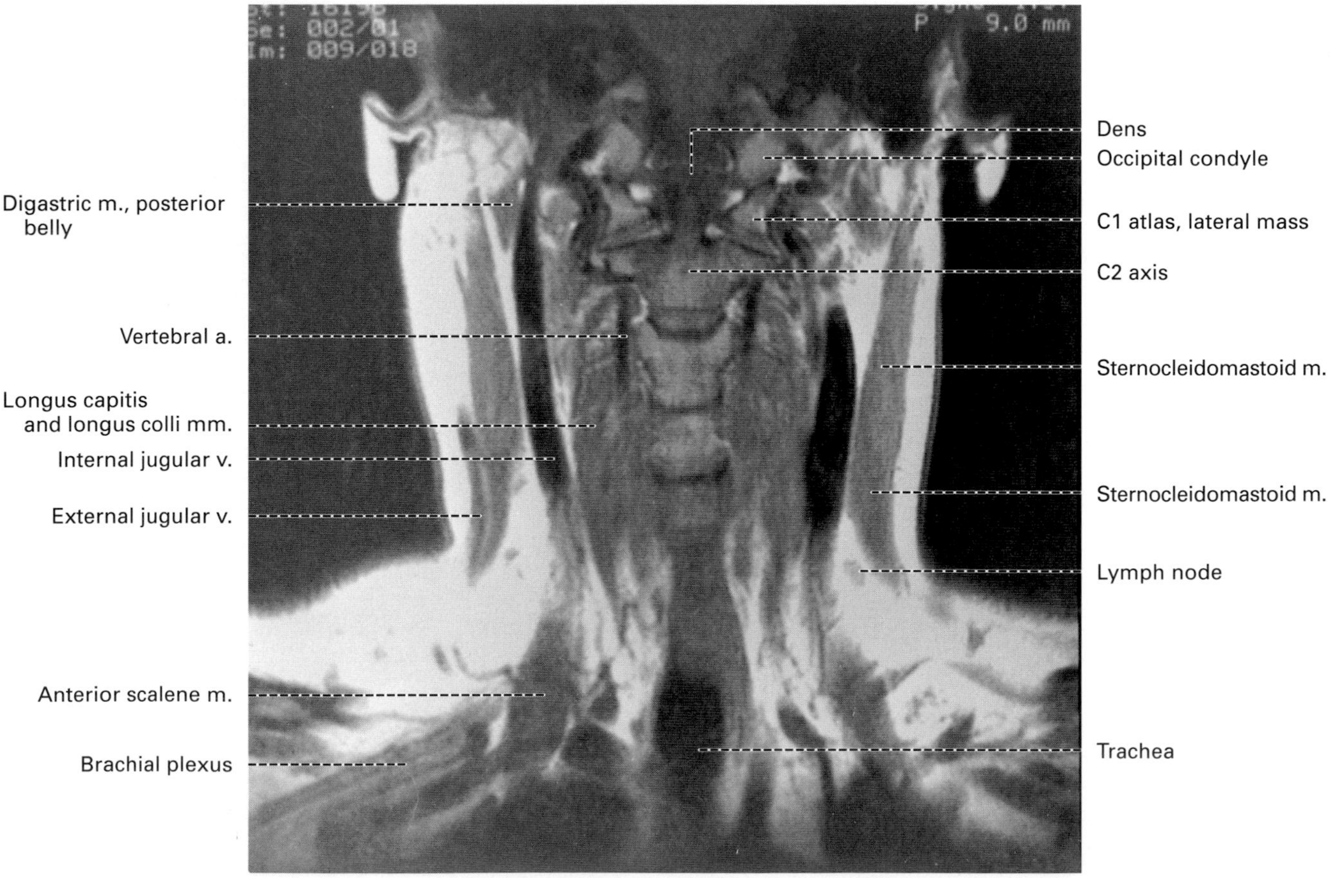
Se: 002/01
Im: 009/018
P 9.0 mm
Digastric m., posterior belly
Vertebral a.
Longus capitis and longus colli mm.
Internal jugular v.
External jugular v.
Anterior scalene m.
Brachial plexus
Dens
Occipital condyle
C1 atlas, lateral mass
C2 axis
Sternocleidomastoid m.
Sternocleidomastoid m.
Lymph node
Trachea

1. The common and internal carotid arteries travel medially to the internal jugular veins.

2. The internal jugular veins are the primary venous drainage route of the intracranial contents.

3. The posterior belly of the digastric muscle travels lateral to the internal jugular vein.

Figure 1.3.10

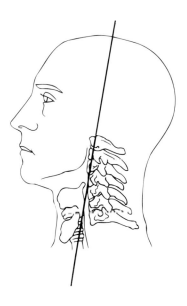

Jugular tubercle	
Hypoglossal canal and n.	
C1, lateral mass	Dens
Digastric m., posterior belly	
	C2 vertebral body
	Longus colli and longus capitis mm.
Sternocleidomastoid m.	
Thyroid gland	
	Internal jugular v.
Trachea	
Internal jugular v.	Common carotid a.
Innominate v.	

Figure 1.3.11

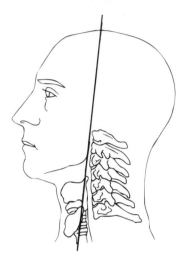

1. The longus capitis and longus colli muscles are prevertebral muscles attached to the anterior lateral surfaces of the cervical vertebrae.

2. The facial nerve (cranial nerve VII), which divides the parotid gland into superficial and deep lobes, passes immediately lateral to the retromandibular vein.

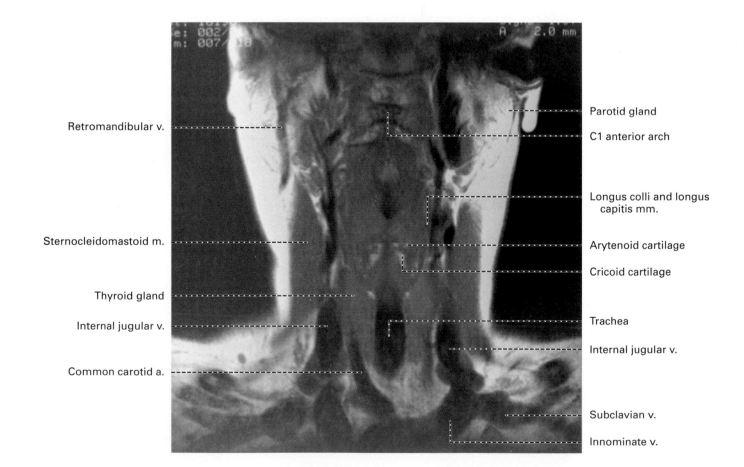

Retromandibular v.

Sternocleidomastoid m.

Thyroid gland

Internal jugular v.

Common carotid a.

Parotid gland

C1 anterior arch

Longus colli and longus capitis mm.

Arytenoid cartilage

Cricoid cartilage

Trachea

Internal jugular v.

Subclavian v.

Innominate v.

1. The thyroid gland is situated medial and deep to the sternocleidomastoid muscles.

Figure 1.3.12

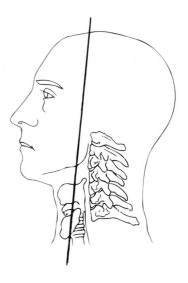

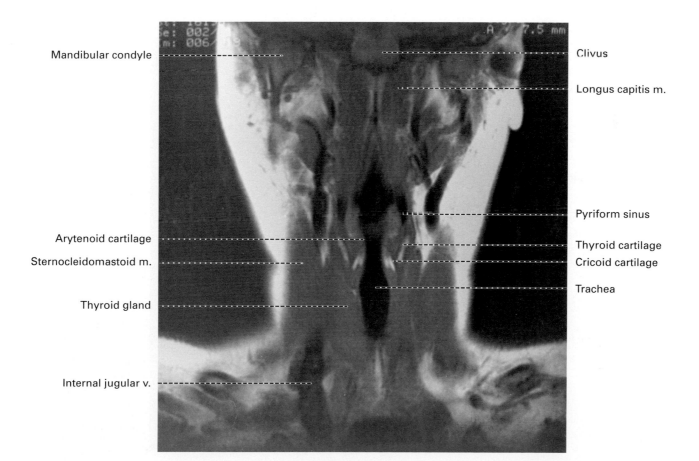

Mandibular condyle

Clivus

Longus capitis m.

Pyriform sinus

Arytenoid cartilage

Thyroid cartilage

Sternocleidomastoid m.

Cricoid cartilage

Trachea

Thyroid gland

Internal jugular v.

Figure 1.3.13

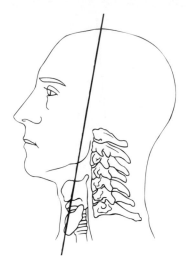

1. The coronal plane depicts the muscles of mastication, which include the masseter, temporalis, and the medial and lateral pterygoid muscles.

2. The sternocleidomastoid muscle has both a medial sternal head and a lateral clavicular head, which subsequently merge to insert on the mastoid process of the temporal bone.

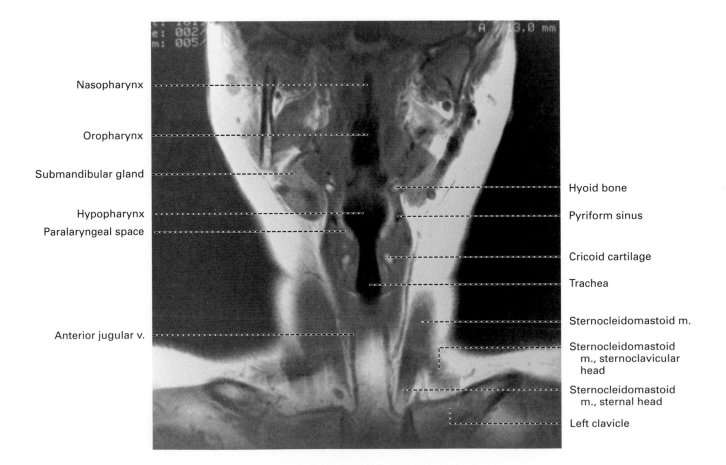

Nasopharynx

Oropharynx

Submandibular gland

Hypopharynx
Paralaryngeal space

Hyoid bone

Pyriform sinus

Cricoid cartilage

Trachea

Sternocleidomastoid m.

Anterior jugular v.

Sternocleidomastoid m., sternoclavicular head

Sternocleidomastoid m., sternal head

Left clavicle

1. The thyroarytenoid muscles form the bulk of the true vocal cords.

2. Although slips of muscle are present within the false cords, the predominant MRI signal of the false cords is that of fat.

3. The parapharyngeal space separates the more medial pharyngeal mucosal space from the masticator and parotid space.

4. The styloglossus muscle forms the inferior boundary of the parapharyngeal space.

Figure 1.3.14

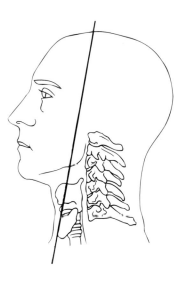

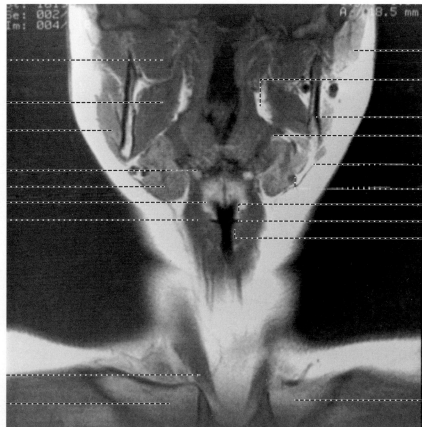

Lateral pterygoid m. — Parotid gland — Parapharyngeal space — Medial pterygoid m. — Masseter m. — Mandible, body — Styloglossus m. — Hyoid bone — Platysma m. — Submandibular gland — Facial v. — Paralaryngeal space — False vocal cords — Infrahyoid m. — Laryngeal ventricle — True vocal cords — Sternocleidomastoid m., sternal head — Right clavicle — Left clavicle

Chapter 2

CERVICAL SPINE

Cervical Spine

The cervical spine is composed of seven vertebral segments: two specialized units and five conventional vertebrae. The C1 unit (the atlas), lacking both a vertebral body and a spinous process, consists of paired lateral masses connected by anterior and posterior arches. The C2 segment has a superior projection of the superior aspect of its vertebral body known as the dens or odontoid process, small paired transverse processes, and conventional posterior elements including paired laminae and a bifid spinous process. The C3 to C7 vertebrae consist of vertebral bodies, paired transverse processes with transverse foramina, paired articular pillars with associated superior and inferior articulating processes, and conventional posterior neural arches consisting of paired laminae joining posteromedially into a spinous process, which is frequently bifid. The superior vertebral body endplates have a cupped appearance with a lateral superior projection known as the uncinate process.

The atlanto-occipital joints allow for slight flexion and extension. The primary rotatory motion in the cervical column occurs at the atlantoaxial joints. The intervertebral discs, interposed between the vertebral bodies from C2 to the sacrum act as shock absorbers, allow for motion of the vertebral column in many directions including flexion, extension, lateral bending, and some rotation. The zygapophyseal joints, also known as facet joints, are arthrodial (gliding) synovial joints that account for the majority of cervical flexion and extension movements. They are oriented in an oblique coronal plane, approximately 45 degrees from vertical.

A complex set of ligaments joins the atlas and axis with the occiput. The dens is linked to the basiocciput via alar and apical ligaments. The transverse ligament, which secures the dens to the anterior arch of C1, is also known as the transverse arm of the cruciate ligament. The vertical arm of the cruciate ligament attaches to the basiocciput beneath the tectorial membrane. The anterior longitudinal ligament is a strong broad-based structure attached to the anterior and anterolateral surfaces of vertebral bodies and intervertebral discs from C1 to the sacrum. The posterior longitudinal ligament is bowstringed along the posterior surfaces of the vertebral bodies and intervertebral discs from C2 to the sacrum. The free portions of the posterior longitudinal ligament at the midvertebral body levels are anchored by a ligament known as the plica mediana dorsalis. The cephalad continuation of the posterior longitudinal ligament to the basiocciput is known as the tectorial membrane. The posterior elements are stablized by the continuous supraspinous ligament as well as the discontinuous interspinous ligaments and ligamentum flavum. The elastic ligamentum flavum connects adjacent laminae.

The spinal cord and thecal sac occupy the bony spinal canal. Ventral roots, which transmit efferent motor impulses, and dorsal roots, which carry afferent sensory input, merge in the lateral portions of the neural foramen to form segmental spinal nerves. Their merger occurs lateral to the dorsal root ganglion, which occupies the midposterior portion of the neural foramen in the cervical spine. The segmental spinal nerves exit over their corresponding pedicles.

The internal vertebral venous plexus occupies a good portion of the epidural space within the bony spinal canal. Connecting veins through neural foramina and between laminae join with the external vertebral venous plexus. The vertebral artery is in intimate contact with the cervical spine as it traverses the foramen transversarium with the cervical column prior to piercing the dura posterolaterally at the level of C1 to C2 to gain entrance to the intracranial space through the foramen magnum.

The suboccipital muscle group, which produces motion at the atlanto-occipital and atlantoaxial joints, consists of the superior and inferior oblique capitis muscles and the rectus capitis posterior major and minor muscles. The posterior cervical spine musculature consists of four primary layers. The deepest layer is the transversospinalis muscle group, which consists of the multifidus, rotatores, and semispinalis capitis and cervicis muscles. The segmental interspinalis muscles can be included in this group. The next layer of posterior muscles is the erector spinae muscle group, consisting of the spinalis cervicis, longissiumus capitis and cervicis, and the iliocostalis cervicis. The erector spinae muscle group, also known as the sacrospinalis group, is the primary posterior muscle group of the thoracic and lumbar spine. The splenius muscles, which are unique to the cervical region, are the next main layer. The most superficial posterior cervical muscle is the trapezius.

1. The basion and opisthion define the anterior and posterior margins of the foramen magnum.

2. Within the cervical and lumbar spines, the intervertebral discs gradually increase in height with caudal progression.

3. The ligamentum nuchae, a posterior midline structure, connects the external occipital crest and protuberance with the C7 spinous process and provides attachment for some of the midline posterior muscles.

Figure 2.1.1A

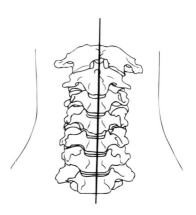

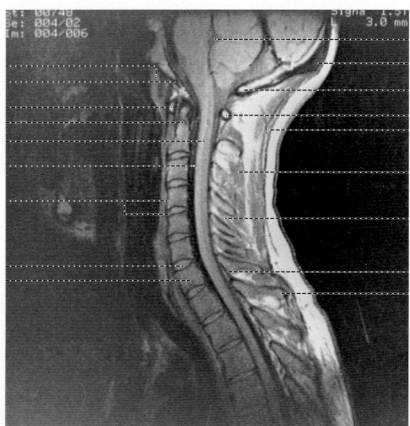

Adenoid tonsils

Basion

C1 anterior arch

Odontoid process

Central gray matter

Anterior subarachnoid space

Anterior longitudinal ligament

C6–C7 intervertebral disc

C7 vertebral body

Fourth ventricle

External occipital protuberance

Opisthion

C1 posterior arch

Ligamentum nuchae

Multifidus m.

Interspinous ligament

Ligamentum flavum

T1 spinous process

Figure 2.1.1B

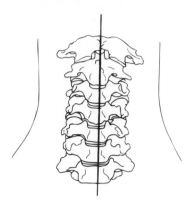

1. This is a midline sagittal T2-weighted fast spin-echo image.

2. The tectorial membrane is the superior continuation of the posterior longitudinal ligament.

3. The supraspinous ligament connects the spinous processes from C2 to the sacrum.

4. The anterior and posterior longitudinal ligaments help to stabilize the vertebral column.

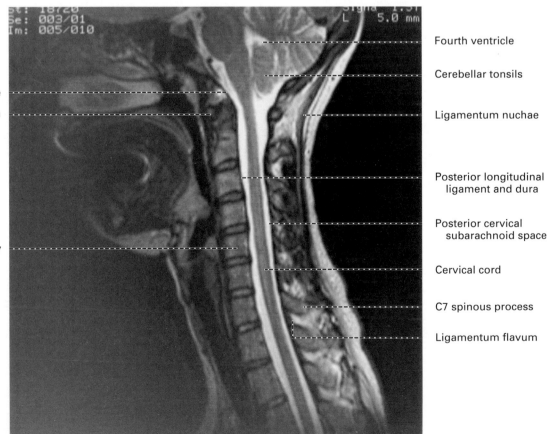

Tentorial membrane

C1 anterior arch

C5 vertebral body

Fourth ventricle

Cerebellar tonsils

Ligamentum nuchae

Posterior longitudinal ligament and dura

Posterior cervical subarachnoid space

Cervical cord

C7 spinous process

Ligamentum flavum

1. The transverse ligament, which can be seen as a focal thickening posterior to the mid dens, is responsible for maintaining the atlantoaxial joint.

2. The position and shape of the paired cerebellar tonsils can best be visualized on paramedian sagittal images.

3. The spinous process of C7 is usually larger and thicker than those at other cervical levels.

Figure 2.1.2

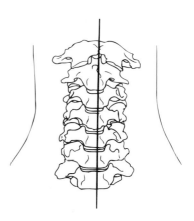

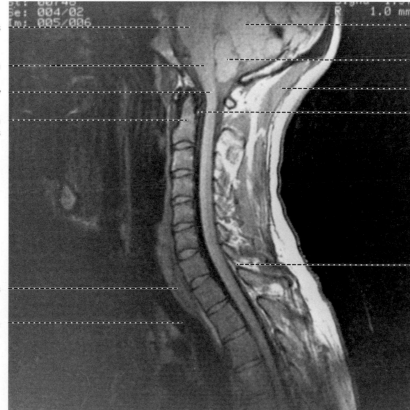

Pons

Medulla

Cervicomedullary junction

Synchondrosis between base of axis and dens

Esophagus

Trachea

Cerebellar vermis

Cerebellar tonsil

Semispinalis capitis m.

Transverse lig.

Ligamentum flavum

Figure 2.1.3

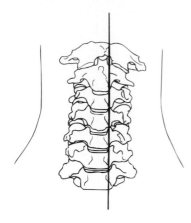

1. On paramedian images, the posterior longitudinal ligament appears as a bowstring over the posterior convex vertebral margins with intervening epidural veins and fat.

2. The four paired suboccipital muscles include the rectus capitis posterior major and minor muscles and the superior and inferior oblique capitis muscles.

3. The suboccipital muscles flex and extend the atlanto-occipital joint and produce rotatory motion at the atlantoaxial joint.

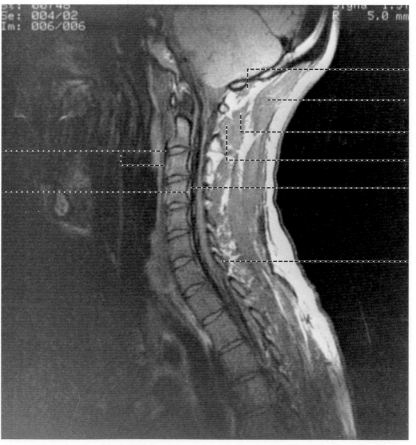

Anterior longitudinal lig.

Anterior epidural fat

Rectus capitis posterior minor m.

Rectus capitis posterior major m.

Superior oblique capitis m.

Inferior oblique capitis m.

Posterior longitudinal ligament

C7 laminae

1. The superior oblique capitis muscle originates on the atlas and inserts on the occipital bone.

2. The inferior oblique muscle originates on the axis and inserts on the atlas.

Figure 2.1.4

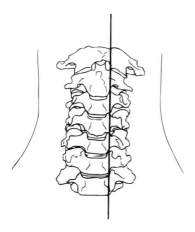

Superior oblique capitis m.

Inferior oblique capitis m.

Pharyngeal constrictor

Longus colli m.

Splenius capitis

Semispinalis cervicis and capitis mm.

Thyroid gland

T3 pedicle

Trapezius m.

Figure 2.1.5

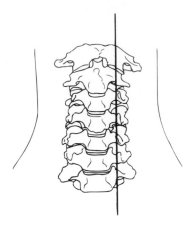

1. Each neural foramen is bordered superiorly and inferiorly by pedicles, anteriorly by an intervertebral disc, and posteriorly by a facet joint.

2. The dorsal root lies superior and posterior to the ventral root within the neural foramen.

3. Within the cervical neural foramina, dorsal root ganglia are positioned lower and closer to the intervertebral disc than in the lumbar spine, where they occupy a more superior position.

4. Fat and a few small veins are present within the upper portion of the cervical neural foramen.

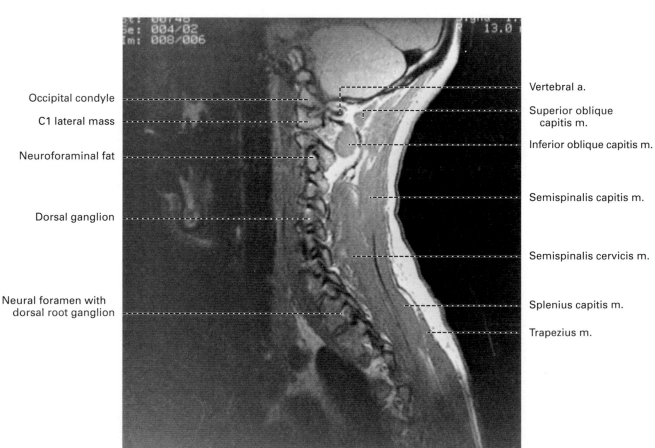

Occipital condyle

C1 lateral mass

Neuroforaminal fat

Dorsal ganglion

Neural foramen with dorsal root ganglion

Vertebral a.

Superior oblique capitis m.

Inferior oblique capitis m.

Semispinalis capitis m.

Semispinalis cervicis m.

Splenius capitis m.

Trapezius m.

1. The articular pillars, with the exception of their intervening facet joints, form a nearly continuous bony column posterior to the neural foramen.

2. The longus colli muscle is the primary anterior vertebral muscle in the cervical region.

3. The vertebral artery passes through the suboccipital triangle.

Figure 2.1.6

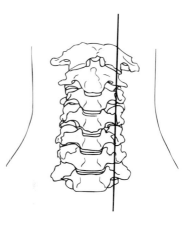

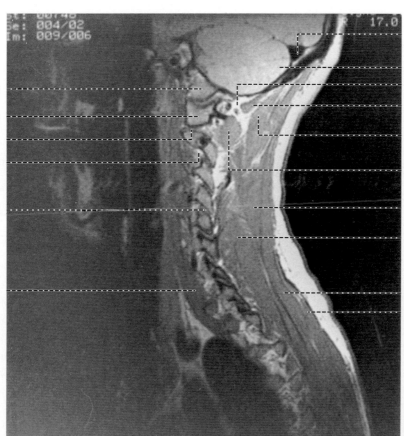

Occipital condyle

C1 lateral mass

Atlantoaxial joint

Neuroforaminal fat

Zygapophyseal joint

Longus colli m.

Transverse venous sinus

Cerebellar hemisphere

Suboccipital triangle

Superior oblique
  capitis m.

Rectus capitis
  posterior major m.

Inferior oblique
  capitis m.

Semispinalis capitis m.

Semispinalis cervicis m.

Splenius capitis m.

Trapezius m.

Figure 2.2.1

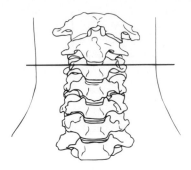

1. The vertebral arteries ascend the neck lateral to the vertebral bodies and pass through the foramina transversarii. The intimate relationship of the vertebral artery with the cervical column predisposes it to injury in the presence of cervical spine trauma.

2. The longus colli muscle forms the bulk of the prevertebral cervical musculature beginning at the C2 level. Above the C2 level, the longus capitis muscle is the visualized prevertebral musculature.

3. The epidural space contains fat and a rich venous plexus known as the internal vertebral venous plexus.

4. The trapezius is innervated by the spinal accessory nerve (cranial nerve XI) after this nerve innervates the sternocleidomastoid muscle.

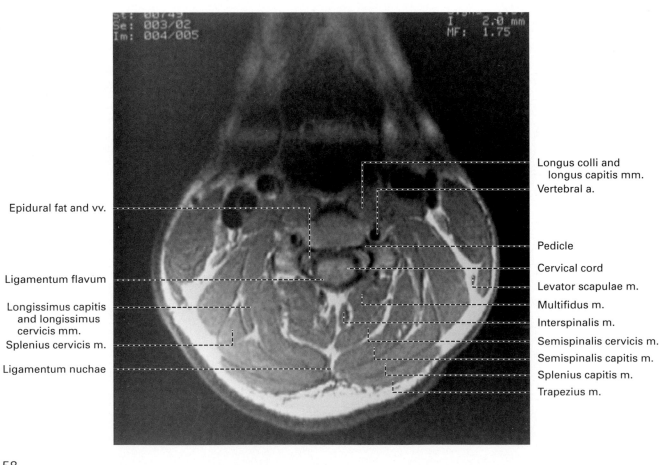

Epidural fat and vv.

Ligamentum flavum

Longissimus capitis and longissimus cervicis mm.

Splenius cervicis m.

Ligamentum nuchae

Longus colli and longus capitis mm.
Vertebral a.

Pedicle

Cervical cord

Levator scapulae m.

Multifidus m.

Interspinalis m.

Semispinalis cervicis m.

Semispinalis capitis m.

Splenius capitis m.

Trapezius m.

1. The ventral roots transmit efferent motor impulses from the spinal cord to the periphery.

2. The dorsal roots channel afferent sensory impulses from the periphery to the spinal cord.

Figure 2.2.2

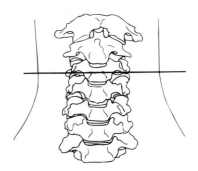

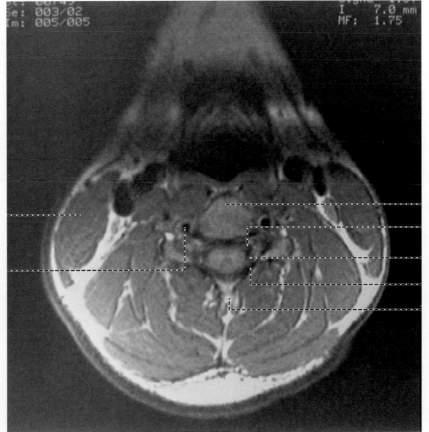

Sternocleidomastoid m.

Vertebral a.

Vertebral body

Ventral n. root

Dorsal n. root

Laminae

Spinous process

Figure 2.2.3

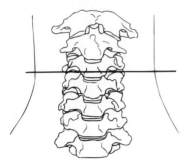

1. The inferior articulating processes are located posterior to the adjacent superior articulating processes.

2. The zygapophyseal joints are diarthrodial (gliding) joints commonly known as facet joints.

3. The cervical facet joints are prone to subluxation or dislocation with trauma owing to their 45-degree orientation in the coronal plane and their relatively redundant joint capsule.

4. The ligamentum nuchae is a thick ligamentous structure providing attachment for many of the posterior cervical muscles.

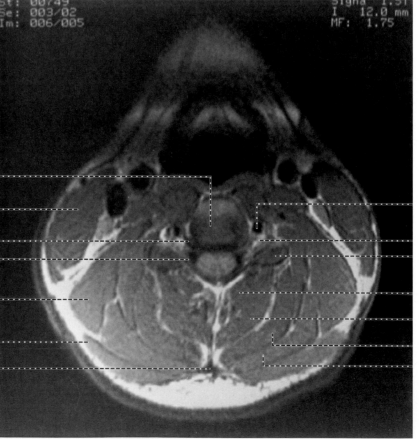

Intervertebral disc

Sternocleidomastoid m.

Anterior epidural v.

Dorsal n. root

Levator scapulae m.

Trapezius m.

Ligamentum nuchae

Vertebral a.

Neuroforaminal fat

Zygapophyseal joint

Multifidus m.

Semispinalis cervicis m.

Semispinalis capitis m.

Splenius capitis m.

1. The dorsal root ganglia are located in the neural foramina in the cervical region lower than in either the thoracic (where they are in the middle portion) or the lumbar region (where they are in the superior portion).

2. The position of the cervical dorsal root ganglia places them in close proximity to the posterolateral margin of the intervertebral disc.

Figure 2.2.4

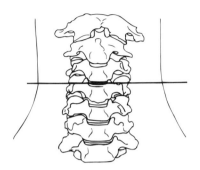

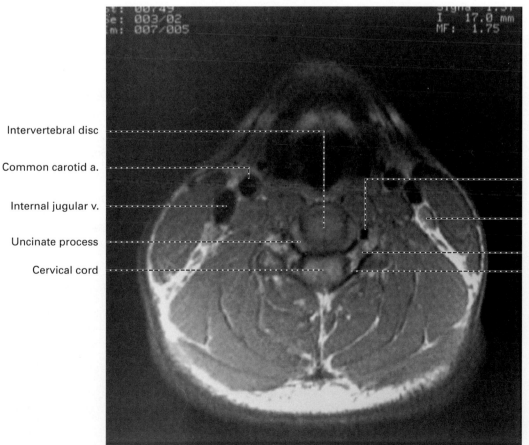

Intervertebral disc

Common carotid a.

Internal jugular v.

Uncinate process

Cervical cord

Vertebral a.

Posterior cervical space lymph node

Dorsal root ganglion

Neuroforaminal fat

CORONAL

Figure 2.3.1

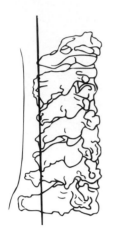

1. The opisthion marks the posterior margin of the foramen magnum.

2. The rectus capitis posterior major and minor muscles are half of the sub-occipital muscle group. The other two members of this group are the inferior and superior oblique capitis muscles.

3. The rectus capitis posterior minor muscle originates from the posterior tubercle of Cl and the rectus capitis posterior major muscle originates from the spinous process of C2. Both muscles insert on the occiput.

4. The trapezius muscle forms the posterolateral roof of the posterior cervical space.

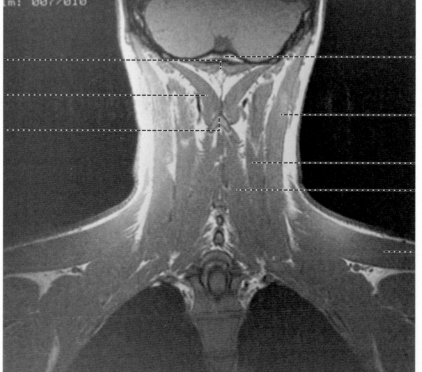

Rectus capitis posterior minor m.

Rectus capitis posterior major m.

C2 spinous process

Opisthion

Splenius capitis m.

Semispinalis capitis m.

Semispinalis cervicis m.

Trapezius m.

1. The superior oblique muscle forms the anterior boundary of the suboccipital triangle on sagittal images.

2. The atlas is made up of two lateral masses, an anterior arch and a posterior arch. The atlas (the C1 segment) does not have a vertebral body or a spinous process.

3. The C2 segment is also known as the axis.

Figure 2.3.2

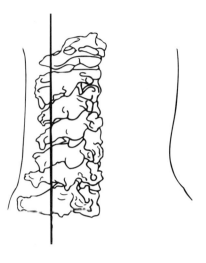

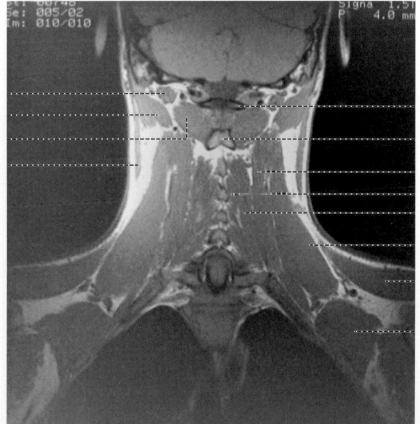

Superior oblique m.

Splenius capitis m.

Inferior oblique m.

Sternocleidomastoid m.

C1 atlas, posterior arch

C2 spinous process

Semispinalis capitis m.

Multifidus m.

Spinalis cervicis m.

Levator scapulae m.

Trapezius m.

Serratus anterior m.

Figure 2.3.3

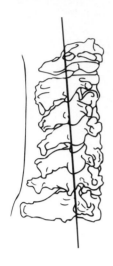

1. The cervical spine laminae, being in close continuity with each other, form a posterolateral bony covering for the spinal cord.

2. The inferior oblique muscle is one of four suboccipital muscle pairs that help to produce atlantoaxial rotatory movement.

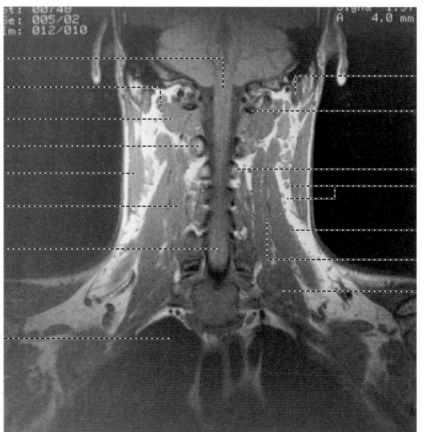

Cervical medullary junction

Superior oblique m.

Inferior oblique m.

C2 laminae

Sternocleidomastoid m.

Splenius cervicis m.

Spinal cord

Lung apex

Digastric m., posterior belly

C1 posterior arch

C3 laminae

Lymph node and fat in posterior cervical space

Levator scapulae m.

Semispinalis capitis m.

Scalene mm.

1. The posterior cervical space is located posteromedial to the sternocleidomastoid muscle; posterior to the internal jugular vein; lateral to the splenius capitiis, levator scapulae, and the middle and posterior scalene muscles; and deep to the trapezius muscle.

2. The posterior cervical space contains spinal accessory lymph nodes, the spinal accessory nerve (cranial nerve XI), and fat.

3. The articular pillars form the lateral margins of the bony cervical spinal canal.

Figure 2.3.4

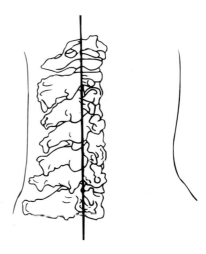

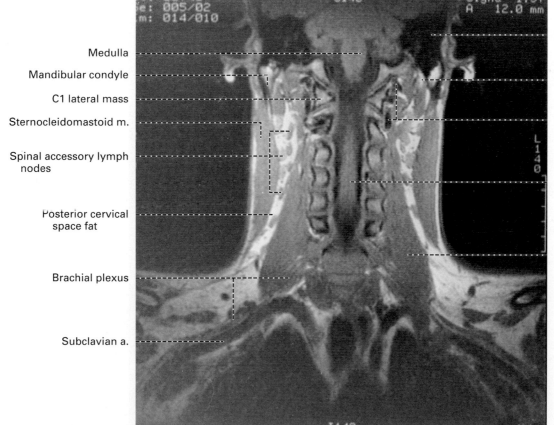

Figure 2.3.5

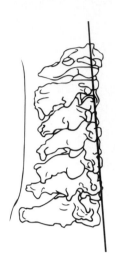

1. The hypoglossal canal, located in the skull base, transmits the hypoglossal nerve (cranial nerve XII).

2. The uncinate processes help to cradle intervertebral discs in the cervical region.

3. The atlantoaxial joints have a normal medial to lateral downslope.

4. The vertebral artery usually enters the spinal column at C6 through the foramen transversarii and ascends superiorly to the C1 level before gaining entrance to the spinal canal above the posterior arch of C1.

5. The odontoid process is thought to represent the C1 vertebral body segment.

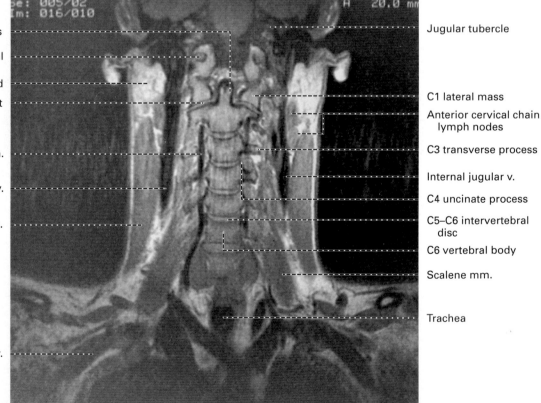

Odontoid process

Hypoglossal canal

Parotid gland

Atlantoaxial joint

Vertebral a.

Internal jugular v.

Sternocleidomastoid m.

Subclavian v.

Jugular tubercle

C1 lateral mass

Anterior cervical chain lymph nodes

C3 transverse process

Internal jugular v.

C4 uncinate process

C5–C6 intervertebral disc

C6 vertebral body

Scalene mm.

Trachea

Chapter 3

THORACIC SPINE

Thoracic Spine

The thoracic spine column comprises twelve structurally similar vertebral segments, each consisting of a body, an arch, a spinous process, and two transverse processes. The height of each vertebral body increases with caudal progression. Each neural arch consists of paired pedicles, laminae, and superior and inferior articulating processes. Each vertebral segment articulates with ribs via arthrodial (gliding) costovertebral joints. The heads of ribs two through ten articulate with two adjacent vertebral bodies via demifacets. Rib heads one, eleven, and twelve articulate only with the upper portions of their respective vertebral bodies. Arthrodial costotransverse articulations are present between the rib tubercles and transverse processes of the rib and vertebral segments one through ten.

The intervertebral discs are sandwiched between flat inferior and superior vertebral endplates without the uncinate processes as seen in the cervical region. The thoracic intervertebral discs are thinner than those in the cervical and lumbar regions. The zygapophyseal joints are oriented in more of a coronal plane than either the cervical or lumbar spine, allowing for significant rotatory movement.

Anterior and posterior longitudinal ligaments secure the vertebral bodies and intervertebral discs. The posterior bony elements are linked and secured by the supraspinous ligament, interspinous ligaments, and the ligamentum flavum.

The thoracic spinal cord usually takes an eccentric anterior position within the thecal sac in the midthoracic bony spinal canal owing to the normal dorsal kyphotic curvature. Ventral (efferent motor) roots and dorsal (afferent sensory) roots join lateral to the dorsal root ganglia to form segmental nerves. In the thoracic and lumbar spine, the segmental nerves exit the neural foramen beneath their corresponding pedicles. The thoracic dorsal root ganglia are centered within the neural foramen on sagittal and axial images.

The internal vertebral venous plexus occupies a portion of the epidural space, particularly anteriorly. The basivertebral venous plexus, located within the posterior central aspect of each vertebral body, drains into the internal vertebral venous plexus. The aorta and inferior vena cava position themselves anterior to the vertebral column in the mid to lower thoracic spine. Intercostal veins, arteries, and nerves maintain a cephalad to caudal relationship in the lateral paraspinal fat at the inferior edge of each rib.

The deep posterior paraspinal muscle group is divided into short-segment transversospinal muscles and the erector spinae muscle group. The transversospinal group in the thoracic region comprises the semispinalis thoracis, the multifidus, the rotatores thoracis, the interspinales, and the intertransversarii muscles. The thoracic spinalis and the longissimus thoracis are the primary thoracic erector muscles.

1. The posterior epidural fat is most abundant at the T6 to T9 levels, opposite the apex of the usual thoracic kyphosis.

2. The primary venous drainage of the hemopoietic vertebral marrow cavities is the basivertebral venous plexus.

3. Postcontrast T1-weighted spine images can be identified by enhancement within the basivertebral plexus.

4. The supraspinous ligament is a continuous (nonsegmental) structure attaching the tips of the spinous processes.

5. The interspinous ligaments are nonsegmental and interconnect adjacent spinous processes.

Figure 3.1.1A

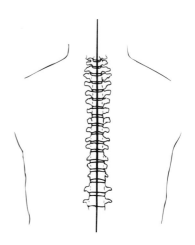

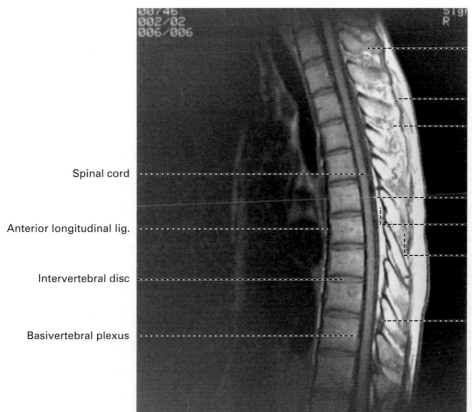

Spinous process

Supraspinous lig.

Interspinous lig.

Posterior subarachnoid space

Posterior epidural fat

Multifidus m.

Ligamentum flavum

Spinal cord

Anterior longitudinal lig.

Intervertebral disc

Basivertebral plexus

Figure 3.1.1B

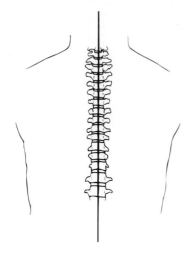

1. This is a fast spin-echo T2-weighted midline image.

2. The intervertebral disc has two primary signal intensities. The central portion of the disc consists of the nucleus pulposus and the inner layer of the anulus fibrosis. The peripheral disc signal is due to the outer layer of the anulus fibrosis.

3. The anterior longitudinal ligament is twice as resistant to tearing than the posterior longitudinal ligament.

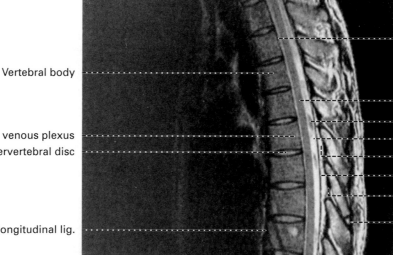

Vertebral body

Basivertebral venous plexus
Intervertebral disc

Anterior longitudinal lig.

Spinous process

Posterior longitudinal lig.

Spinal cord
Cerebrospinal fluid flow artifact
Posterior subarachnoid space
Posterior epidural fat
Dura
Ligamentum flavum
Supraspinous lig.

1. The ligamentum flavum connects the anterior surface of the upper lamina to the posterior surface of the next lower lamina.

2. The thoracic spine has a normal kyphotic curvature.

3. The trapezius muscle is innervated by the spinal accessory nerve (cranial nerve XI).

4. The thoracic spine is essentially devoid of anterior paraspinal musculature. From a mechanical standpoint, the thoracic kyphotic curvature and rib cage stabilization effect on the thoracic spine make anterior paraspinal musculature unnecessary in this region.

Figure 3.1.2

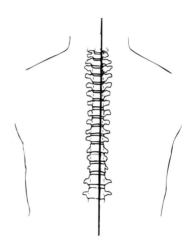

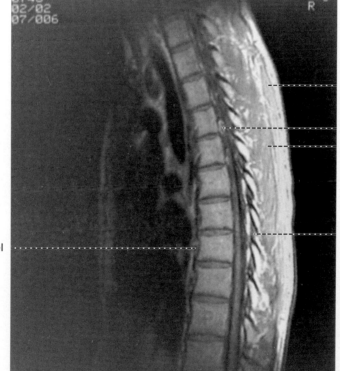

Trapezius m.

Segmental n. root

Spinalis thoracis m.

Ligamentum flavum

Intercostal vessel

Figure 3.1.3

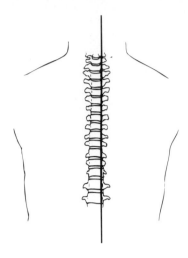

1. The gliding motion of the zygapophyseal joints is due to the redundant ligaments at the superior and inferior poles of the joints.

2. The lateral extension of the ligamentum flavum forms the anterior capsular ligament.

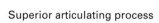

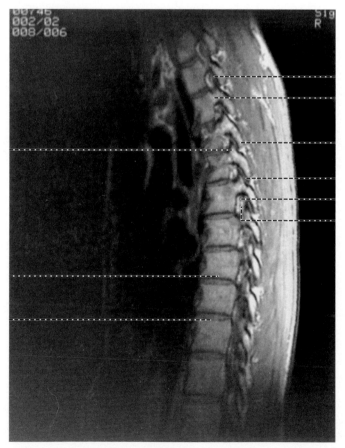

Superior articulating process

Inferior vertebral body endplate

Superior vertebral body endplate

Dorsal root ganglion

Pedicle

Inferior articulating process

Zygapophyseal joint, facet

Dorsal root ganglion

Radicular a.

1. The superior articulating process of the lower vertebral segment is located anterior to the inferior articulating process of the upper vertebral segment.

2. The anterior boundaries of the neural foramen include the lower postero-lateral aspect of the vertebral body of the intervertebral disc.

3. Adjacent pedicles provide the superior and inferior borders of the neural foramen.

Figure 3.1.4

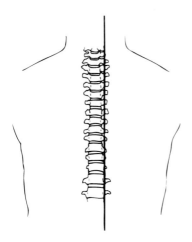

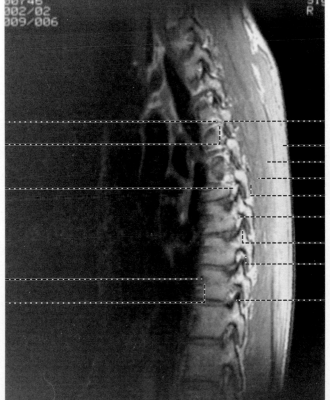

Radicular v. .... Dorsal root ganglion

Radicular a. .... Trapezius m.

Longissimus thoracis m.

Spinalis thoracis m.

Neuroforaminal fat .... Multifidus m.

Spinal n.

Superior articulating process

Inferior articulating process

Radicular v. ....

Radicular a. .... Zygapophyseal joint

Figure 3.1.5

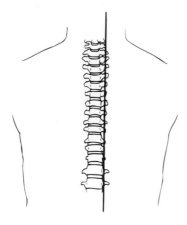

1. The costovertebral articulations are anterior to the thoracic transverse processes. These articulations and the ribs help stabilize thoracic motion segments and limit flexion, extension, and lateral bending in this region.

2. The transverse processes serve as bony attachment for several muscles, including the longissimus, spinalis thoracis, multifidus, rotatores, and intertransversarii.

3. The circumferential vessels represent anterior external vertebral veins (including intercostal veins) and intercostal arteries.

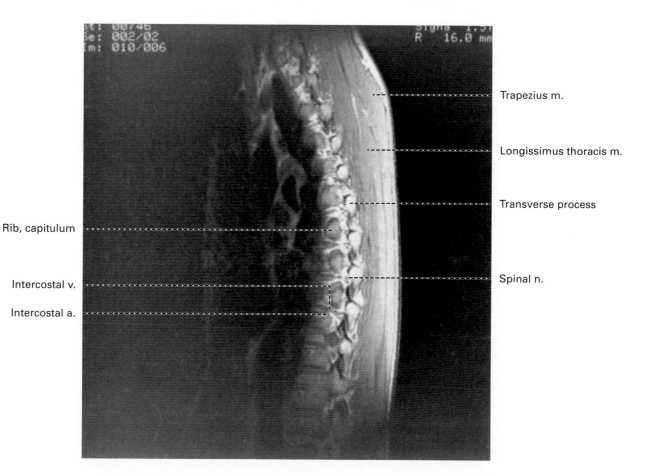

1. The opening between the rib and the transverse process is known as the costotransverse foramen.

2. The ribs stabilize the thoracic spine via the costovertebral and costotransverse articulations.

3. The epidural space contains fatty tissue and the internal vertebral venous plexus.

4. The longissimus thoracis muscle originates from the upper and midthoracic transverse processes and inserts on the sacrum, ilium, and lumbar spinous processes via distal tendons and the aponeurosis of the erector spinae muscles.

Figure 3.2.1

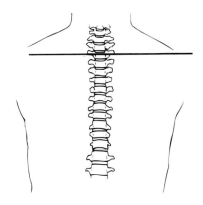

	Se: 004/04 Im: 005/005 S 27.0 mm MF: 1.5

T6 vertebral body near superior endplate

Costovertebral joint

Sixth rib, capitulum

Costotransverse foramen

T6 transverse process

Spinalis thoracis m.

Longissimus thoracis m.

Thoracolumbar fascia, posterior layer

Aorta

Hemiazygous v.

Intercostal a.

Spinal cord

T6 pedicle

Epidural fat

T6 costotransverse joint

Multifidus m.

T5 spinous process

Supraspinous lig.

Trapezius m.

Figure 3.2.2

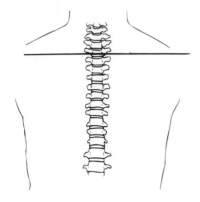

1. The thoracic zygapophyseal joints are oriented in a coronal plane. Their orientation allows significant rotatory thoracic movement.

2. The neural elements in the thoracic region are smaller than those in the lumbar region.

3. The sympathetic trunk lies lateral to the pedicles in the thoracic spine.

4. The eccentric anterior position of the spinal cord within the thecal sac is due to the usual thoracic kyphotic curve.

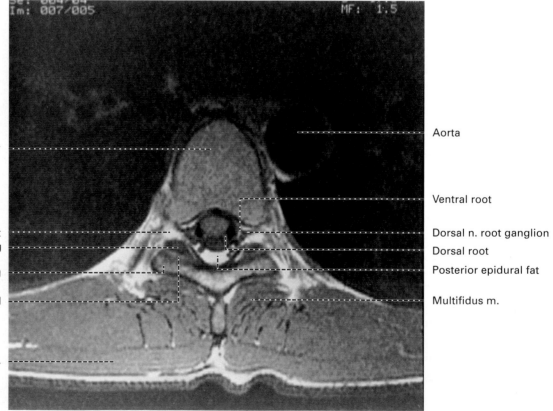

T6 vertebral body, near inferior endplate

Neuroforaminal fat
T7 superior articulating process
T6 inferior articulating process
T6–T7 zygapophyseal joint

Trapezius m.

Aorta

Ventral root

Dorsal n. root ganglion
Dorsal root
Posterior epidural fat

Multifidus m.

1. The erector spinae and the transversospinalis muscles fill the posterior paraspinal space between the ribs and the spinous processes of the vertebral bodies.

2. The erector spinae muscle group in the thoracic and lumbar regions consists of the medially located spinalis thoracis muscle, the longissimus thoracis muscle, and the laterally located iliocostalis muscle.

3. The transversospinalis muscle group is composed of short muscles attached to the posterior vertebral elements. This group comprises interspinalis, rotatores, multifidus, semispinalis, and intertransversarii muscles.

Figure 3.2.3

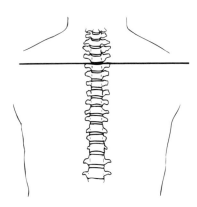

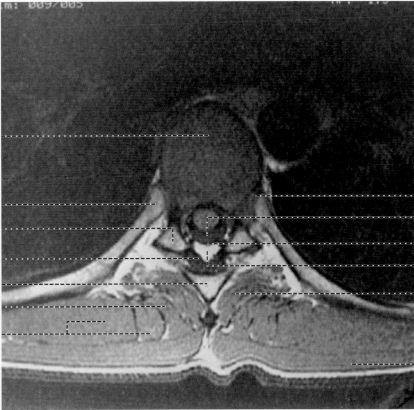

T6–T7 intervertebral disc

Seventh rib

T7 superior articulating process

Ligamentum flavum

T6 spinous process

Spinalis thoracis m.

Longissimus thoracis m.

Subarachnoid space

Costovertebral joint

Dura

Posterior epidural fat

Multifidus m.

Trapezius m.

Figure 3.3.1

1. The intercostal vein, artery, and nerve maintain a constant superior to inferior relationship upon the inferior undersurface of the rib.

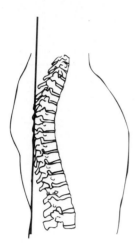

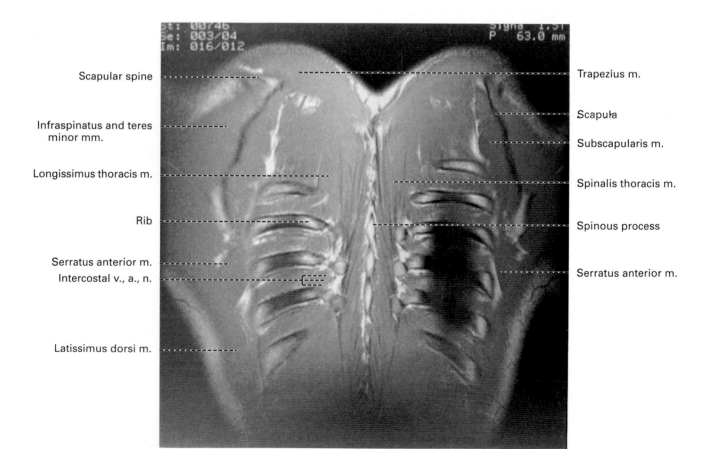

Scapular spine

Infraspinatus and teres minor mm.

Longissimus thoracis m.

Rib

Serratus anterior m.

Intercostal v., a., n.

Latissimus dorsi m.

Trapezius m.

Scapula

Subscapularis m.

Spinalis thoracis m.

Spinous process

Serratus anterior m.

1. The multifidus muscles originate on the transverse processes and insert superiorly on spinous processes two to four levels above.

Figure 3.3.2

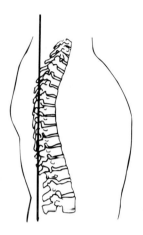

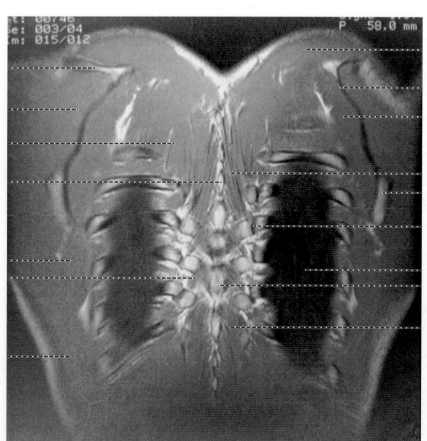

Scapular spine

Infraspinatus and teres minor mm.

Longissimus thoracis m.

Spinous process

Serratus anterior m.

Multifidus m.

Latissimus dorsi m.

Trapezius m.

Scapula

Subscapularis m.

Spinalis thoracis m.

Scapula

Costotransverse joint

Left lung

Laminae

Spinalis thoracis m.

Figure 3.3.3

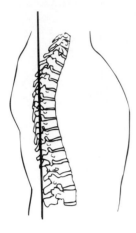

1. The thoracic zygapophyseal joints are usually not visualized on coronal images as they are oriented in a coronal plane.

2. The superior and inferior articulating processes of a single vertebral segment are well outlined in this imaging plane.

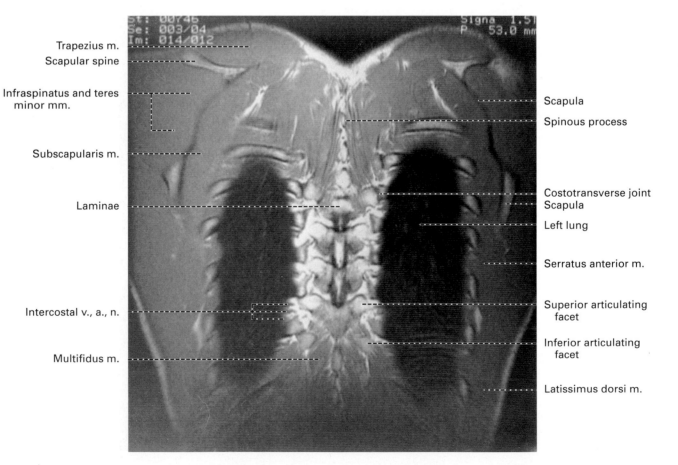

Trapezius m.
Scapular spine
Infraspinatus and teres minor mm.
Subscapularis m.
Laminae
Intercostal v., a., n.
Multifidus m.

Scapula
Spinous process
Costotransverse joint
Scapula
Left lung
Serratus anterior m.
Superior articulating facet
Inferior articulating facet
Latissimus dorsi m.

1. The high-signal-intensity neuroforaminal fat helps to outline neural elements and vascular structures within the neural foramen.

Figure 3.3.4

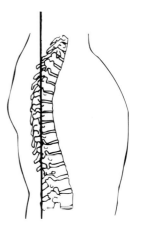

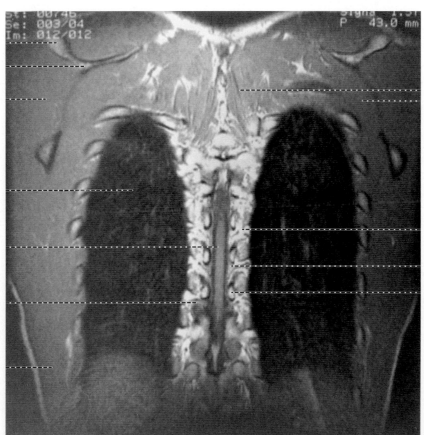

Supraspinatus m.

Scapular spine

Infraspinatus and teres minor mm.

Right lung

Spinal cord

Segmental n.

Latissimus dorsi m.

Semispinalis cervicis m.
Subscapularis m.

Neuroforaminal fat

Dorsal root ganglion

Pedicle

Figure 3.3.5

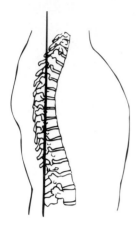

1. The high-signal intensity surrounding the basivertebral venous plexus is due to marrow fat.

2. The basivertebral plexus is the principal venous drainage of the vertebral bodies.

3. The dorsal root ganglia are located immediately caudal to the corresponding segmental pedicle in the thoracic and lumbar regions.

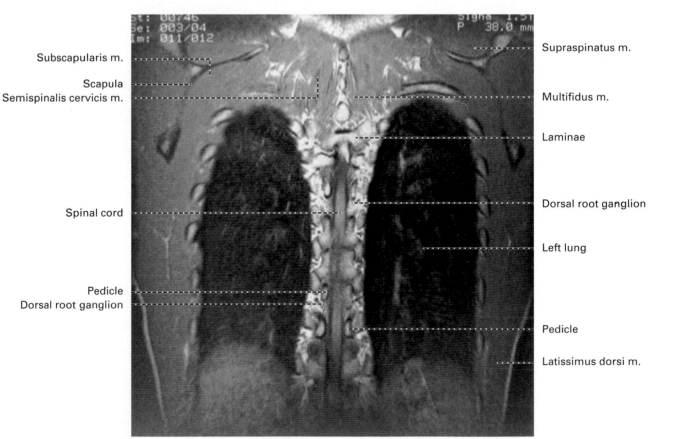

1. The psoas major muscle attaches laterally to vertebral segment T12 and inserts on the lesser trochanter of the femur. Thoracic infections can migrate along the psoas sheath to the hip joint.

2. The anterior median fissure is a small groove on the anterior surface of the spinal cord.

3. Paired ascending lumbar veins are visualized anterior to the transverse processes in the lower thoracic region. They eventually become the azygous and hemiazygous veins.

Figure 3.3.6

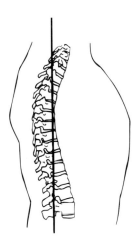

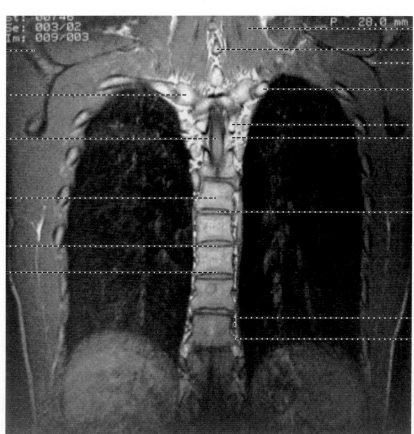

Scapular spine

Transverse process

Anterior median fissure of spinal cord

Vertebral body, marrow

Superior vertebral endplate

Inferior vertebral endplate

Semispinalis capitis m.

Spinous process
Scapula

Rib

Pedicle
Neuroforaminal perineural fat

Intervertebral disc

Intercostal v.

Intercostal a.

Chapter 4

LUMBAR SPINE

Lumbar Spine

The lumbar vertebral column usually consists of five conventional vertebral segments, each containing a vertebral body, an arch, a spinous process, and paired transverse processes. A transitional vertebral segment at the lumbosacral junction is not uncommon. Like the thoracic spine, lumbar vertebral body heights increase with caudal progression. The lumbar vertebrae are larger than thoracic and cervical vertebrae and compensate for great weightbearing stresses. The costal elements that produce ribs in the thoracic region form the bulk of the lumbar transverse process. The original transverse processes form rudimentary posteriorly projecting accessory processes in the lumbar region. The mamillary processes, posterior bony projections forming the lumbar articular facets, serve as origins for many deep back muscles. The interarticular part joins the articular processes to the pedicles.

The lumbar intervertebral disc spaces increase in height with caudal progression with the frequent exception of disc L5 to S1. The zygapophyseal joints are oriented in a slightly oblique sagittal plane. With the superior articulating processes facing medially and the inferior articulating processes facing laterally, the primary lumbar motion is flexion and extension.

The primary ligaments in the lumbar spine are the anterior and posterior longitudinal ligaments, the ligamentum flavum, interspinous ligaments, and the supraspinous ligaments. Through the spinal column, the posterior longitudinal ligament is fixed along the outer annular fibers of the intervertebral discs and the superior and inferior vertebral margins, producing a bowstring appearance within the lumbar spine. A midline ligamentous thickening called the plica mediana dorsalis connects the free edge of the posterior longitudinal ligament to the posterior vertebral body at midlevel, bisecting the anterior epidural space.

The conus medullaris, the terminal end of the spinal cord, is usually located at the L1 to L2 level in adults. The filum terminale and cauda equina occupy the lumbar thecal sac below the level of the conus medullaris. The dorsal root ganglia in the lumbar region occupy the superior portion of neural foramina.

The internal vertebral venous plexus occupies a portion of the epidural space with connecting veins traversing the neural foramina. Circumferential lumbar veins surround the vertebral column and interconnect the anterior external venous plexus with the internal vertebral venous plexus. The basivertebral venous plexus, which is the primary venous outflow for each vertebra, occupies the posterior central portion of each vertebral body.

The paired psoas muscles account for the anterolateral paraspinal lumbar muscles. The primary deep back muscles are composed of two main groups: the short segment transversospinalis muscle group and the longer, more superficial, erector spinae muscle group. The transversospinalis muscle group consists of the multifidus, rotatores, interspinales, and intertransversarii muscles. In the lumbar region, the primary erector spinae muscles are the longissimus and the iliocostalis muscles.

Figure 4.1.1A

1. The posterior epidural fat is most prominent in the midline, where it helps define the posterior dural margin and the anterior surface of the ligamentum flavum.

2. In the midline plane, the ligamentum flavum appears as an oblique linear band of low to intermediate signal that spans the anterior borders of the adjacent spinous processes.

3. The adjacent spinous processes are also united by segmental interspinous ligaments and the intersegmental supraspinous ligament.

4. The thecal sac extends caudally in most individuals to the S2 level.

5. The anterior and posterior longitudinal ligaments connect the vertebral bodies and discs from the skull base to the sacrum.

6. The anterior longitudinal ligament is firmly bound anterior and anterolateral to both the vertebral body and disc, whereas the posterior longitudinal ligament forms a bowstring across the posterior vertebral body with the anterior epidural space interposed between it and the posterior vertebral margin.

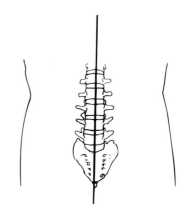

L1 vertebral body, marrow space

Basivertebral v.

Anterior external vertebral venous plexus

Anterior longitudinal lig. and outer annular fibers

Anterior epidural fat

S2 vertebral segment

Presacral fat

Conus medullaris

Ligamentum flavum

Supraspinous lig.

L3 spinous process

Posterior epidural fat

Posterior longitudinal lig. and dura

Termination of thecal sac

Figure 4.1.1B

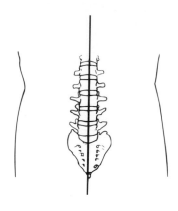

1. This is a midline sagittal T2-weighted fast spin-echo image.

2. The contents within the bony spinal canal are divided into epidural (extradural) and intradural regions.

3. The epidural space contains primarily fat and the internal vertebral venous plexus.

4. The intradural space in the lumbar region contains the conus medullaris, cauda equina, and cerebrospinal fluid.

5. The preservation of the fat signal with this technique combined with the high-signal cerebrospinal fluid delineates the dural margins, allowing distinction between the epidural and intradural spaces.

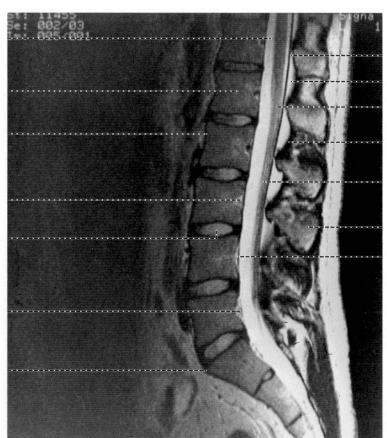

Anterior subarachnoid space

L1 vertebral body marrow space

Anterior longitudinal lig. and anterior vertebral cortex

Basivertebral venous plexus

L3–L4 intervertebral disc

Anterior epidural space

Presacral promontory

Posterior dura

Posterior epidural fat

Conus medullaris

Ligamentum flavum

Cauda equina

L3 spinous process

Posterior longitudinal lig. and anterior dura

1. The high-signal-intensity tissue posterior to the vertebral bodies represents fat and epidural veins.

2. Note the slight physiologic bulging of the intervertebral discs.

3. Note the gradual increase in height of the intervertebral discs from T12 to L5. The intervertebral disc usually accounts for 20 percent of adult spine height.

4. On paramedian sections, the ligamentum flavum is thick and triangular with a wide cranial base as it interconnects adjacent laminae.

5. The ligamentum flavum appears brighter than the anterior and posterior longitudinal ligaments on both T1- and T2-weighted sequences because it is composed primarily of elastin rather than collagen.

Figure 4.1.2

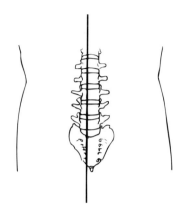

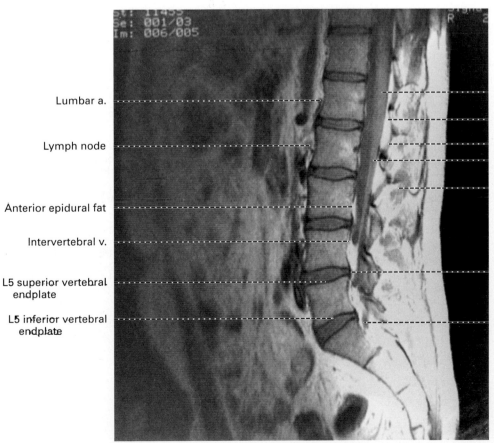

Lumbar a. — Conus medullaris

Posterior epidural fat

Lymph node — Ligamentum flavum

Cauda equina

Interspinous m.

Anterior epidural fat

Intervertebral v.

L5 superior vertebral endplate — Posterior longitudinal lig. and outer annular fibers

L5 inferior vertebral endplate — S1 n. root sheath

Figure 4.1.3

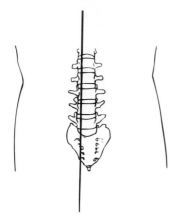

1. The lateral recess can be depicted on sagittal images by identifying dura-invested segmental nerves surrounded by epidural fat.

2. Longitudinally oriented ventral veins run anterior to the segmental nerve within the lateral recess, connecting the basivertebral plexuses.

3. The pars interarticulares, which connects the articular pillar to the facet joint, is best visualized on sagittal images.

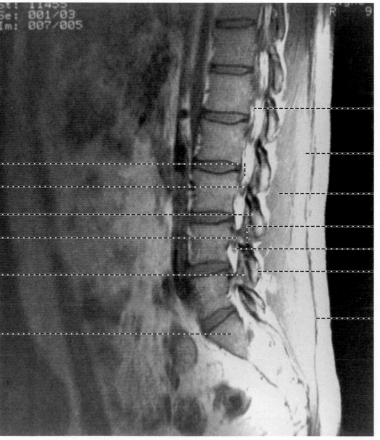

Ventral internal vertebral v.

L3 n. in lateral recess

L3–L4 zygapophyseal joint

L4 pedicle

L5 superior articulating process

S1 vertebral segment

Ventral internal vertebral v.

Longissimus thoracis m., lumbar part

Multifidus m.

L4 pars interarticularis

L4 dorsal root ganglion

L4 inferior articulating process

Thoracolumbar fascia, posterior layer

1. This parasagittal image is through the pedicles and neural foramina.

2. The dorsal root ganglion, sinovertebral nerve, and segmental artery occupy the superior portion of the neural foramen in the lumbar spine.

3. At the neural foramen level, the ligamentum flavum forms the anterior capsule of the lower facet joint.

4. The superior articulating process and the ligamentum flavum form the posterior border of the neural foramen.

5. From medial to lateral, the segmental nerves descend in an anterior and inferior direction within the neural foramina.

Figure 4.1.4

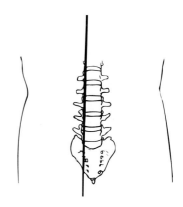

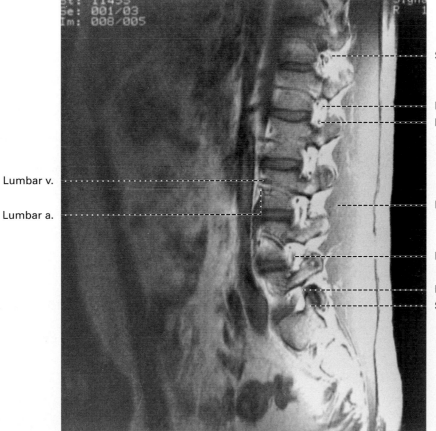

Segmental spinal a.

L1 dorsal root ganglion
Radicular v.

Lumbar v.

Lumbar a.

Longissimus thoracis m.,
lumbar part

L4 segmental n.

Ligamentum flavum
S1 superior articulating
process

Figure 4.1.5

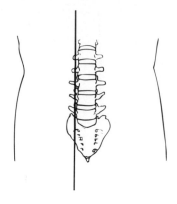

1. The posterior layer of the thoracolumbar fascia clearly separates the posterior paraspinal muscles from the subcutaneous fat.

2. Circumferential lumbar veins connect the rich venous plexus with the lateral neural foramina.

3. The lateral intertransversarii muscles insert on adjacent transverse processes.

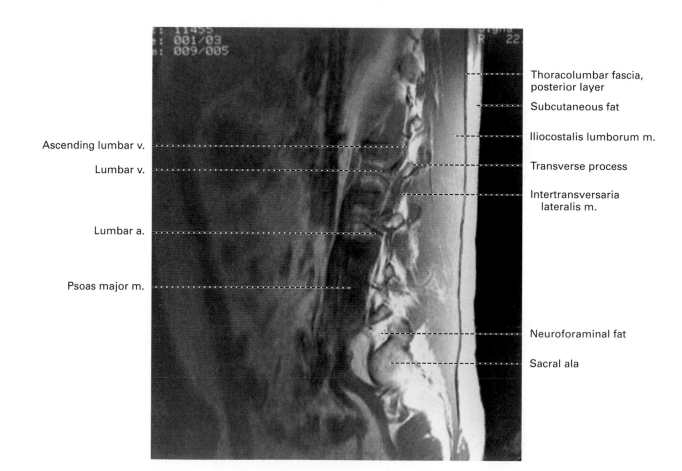

1. The paired sympathetic trunks lie in paramedian locations anterior to the vertebral column and posterior to the aorta and vena cava.

2. Although they are transversospinal muscles, both the rotatores and multifidus muscles originate in the lumbar spine from the mamillary processes to the superior articular facets rather than the transverse processes.

3. The rotatores muscles insert on spinous processes one to two levels above their point of origin, whereas the multifidus muscles insert on spinous processes two to four levels above their origin.

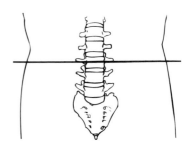

Figure 4.2.1

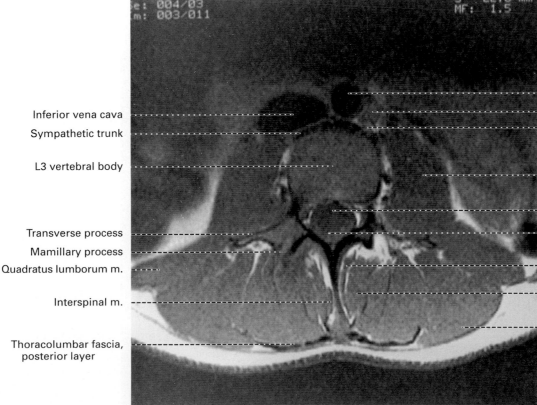

Inferior vena cava
Sympathetic trunk

L3 vertebral body

Transverse process
Mamillary process
Quadratus lumborum m.

Interspinal m.

Thoracolumbar fascia,
posterior layer

Aorta
Lymph node
Sympathetic trunk

Psoas major m.

Thecal sac
Cauda equina

Rotatores m.

Multifidus m.

Iliocostalis lumborum

Figure 4.2.2

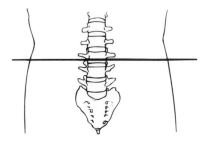

1. The ligamentum flavum is a segmental structure; hence, it is absent from the anterior surfaces of the laminae and the adjacent pars interarticularis.

2. The interspinal muscles are paired short fascicles that connect spinous processes from C2 to the lumbar spine. They are frequently duplicated in the cervical region (because of the cervical bifid spinous processes) and may be absent in the thoracic region.

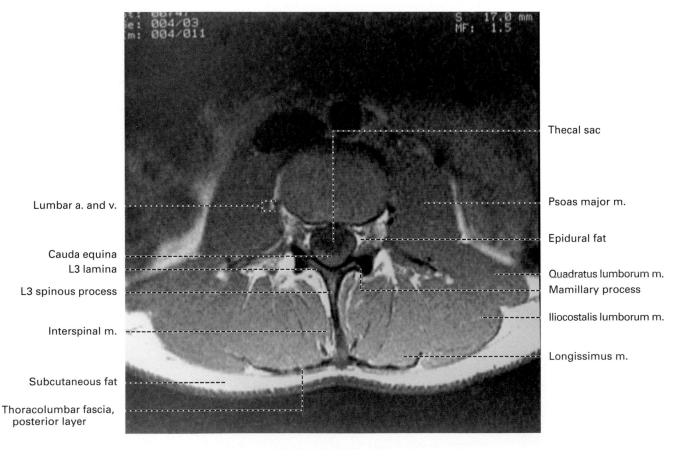

1. The anterior longitudinal ligament is indistinguishable from the anterior disc margins and the anterior cortex of the vertebral bodies in all pulse sequences.

2. The posterior longitudinal ligament has a narrow retrovertebral body segment and a wide retrodiscal segment that fans out to cover the posterior disc margin.

3. The quadratus lumborum muscle is sandwiched between the anterior and middle layers of the thoracolumbar fascia.

4. The dorsal root ganglion is situated in the superior neural foramen between the facet joint capsule posteriorly and the posterolateral cortex of the lower portion of the vertebral body.

5. The lateral course of the transvertebral (radicular) veins distinguishes them from the spinal nerve roots, which proceed in an anterolateral direction from the spinal canal.

Figure 4.2.3

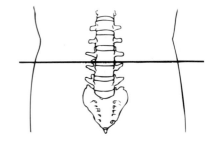

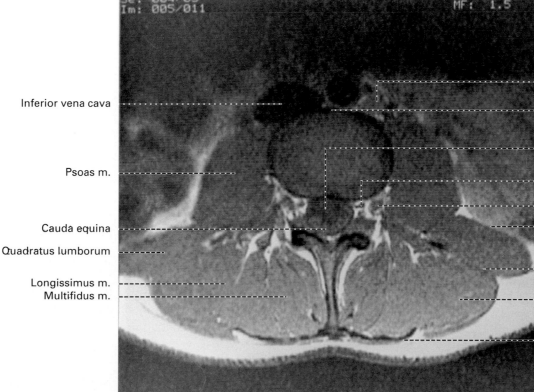

Inferior vena cava

Psoas m.

Cauda equina

Quadratus lumborum

Longissimus m.
Multifidus m.

Lymph node

Anterior longitudinal lig. and anterior vertebral cortex

Thecal sac

Radicular v.

L3 dorsal root ganglion

Thoracolumbar fascia, anterior layer

Thoracolumbar fascia, middle layer

Iliocostalis lumborum m.

Thoracolumbar fascia, posterior layer

Figure 4.2.4

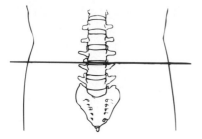

1. The deep muscles of the back consist mainly of the erector spinae group (iliocostalis lumborum and longissimus thoracis [lumbar portion]) and the transversospinalis group (multifidus and rotatores).

2. The fat, posterior to every lamina, is located in the extracapsular inferior recess of the superior facet joint.

3. This retrolaminar fat is enclosed by the insertions of the multifidus muscle.

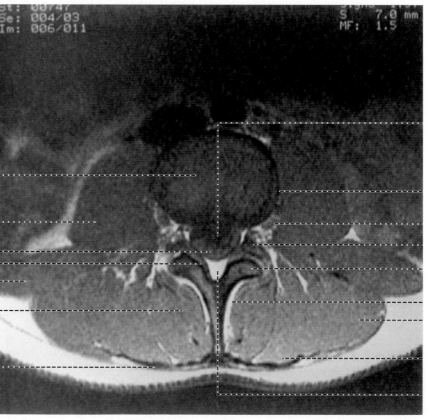

L3–L4 intervertebral disc, nucleus pulposus

Psoas m.

Cauda equina
Ligamentum flavum

Quadratus lumborum m.

Multifidus m.

Thoracolumbar fascia, posterior layer

Thecal sac

L3–L4 intervertebral disc, annulus fibrosis

L3 segmental n.

L4 superior articulating process

L3 inferior articulating process

Retrolaminar fat

Iliocostalis lumborum m.

Longissimus m.

Posterior epidural fat

1. The psoas muscles lie along the sides of the lumbar vertebral column.

2. The anterior layer of the thoracolumbar fascia, also known as the internal abdominal layer, envelops the psoas muscles anteriorly.

Figure 4.2.5

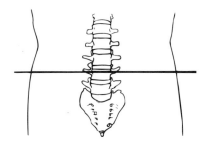

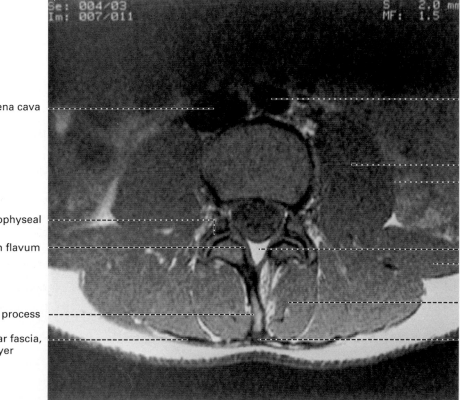

Inferior vena cava

L3–L4 zygapophyseal joint

Ligamentum flavum

L3 spinous process

Thoracolumbar fascia, posterior layer

Aortic bifurcation

Psoas major m.

Thoracolumbar fascia, anterior layer

Posterior epidural fat

Quadratus lumborum m.

Multifidus m.

Supraspinous lig.

Figure 4.2.6

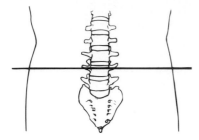

1. The anterior epidural space, defined as the region between the posterior body margin and the thecal sac, contains a venous network embedded in fat and connective tissue, the posterior longitudinal ligament, the midline septum, and the lateral membranes.

2. The lateral membranes, which are very thin and translucent, connect the free edge of the posterior longitudinal ligament to the lateral spinal canal.

3. Besides channeling venous circulation from hematopoiesis-producing vertebral marrow cavities, the epidural space functions to facilitate the mechanical interaction between the spine and thecal sac.

4. The epidural venous plexus consists of valveless, thin-walled veins through which tumor cells may readily migrate from the sacrum to the occiput.

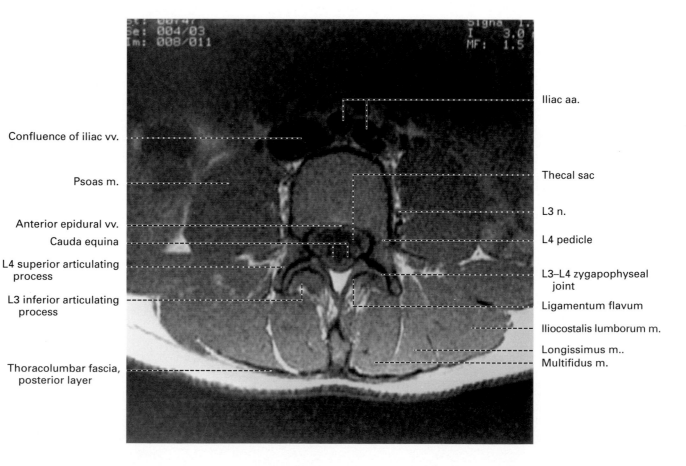

Confluence of iliac vv.

Psoas m.

Anterior epidural vv.

Cauda equina

L4 superior articulating process

L3 inferior articulating process

Thoracolumbar fascia, posterior layer

Iliac aa.

Thecal sac

L3 n.

L4 pedicle

L3–L4 zygapophyseal joint

Ligamentum flavum

Iliocostalis lumborum m.

Longissimus m..

Multifidus m.

Figure 4.2.7

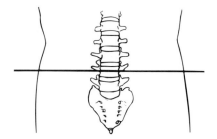

1. The quadratus lumborum muscle is located anterior to the lumbar aponeurosis and the middle layer of the thoracolumbar fascia.

2. The dorsal spine musculature is bounded anteriorly by the transverse processes, the middle layer of the thoracolumbar fascia, and the lumbar aponeurosis.

3. The lumbar aponeurosis forms a strong membrane from the twelfth rib to the iliac crest.

4. The posterior layer of the thoracolumbar fascia forms the posterior boundary of the dorsal spinal musculature.

5. The multifidus muscles originate from the mamillary processes within the lumbar spine.

6. The ureters descend along the anterior surface of the psoas muscles.

7. The epidural venous plexus consists of valveless, thin-walled veins through which tumor cells may readily migrate from the sacrum to the occiput.

8. The left ascending lumbar vein is connected to the common iliac vein by a segmental lumbar vein.

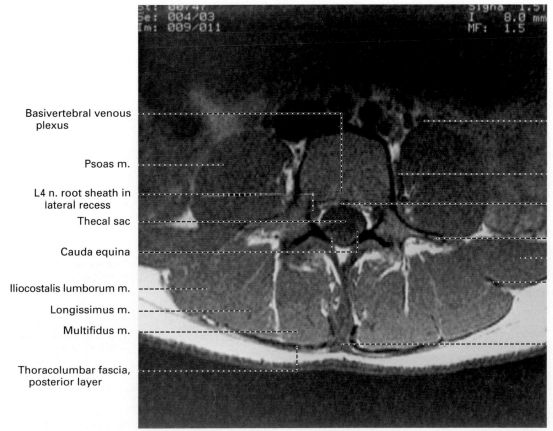

Basivertebral venous plexus

Psoas m.

L4 n. root sheath in lateral recess

Thecal sac

Cauda equina

Iliocostalis lumborum m.

Longissimus m.

Multifidus m.

Thoracolumbar fascia, posterior layer

Ureter

Lumbar v.

Posterior longitudinal lig. and dura

L4 transverse process

Quadratus lumborum m.

Thoracolumbar fascia, middle layer

Supraspinous lig.

Figure 4.2.8

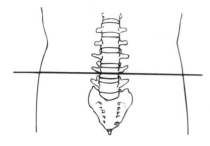

1. The midline septum, which splits the anterior epidural space, connects the posterior longitudinal ligament to the convex portion of the vertebral body. It is also known as the plica mediana dorsalis.

2. The presence of the plica mediana dorsalis accounts for the predominantly paramedian location of extruded disc fragments.

3. Although present throughout the spinal canal, the plica or midline septum is most easily visualized in the lower lumbar where the retrovertebral posterior longitudinal ligament is farthest from the vertebral body.

4. The intertransverse process ligaments are continuous laterally with the lumbar aponeurosis.

5. The lateral raphe joins the middle and posterior layers of the thoracolumbar fascia.

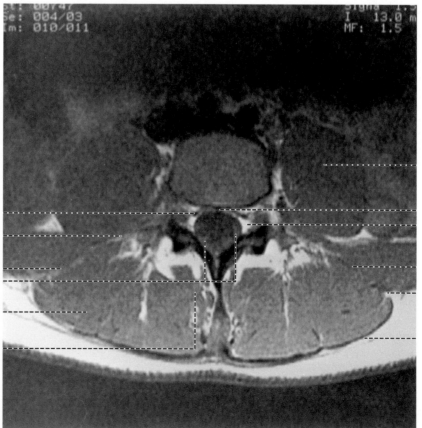

Anterior internal venous plexus

Intertransverse process ligs.

Lumbar aponeurosis
Cauda equina

Iliocostalis lumborum m.

Multifidus m.

Psoas m.

Plica mediana dorsalis
Epidural fat

Thoracolumbar fascia, middle layer
Lateral raphe

Thoracolumbar fascia, posterior layer

1. The ligamentum flavum, which merges into the anterior capsule of the facet joint, forms the posterior boundary of the neural foramen.

2. The ventral and dorsal roots unite to form a segmental nerve lateral to the dorsal root ganglion.

3. The ventral roots are approximately three times thinner than the dorsal roots.

Figure 4.2.9

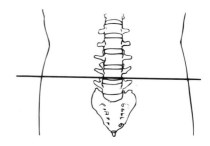

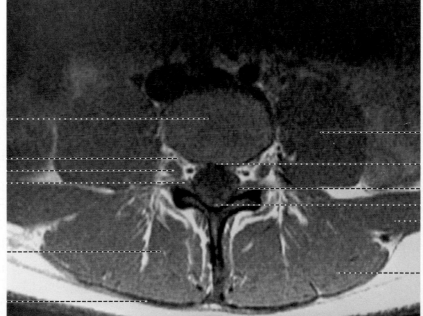

L4 vertebral body

L4 ventral root
L4 dorsal root ganglion
Ligamentum flavum

Longissimus m.

Thoracolumbar fascia,
posterior layer

Psoas m.

Posterior longitudinal
lig. and dura
Dura
Cauda equina
Quadratus lumborum m.

Iliocostalis lumborum
m.

Figure 4.2.10

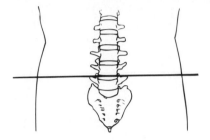

1. The segmental nerve has efferent motor fibers and afferent sensory fibers.

2. The lumbosacral plexus forms adjacent to and within the psoas musculature.

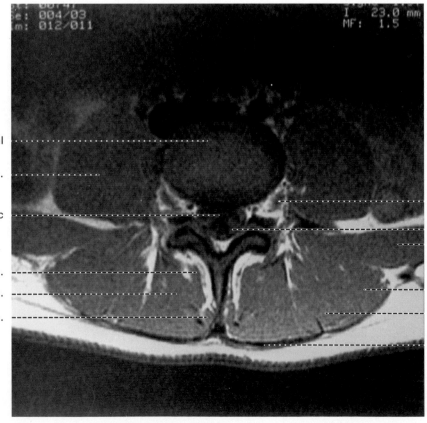

L4 inferior vertebral endplate

Psoas major m.

Thecal sac

Rotatores m.

Multifidus m.

Interspinal m.

L4 segmental n. root

Cauda equina

Quadratus lumborum m.

Iliocostalis lumborum m.

Longissimus m.

Thoracolumbar fascia, posterior layer

1. Because the superior articular processes face medially and the inferior articular processes face laterally, movement in the lumbar spine is primarily that of flexion and extension.

2. The lumbar spinal canal loses its ovoid shape in the lower lumbar region and becomes more triangular due to mild posterolateral indentations by the superior articular processes.

Figure 4.2.11

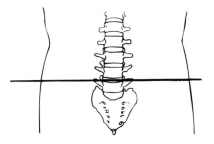

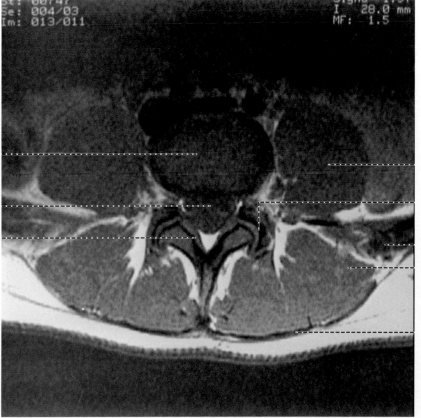

L4–L5 intervertebral disc

Thecal sac

Ligamentum flavum

Psoas m.

L4–L5 zygapophyseal joint

Quadratus lumborum m.

Iliocostalis lumborum m.

Thoracolumbar fascia, posterior layer

Figure 4.3.1

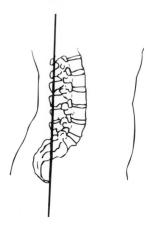

1. This coronal image is through the posterior lumbar musculature.

2. A fat plane separates the multifidus muscles from the erector spinae muscle group.

3. The primary erector spinae muscles in the lumbar region are the longissimus and the iliocostalis.

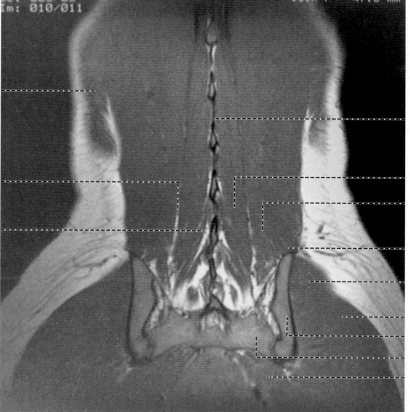

Latissimus dorsi m.

Fat pad between multifidus and erector spinae group

Multifidus m., short fascicle

Interspinal lig.

Multifidus m.

Longissimus thoracis m., lumbar part

Iliocostalis lumborum m.

Gluteus medius m.

Gluteus maximus m.

Ilium

Sacrum

Piriformis m.

1. The ligamentum flavum connects adjacent laminae.

2. Made from elastic fibers, the ligamentum flavum can increase in length and flexion by up to 70 percent in a young adult.

3. The elastic properties of the ligmentum flavum diminish with aging. In a 70-year-old adult, the ligamentum flavum will only increase in length up to 30 percent before rupturing.

4. The L4 to L5 and L5 to S1 zygapophyseal joints are the largest of the posterior articular joints and support the most weight. The normal lumbar lordosis exacerbates the stress on these lower lumbar facet joints.

5. Although the lumbar zygapophyseal joints are vertically oriented in the coronal plane, the articulation is actually curved, usually resulting in a 45-degree angulation in the sagittal plane.

Figure 4.3.2

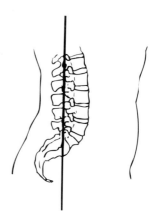

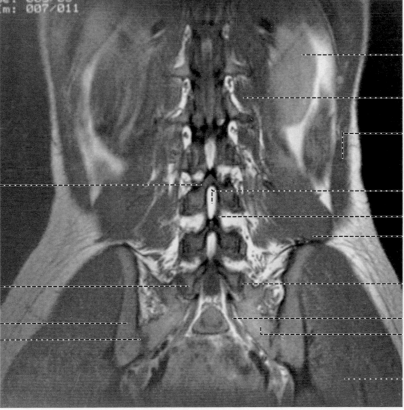

Left kidney

Intertransverse m.

Internal and external oblique and transversus abdominis mm.

Posterior epidural fat

Ligamentum flavum m.

Quadratus lumborum m.

L5–S1 zygapophyseal joint

S1 n. root

Sacrum

Gluteus medius m.

L3 lamina

L5 superior articulating process

Ilium

Sacroiliac joint

Figure 4.3.3

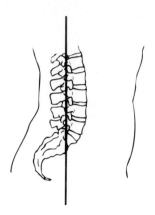

1. The conus medullaris is usually located at the L1 to L2 level.

2. The intertransversarii muscles are slender muscles that originate from and insert on adjacent transverse processes.

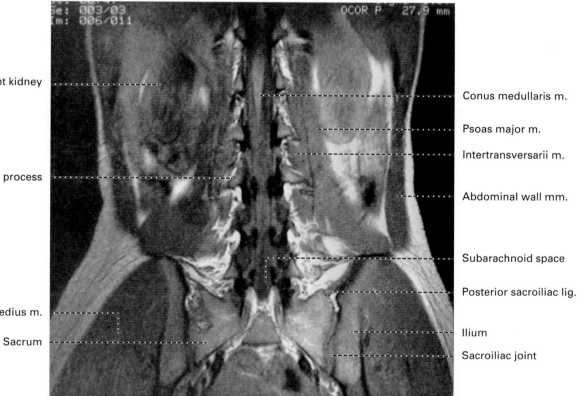

Right kidney

L3 transverse process

Gluteus medius m.

Sacrum

Conus medullaris m.

Psoas major m.

Intertransversarii m.

Abdominal wall mm.

Subarachnoid space

Posterior sacroiliac lig.

Ilium

Sacroiliac joint

1. The anterior portion of the sacroiliac joint is synovial, in contrast to the fibrous or ligamentous posterior portion.

Figure 4.3.4

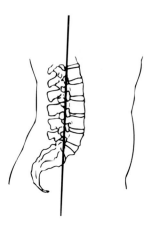

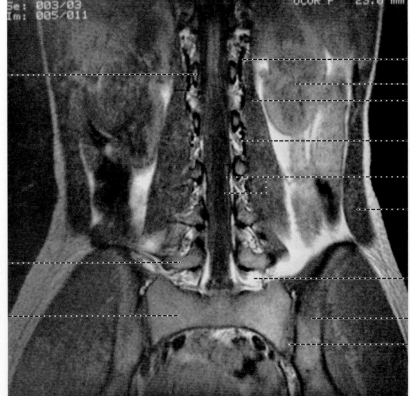

L1 pedicle

L5 transverse process

Sacral ala

Ascending lumbar v.

Left kidney
Psoas major m.

L2 n. root

Cauda equina n. roots

Abdominal wall mm.

Neuroforaminal fat

Ilium

Sacroiliac joint

Figure 4.3.5

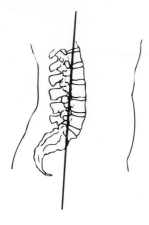

1. The dorsal root ganglion receives sensory input from the periphery and relays it to the spinal cord via dorsal roots.

2. The dorsal root ganglion is located in the superior portion of the lumbar neural foramen.

3. The ventral roots conduct motor impulses.

4. The ventral and dorsal roots join distal to the dorsal root ganglion to form a segmental nerve.

5. In the thoracic and lumbar regions, the numbering system is such that a segmental nerve exits beneath a pedicle of the same number. For example, the L5 nerve root exits beneath the L5 pedicle.

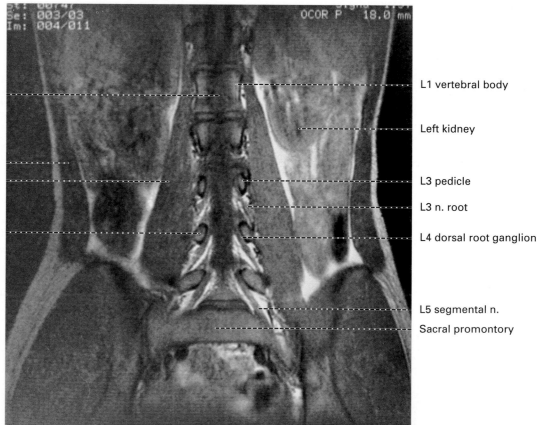

1. The psoas major muscle originates from the lateral aspects of the vertebral bodies and intervertebral discs from T12 to L5 and inserts on the lesser trochanter of the femur.

2. The psoas major muscle sheath can serve as a conduit for spreading thoracic spine infections to the hip joint.

3. Only 50 percent of individuals have a psoas minor muscle, which is a small muscle originating from the anterior aspect of the lumbar vertebral bodies.

4. The asymmetric thickness between inferior and superior vertebral endplates is due to a chemical shift artifact.

Figure 4.3.6

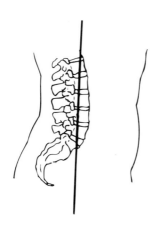

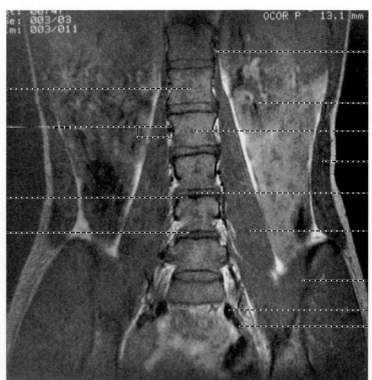

T12 vertebral body

Lumbar v., a.

Superior vertebral endplate

Inferior vertebral endplate

Crus of diaphragm

Left kidney

Basivertebral v.

Abdominal wall mm.

Intervertebral disc

Psoas major m.

Iliacus m.

Common iliac v.
Common iliac a.

Chapter 5

SHOULDER

Musculature of the Shoulder

The muscles arising from the anterior thoracic region are pectoralis major, pectoralis minor, and subclavius.

The largest and most superficial of the three is pectoralis major. This triangular muscle arises from the medial half of the clavicle, sternum, and second through sixth ribs and inserts onto the lateral lip of the intertubercular sulcus of the humerus. Its lateral margin adjoins the ventral margin of the deltoid, from which it is separated only by the cephalic vein.

Pectoralis minor is covered by pectoralis major. This smaller triangular muscle arises from the second through fifth ribs and inserts onto the tip of the coracoid process of the scapula.

The small subclavius muscle lies below the clavicle and arises from the first rib upward and medially to insert onto the clavicle.

Pectoralis major adducts and flexes the arm and rotates it medially. Pectoralis minor protracts, depresses, and rotates the shoulder girdle downward, moving the inferior angle of the scapula medially. Subclavius depresses the shoulder girdle and keeps the clavicle and sternum in apposition. With the clavicle fixed, the muscle can assist in respiratory movements of the rib cage.

Pectoralis major is innervated by the lateral and medial pectoral nerves. Pectoralis minor is also supplied by the lateral and medial pectoral nerves. Subclavius is supplied by the nerve to subclavius, usually derived from the superior trunk of the brachial plexus.

The muscles of the shoulder region include deltoid, teres minor, infraspinatus, supraspinatus, latissimus dorsi, teres major, and subscapularis.

The muscles of the shoulder are innervated by nerves arising from the dorsal divisions of the brachial plexus. The muscles are innervated by suprascapular, subscapular, axillary, and radial nerves.

The deltoid muscle is large and shaped like a shield. The muscle arises from the spine of the scapula, acromion, and the lateral third of the clavicle. It inserts onto the deltoid tuberosity of the humerus. The muscle abducts, adducts, extends, flexes, and rotates the arm.

Teres minor, infraspinatus, and supraspinatus as a group arise from the back of the scapula, the tendons of which pass over the capsule of the shoulder joint and are attached to it, and course under the deltoid muscle to insert onto the top and dorsal margin of the greater tubercle of the humerus. Teres minor is rounded and originates from the upper two-thirds of the axillary border of the scapula. Infraspinatus is triangular in shape and originates from the entire infraspinous fossa of the scapula, with the exception of the neck and axillary border. Infraspinatus inserts above teres minor on the greater tubercle. Supraspinatus is pyramidal in shape and arises under the cover of trapezius from the supraspinous fossa. Supraspinatus inserts above infraspinatus at the highest point of the greater tubercle.

Teres minor and infraspinatus act as lateral rotators of the arm, supraspinatus along with the upper part of infraspinatus abducts the arm, and the lower part of infraspinatus and teres minor adduct the arm.

Latissimus dorsi, teres major, and subscapularis form a group of muscles that insert onto the lesser tubercle of the humerus and onto the crest or ridge of bone that extends distally from this tubercle on the medial side, as well as into the intertubercular groove.

Latissimus dorsi is a large flat triangular muscle originating from an aponeurosis that covers the lumbar and lower half of the thoracic regions of the back and from the posterior part of the iliac crest. The muscle inserts into the intertubercular groove.

Teres major is a round, thick muscle that originates from the dorsal surface of the inferior angle of the scapula. The muscle inserts behind latissimus dorsi onto the crest of the lesser tubercle of the humerus.

Subscapularis is also a thick muscle but triangular in shape; it extends from the subscapular fossa to the lesser tubercle of the humerus.

These muscles adduct the arm and rotate it medially. Latissimus dorsi is also the primary extensor of the arm.

Latissimus dorsi, teres major, and subscapularis form the posterior wall of the axillary fossa. Near their insertions, they are crossed by the blood supply and nerves of the arm, by the short head of biceps brachii, and by coracobrachialis.

Supraspinatus and infraspinatus are innervated by the suprascapular nerve; deltoid and teres minor are innervated by the axillary nerve; and subscapularis, teres major, and latissimus dorsi are innervated by subscapular nerves. Subscapularis is innervated by the upper and lower subscapular nerves. Teres major is innervated by the lower subscapular nerve. The middle or long subscapular nerve that supplies the latissimus dorsi is known as the thoracodorsal nerve.

Table 5-1. Anterior Thoracic Region

Muscle	Origin	Insertion	Nerve Supply	Arterial Supply
Pectoralis major	Medial half of anterior surface of the clavicle, side and front of the sternum as far as the 6th costal cartilage, front and surfaces of the cartilage of the 2nd through 6th ribs, osseous ends of the 6th and 7th ribs, and aponeurosis of external abdominal oblique	Crest of the greater tubercle of the humerus, lateral lip of intertubercular groove, deltoid tubercle, and fibrous periosteum of the intertubercular sulcus	Lateral and medial pectoral nerves (C5 and C6 for the clavicular part, and C7, C8, and T1 for the sternocostal part)	Axillary branches including supreme thoracic, thoracoacromial, thoracodorsal, anterior circumflex humeral, and subclavian by its internal thoracic and internal thoracic perforating branches
Pectoralis minor	Aponeurotic slips from the 2nd through 5th ribs, near costal cartilages	Anterior half of the medial border and upper surface of the coracoid process of the scapula	Medial and lateral pectoral nerves (C6, C7, C8)	Pectoral branches from the thoracoacromial, lateral thoracic, and thoracodorsal
Subclavius	First rib and its cartilage	Inferior surface of the clavicle between the costal and coracoid tuberosities	Nerve to subclavian (C5 or C5 and C6)	Thoracoacromial
Deltoid	Lateral border and upper surface of the lateral third of the clavicle, the acromion, and the scapular spine	Deltoid tuberosity of the humerus	Axillary n. (C5, C6)	Deltoid branch of thoracoacromial and posterior circumflex humeral
Teres minor	Upper two-thirds of the axillary border of the scapula	Shoulder capsule and the inferior facet of the greater tubercle of the humerus	Axillary n. (C4, C5, C6)	Circumflex scapular branch of subscapular; suprascapular and dorsal scapular may also contribute
Infraspinatus	Infraspinous fossa, scapular spine, investing (deep) fascia, and adjacent aponeurotic septa	Shoulder capsule and the middle facet of the greater tubercle of the humerus	Suprascapular n. (C4, C5, C6)	Circumflex scapular; suprascapular and dorsal scapular may also contribute
Supraspinatus	Supraspinous fossa and investing fascia	Shoulder capsule and the superior facet of the greater tubercle of the humerus	Suprascapular n. (C4, C5, C6)	Superficial branch of transverse cervical
Latissimus dorsi	Spines and interspinous ligaments of the lower five or six thoracic vertebrae, upper lumbar vertebrae, thoracodorsal fascia, posterior third of the crest of the ilium, and the lateral surface and upper edge of the lower three or four ribs	The muscle tendon inserts onto the ventral side of the crest of the lesser tubercle of the humerus and onto the floor of the intertubercular groove ventral to the tendon of teres major. The tendon may extend to the greater tubercle of the humerus	Thoracodorsal n. (C6, C7, C8)	Thoracodorsal branch of the subscapular
Teres major	Inferior angle of scapula	Medial lip of intertubercular groove of humerus	Lower subscapular n. (C6, C7)	Subscapular, lesser supply by circumflex scapular and posterior circumflex humeral
Subscapularis	Subscapularis fossa	Shoulder capsule and lesser tubercle of humerus and its shaft immediately below the tubercle	Two or three subscapular branches from posterior cord and upper and lower subscapular nerves (C5, C6, C7)	Dorsal scapular, with the suprascapular and axillary

113

Figure 5.1.1

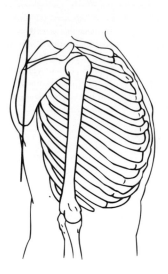

1. This oblique coronal section is through the posterior muscles of the shoulder girdle.

2. Note the trapezius muscle forming the superior aspect of the shoulder and covering the supraspinous fossa and supraspinatus muscle.

3. The middle fibers of the deltoid muscle are depicted here. This portion of the deltoid and the supraspinatus act as abductors of the arm.

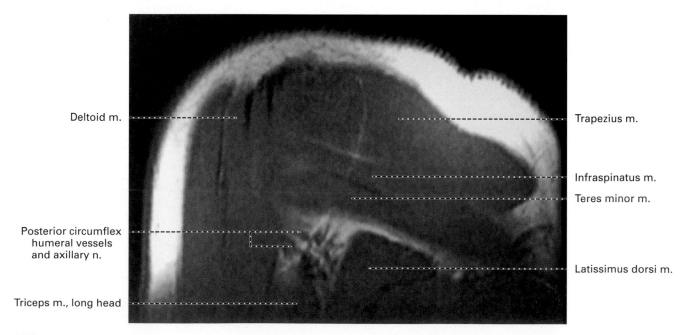

Deltoid m.

Posterior circumflex humeral vessels and axillary n.

Triceps m., long head

Trapezius m.

Infraspinatus m.

Teres minor m.

Latissimus dorsi m.

1. Note the posterior humeral circumflex vessels. They reach the posterior aspect of the shoulder by passing through the quadrangular space.

2. The anterior and posterior circumflex humeral arteries are branches of the axillary artery. They anastomose around the surgical neck of the humerus.

3. The axillary nerve also exits through the quadrangular space and innervates the teres minor and deltoid muscles.

4. Some fibers of the axillary nerve supply the shoulder joint and skin over the shoulder.

5. The long head of the triceps is the most medial portion of this muscle. It originates from the infraglenoid tubercle.

Figure 5.1.2

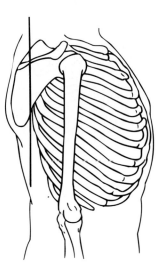

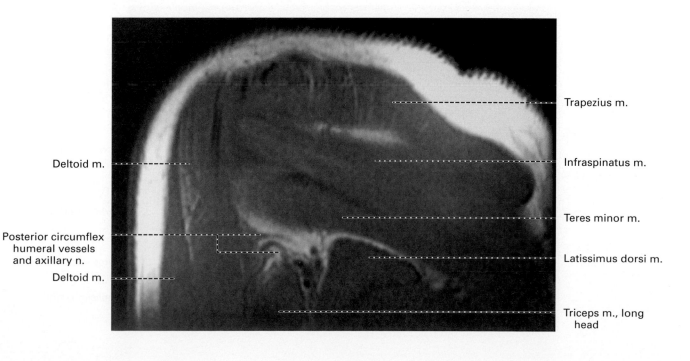

Deltoid m.

Posterior circumflex humeral vessels and axillary n.

Deltoid m.

Trapezius m.

Infraspinatus m.

Teres minor m.

Latissimus dorsi m.

Triceps m., long head

Figure 5.1.3

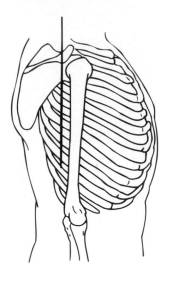

1. Note the insertion of the trapezius muscle on the spine of the scapula.

2. The teres major and latissimus dorsi muscles form the posterior axillary fold. Along with the subscapularis muscle, they form the posterior wall of the axilla.

3. The radial nerve, which supplies the triceps muscle, courses distally with the profunda brachii artery in what is called the spiral groove of the humerus.

4. The spiral groove of the humerus is located between the origins of the medial and lateral heads of the triceps.

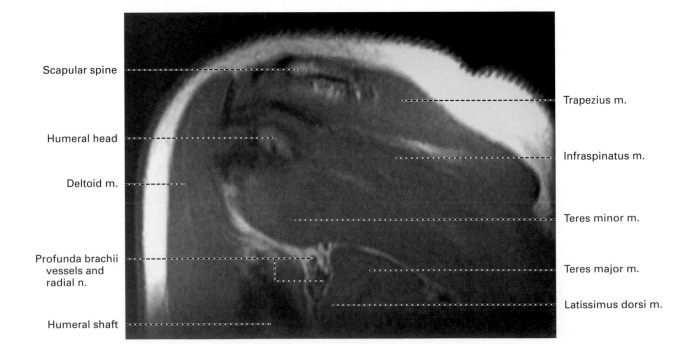

Scapular spine

Humeral head

Deltoid m.

Profunda brachii vessels and radial n.

Humeral shaft

Trapezius m.

Infraspinatus m.

Teres minor m.

Teres major m.

Latissimus dorsi m.

1. The teres major and teres minor muscles originate from the axillary border of the scapula.

2. The flat infraspinatus muscle originates from the infraspinous fossa.

3. Both the deltoid and trapezius muscles attach to the spine of the scapula, the acromion, and the lateral third of the clavicle.

Figure 5.1.4

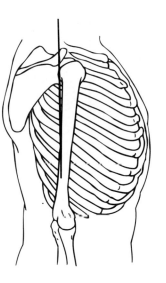

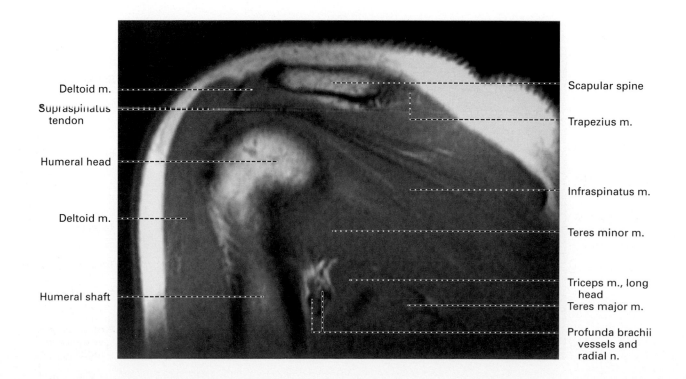

Figure 5.1.5

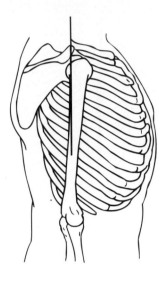

1. Note the supraspinatus tendon as it courses laterally to insert on the greater tuberosity of the humerus.

2. The space containing the distal third of the supraspinatus muscle and tendon is called the coracoacromial arch, or supraspinatus outlet.

3. The coracoacromial arch is formed by the coracoid process, coracoacromial ligament, and acromion.

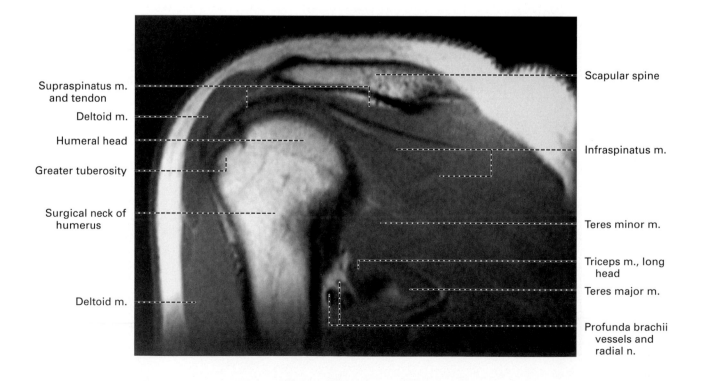

Supraspinatus m. and tendon
Deltoid m.
Humeral head
Greater tuberosity
Surgical neck of humerus
Deltoid m.

Scapular spine
Infraspinatus m.
Teres minor m.
Triceps m., long head
Teres major m.
Profunda brachii vessels and radial n.

1. The acromion process is a continuation of the scapular spine. It provides muscle attachments for the trapezius and deltoid muscles.

2. The scapular spine divides the posterior surface of the scapula into the supraspinous and infraspinous fossae.

3. Note that the long head of the triceps muscle originates from the infraglenoid tuberosity.

4. The four muscles of the rotator cuff, subscapularis, supraspinatus, interspinatus, and teres minor muscles, surround the glenohumeral joint. The tendons of these muscles blend with the joint capsule.

Figure 5.1.6

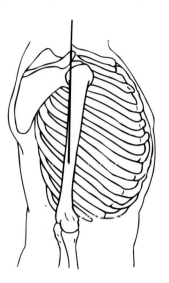

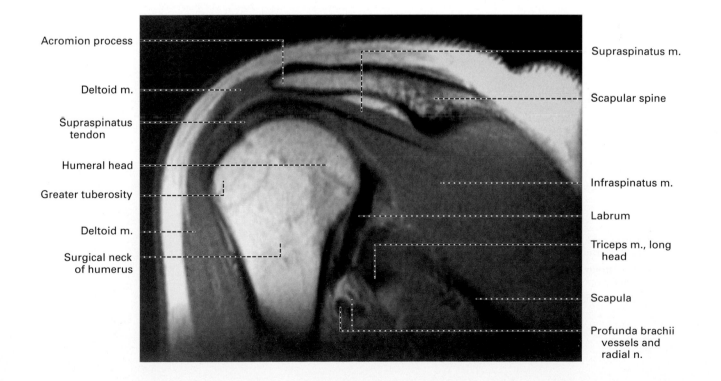

Acromion process

Deltoid m.

Supraspinatus tendon

Humeral head

Greater tuberosity

Deltoid m.

Surgical neck of humerus

Supraspinatus m.

Scapular spine

Infraspinatus m.

Labrum

Triceps m., long head

Scapula

Profunda brachii vessels and radial n.

Figure 5.1.7

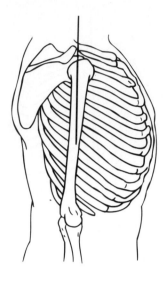

1. The greater tuberosity of the humerus provides insertion sites for the supraspinatus, infraspinatus, and teres minor muscles.

2. The posterior circumflex artery along with the axillary nerve curves around the surgical neck of the humerus by passing through the quadrangular space.

3. The space separating the acromion process and deltoid from the supraspinatus tendon contains the subacromial subdeltoid bursa.

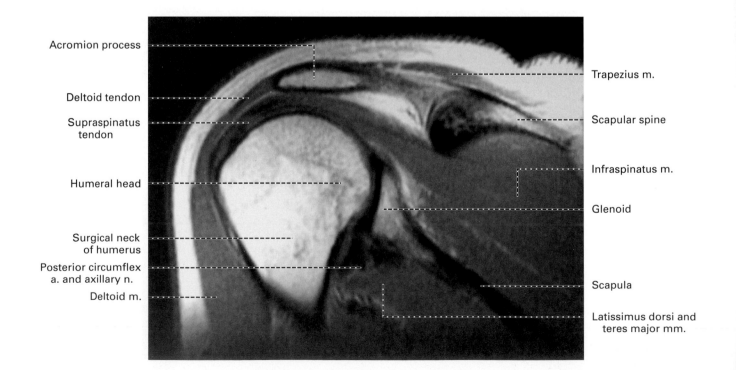

Acromion process

Deltoid tendon

Supraspinatus tendon

Humeral head

Surgical neck of humerus

Posterior circumflex a. and axillary n.

Deltoid m.

Trapezius m.

Scapular spine

Infraspinatus m.

Glenoid

Scapula

Latissimus dorsi and teres major mm.

1. Note the supraclavicular artery running in the retroclavicular space before crossing over the suprascapular ligament.

2. The suprascapular nerve usually crosses under the suprascapular ligament and the suprascapular artery usually crosses over this ligament.

3. The suprascapular nerve innervates the supraspinatus and infraspinatus muscles.

Figure 5.1.8

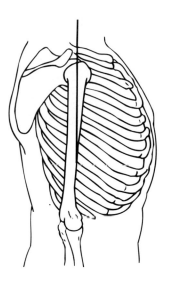

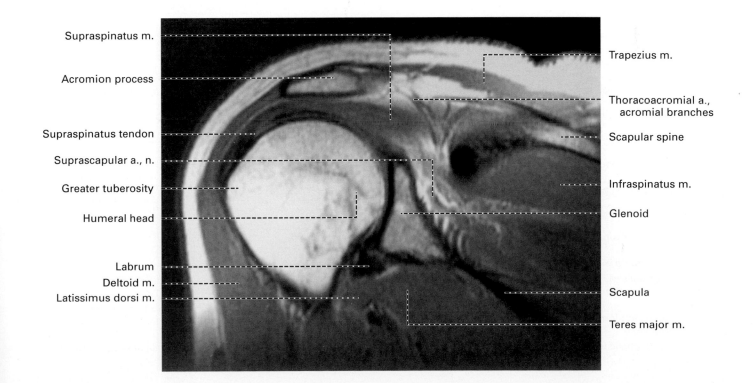

Supraspinatus m.

Acromion process

Supraspinatus tendon

Suprascapular a., n.

Greater tuberosity

Humeral head

Labrum
Deltoid m.
Latissimus dorsi m.

Trapezius m.

Thoracoacromial a., acromial branches

Scapular spine

Infraspinatus m.

Glenoid

Scapula

Teres major m.

Figure 5.1.9

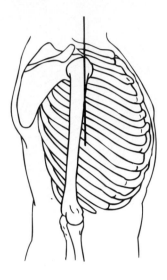

1. This section is through the scapular notch, which usually admits the supra-scapular nerve.

2. Note that the shallow glenoid cavity is deepened by the glenoid labrum.

3. The long head of the biceps is depicted in this section as it descends in the bicipital groove.

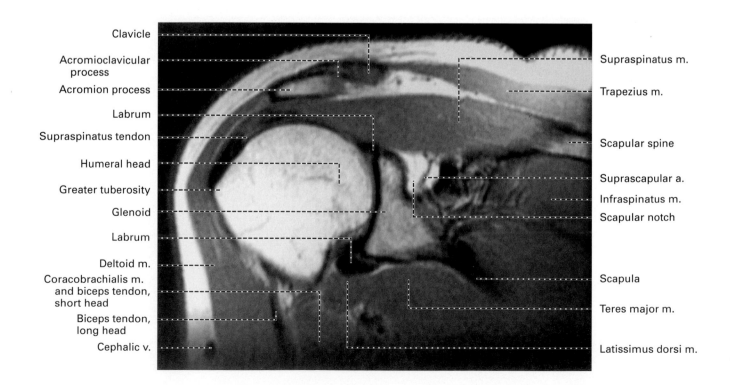

1. This section is through the acromioclavicular joint.

2. Stability for the acromioclavicular joint is provided by the coracoclavicular ligament (conoid and trapezoid portions).

3. The subscapularis muscle originates from the subscapularis fossa on the anterior surface of the scapula.

4. Note the tendon of the supraspinatus muscle as it inserts on the greater tuberosity of the humerus.

Figure 5.1.10

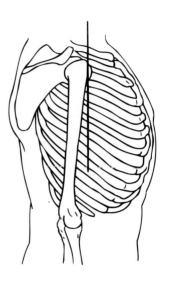

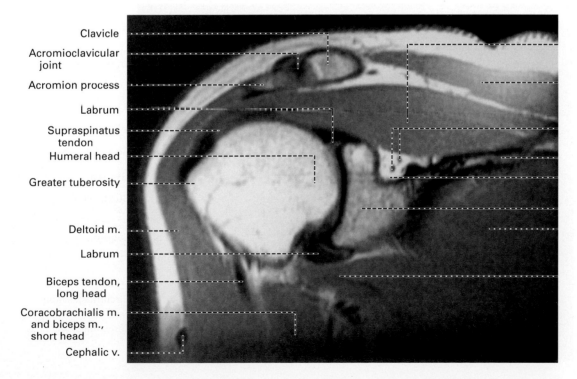

Clavicle
Acromioclavicular joint
Acromion process
Labrum
Supraspinatus tendon
Humeral head
Greater tuberosity
Deltoid m.
Labrum
Biceps tendon, long head
Coracobrachialis m. and biceps m., short head
Cephalic v.

Supraspinatus m.
Trapezius m.
Suprascapular a., n.
Scapular spine
Scapular notch
Glenoid
Subscapularis m.
Latissimus dorsi m.

Figure 5.1.11

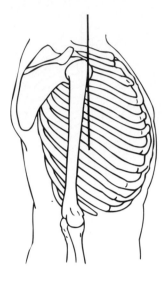

1. Note that both the trapezius and deltoid muscles have muscular attachments on the lateral third of the clavicle.

2. The greater tuberosity, lesser tuberosity, and bicipital groove are demonstrated on this section.

3. The supraspinatus muscle originates from the medial portion of the supraspinous fossa. Its tendon courses under the coracohumeral arch to insert on the superior aspect of the greater tuberosity of the humerus.

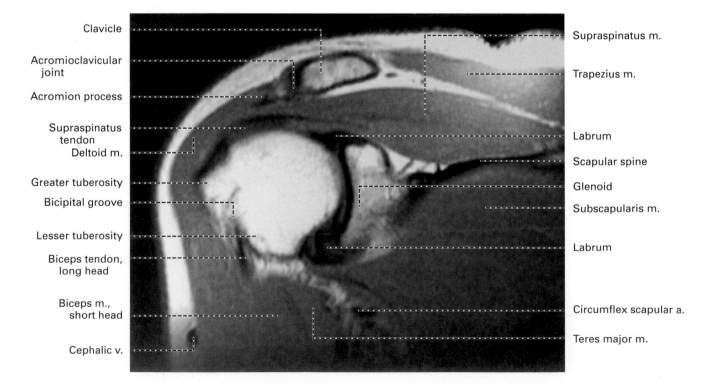

Clavicle

Acromioclavicular joint

Acromion process

Supraspinatus tendon
Deltoid m.

Greater tuberosity

Bicipital groove

Lesser tuberosity

Biceps tendon, long head

Biceps m., short head

Cephalic v.

Supraspinatus m.

Trapezius m.

Labrum

Scapular spine

Glenoid

Subscapularis m.

Labrum

Circumflex scapular a.

Teres major m.

1. The long head of the biceps tendon is depicted between the lesser and greater tuberosities.

2. The biceps and coracobrachialis muscles of the anterior compartment are seen along the anterior and anteromedial part of the shaft of the humerus.

3. All the muscles of the anterior compartment are innervated by the musculocutaneous nerve.

Figure 5.1.12

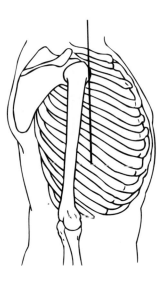

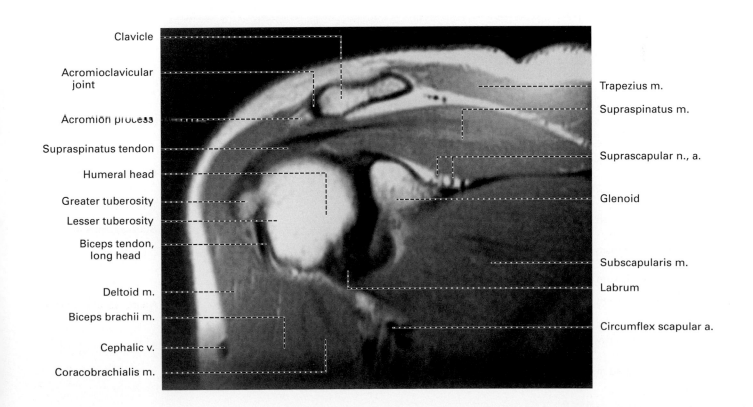

Figure 5.1.13

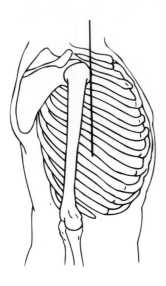

1. This section is through the base of the coracoid process.

2. In its course, the long head of the biceps tendon passes over the humeral head. It originates on the labrum and supraglenoid tuberosity.

3. Note the insertion of the subscapularis on the lesser tuberosity of the humerus of the scapula.

4. Immediately inferior to the insertion of the subscapularis muscle, the teres major and latissimus dorsi muscles insert on the humerus.

5. The axillary vein courses anterior and medial to the axillary artery.

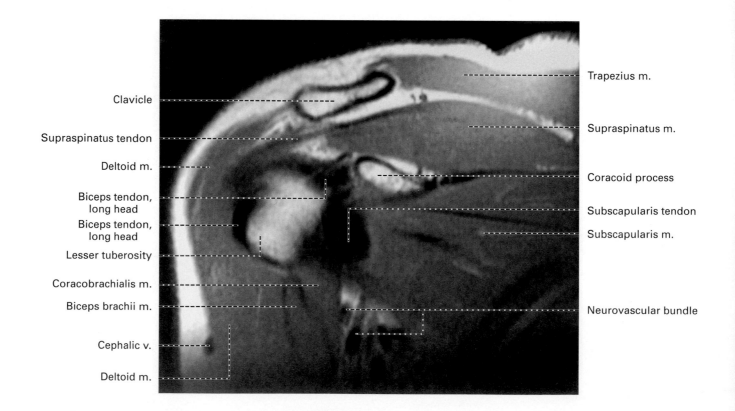

1. The subscapularis, teres major, and latissimus dorsi muscles form the posterior wall of the axilla.

2. This section depicts the lateral fibers of the deltoid. These fibers along with the supraspinatus act as abductors of the arm.

3. The latissimus dorsi and teres major muscles insert on the crest of the lesser tuberosity just inferior to the insertion of the subscapularis.

Figure 5.1.14

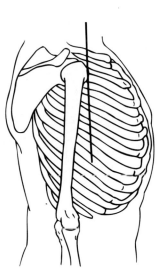

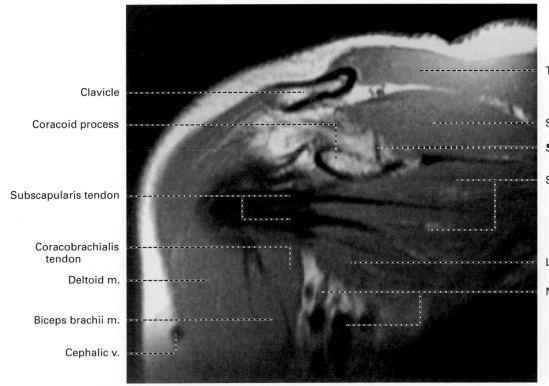

Clavicle

Coracoid process

Subscapularis tendon

Coracobrachialis tendon

Deltoid m.

Biceps brachii m.

Cephalic v.

Trapezius m.

Supraspinatus m.

Suprascapular a.

Subscapularis m.

Latissimus dorsi and teres major mm.

Neurovascular bundle

Figure 5.1.15

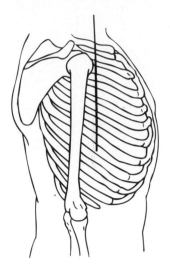

1. The trapezoid portion of the coracoclavicular ligament is clearly depicted on this section.

2. The coracoclavicular ligament is important in maintaining the stability of the acromioclavicular joint.

3. The axillary artery continues as the brachial artery at the level of the teres major muscle.

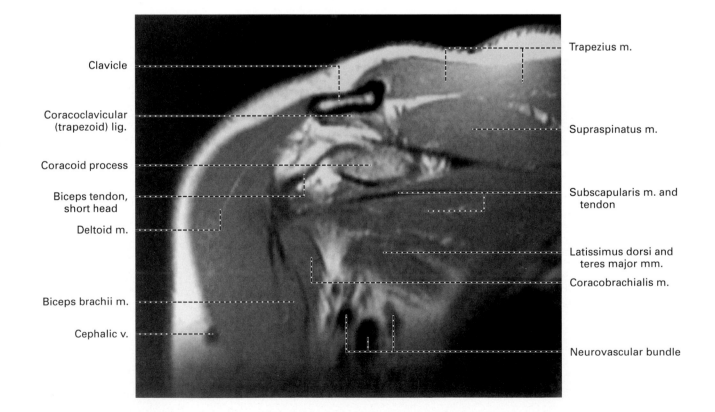

Clavicle

Coracoclavicular (trapezoid) lig.

Coracoid process

Biceps tendon, short head

Deltoid m.

Biceps brachii m.

Cephalic v.

Trapezius m.

Supraspinatus m.

Subscapularis m. and tendon

Latissimus dorsi and teres major mm.

Coracobrachialis m.

Neurovascular bundle

1. Note the origin of the short head of the biceps and coracobrachialis muscles from the tip of the coracoid process.

2. Both the trapezoid and conoid portions of the coracoclavicular ligament are depicted in this section.

3. The neurovascular bundle courses distally alongside the coracobrachialis muscle.

Figure 5.1.16

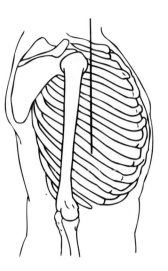

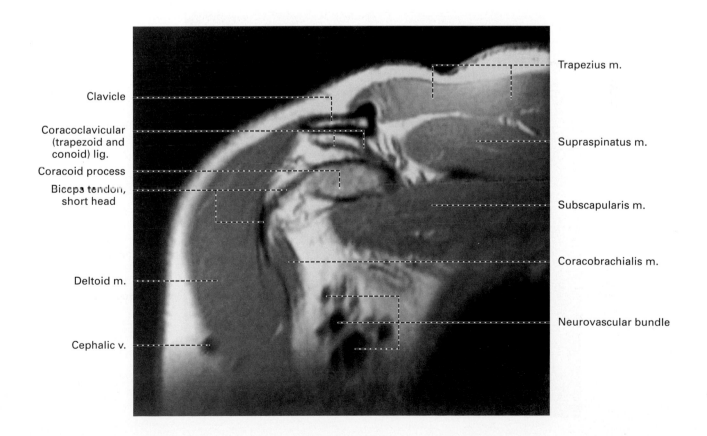

Figure 5.1.17

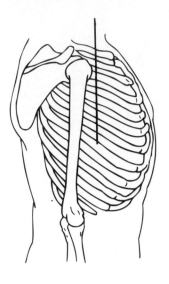

1. This section goes through the tip of the coracoid.

2. Note the serratus anterior muscle, which originates as fleshy digitations from the upper eight or nine ribs. It inserts on the medial border of the scapula.

3. The serratus anterior muscle forms the medial wall of the axilla.

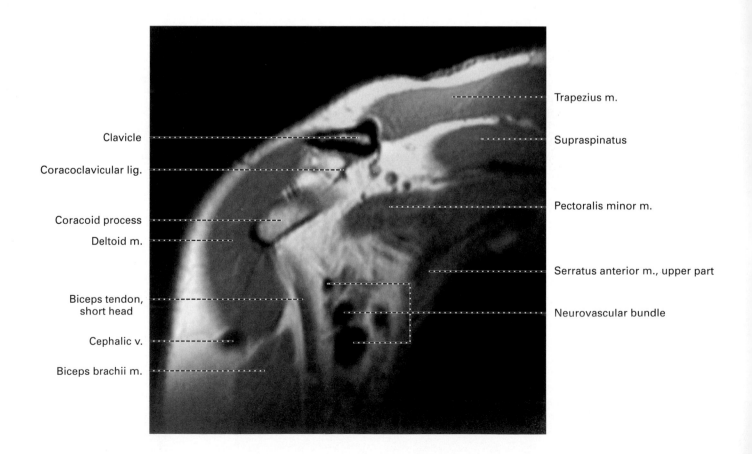

1. Both the deltoid and trapezius muscles are seen attaching to the lateral third of the clavicle.

2. The short head and long head of the biceps join on the anterior aspect of the arm to form a single muscle mass.

Figure 5.1.18

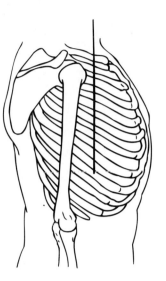

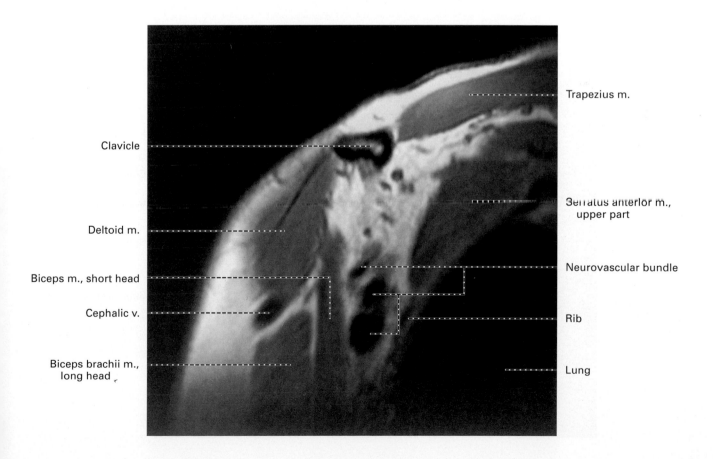

Trapezius m.

Clavicle

Serratus anterior m., upper part

Deltoid m.

Neurovascular bundle

Biceps m., short head

Cephalic v.

Rib

Biceps brachii m., long head

Lung

Figure 5.2.1

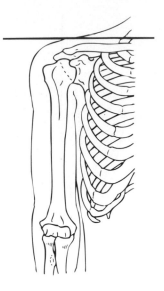

1. This section is through the superior aspect of the shoulder.

2. The trapezius is well seen. Its most superior fibers insert on the posterior aspect of the lateral third of the clavicle. Lower cervical and upper thoracic fibers insert on the acromion process and upper border of the scapular spine. The rest of its fibers arise from the thoracic region and course laterally and superiorly to insert along the spine of the scapula.

3. Levator scapulae arises from the transverse process of the first four cervical vertebrae and inserts on the superior angle of the scapula.

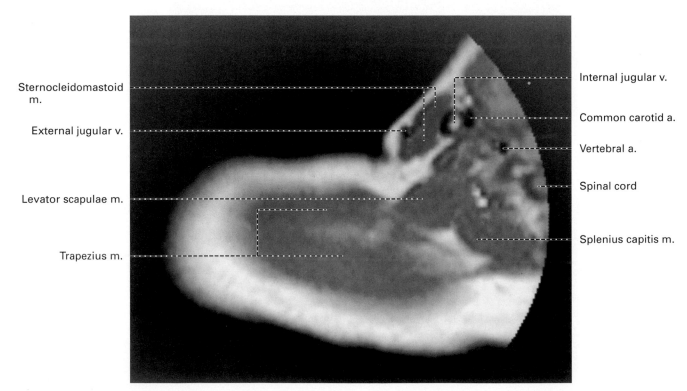

Sternocleidomastoid m.

External jugular v.

Levator scapulae m.

Trapezius m.

Internal jugular v.

Common carotid a.

Vertebral a.

Spinal cord

Splenius capitis m.

1. The portions of the trapezius inserting on the clavicle and scapula are distinctly separated.

2. The sternocleidomastoid is seen on the anterior aspect of the neck.

3. Beneath sternocleidomastoid are the internal jugular vein and common carotid artery.

Figure 5.2.2

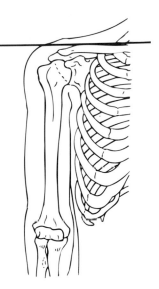

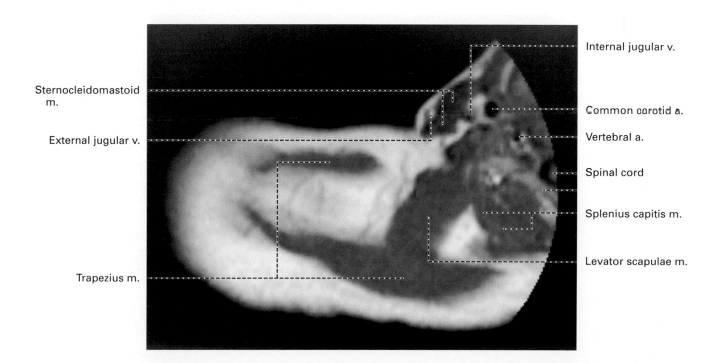

Figure 5.2.3

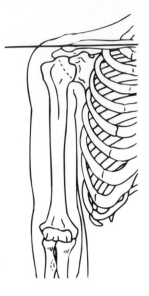

1. This section is through the superior aspect of the acromioclavicular joint.

2. The trapezius inserts on the lateral third of the clavicle, acromion process, and spine of the scapula.

3. The stability of the acromioclavicular joint is provided by the coracoclavicular ligaments. These ligaments are demonstrated on the coronal sections of the shoulder.

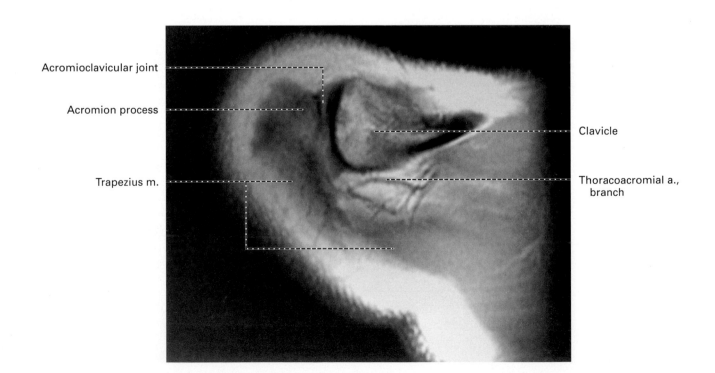

1. Note that the lateral third of the clavicle is convex posteriorly.

2. The portion of the scapula superior to the spine is the supraspinous fossa, which houses the supraspinatus muscle.

3. The anterior part of the deltoid is seen originating from the lateral third of the clavicle.

4. The spine of the scapula continues laterally and anteriorly to become the acromion process.

Figure 5.2.4

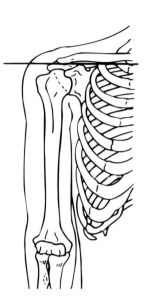

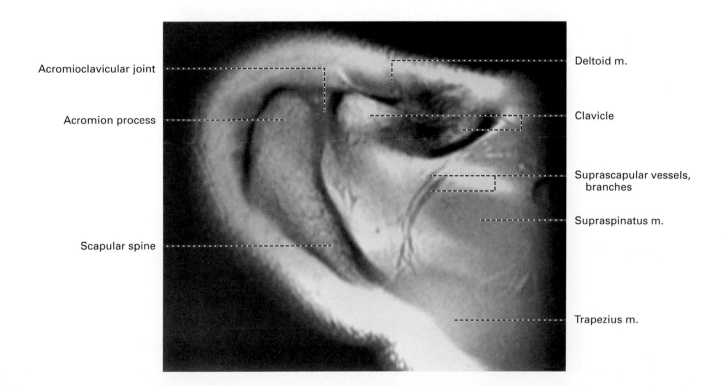

Acromioclavicular joint

Acromion process

Scapular spine

Deltoid m.

Clavicle

Suprascapular vessels, branches

Supraspinatus m.

Trapezius m.

Figure 5.2.5

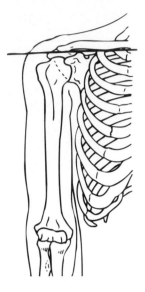

1. The supraspinatus courses below the acromion process to insert on the superior aspect of the greater tuberosity of the humerus.

2. The acromion, coracoid, and coracoacromial ligament form the coracoacromial arch, through which the supraspinatus tendon passes to insert on the greater tuberosity of the humerus.

3. Note the multipennate structure of the deltoid, which is well demonstrated on this section.

4. The medial portion of the clavicle is convex anteriorly.

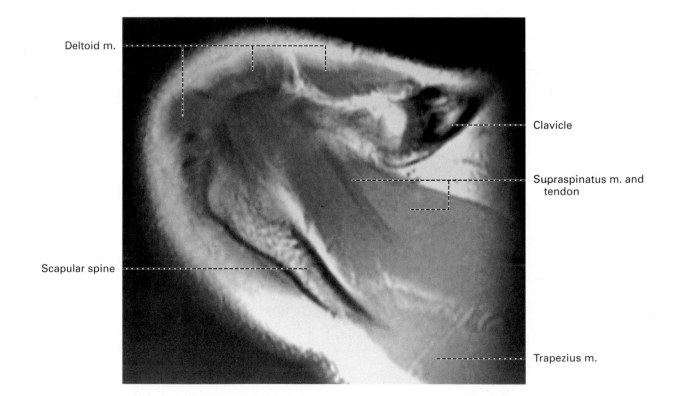

1. The lateral portion of the deltoid originates from the acromion process and the posterior portion from the spine of the scapula.

2. The supraspinatus tendon is clearly depicted in this section.

3. The four rotator cuff muscles surround the shoulder joint and blend with the joint capsule. They help in maintaining contact between the humeral head and the glenoid cavity.

Figure 5.2.6

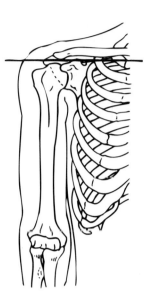

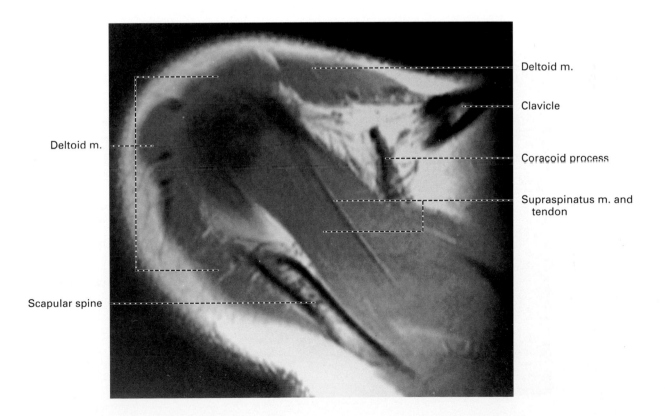

Deltoid m.

Clavicle

Coracoid process

Supraspinatus m. and tendon

Deltoid m.

Scapular spine

Figure 5.2.7

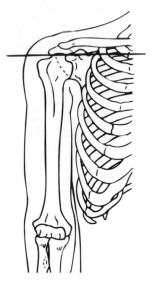

1. Inferior to the scapular spine is the infraspinatus fossa, which houses the infraspinatus muscle.

2. The suprascapular artery, which is depicted in this section, travels with the suprascapular nerve and innervates the supraspinatus and infraspinatus muscles.

3. Note the extent and size of the deltoid. It completely covers the rotator cuff muscles around the shoulder joint.

4. Each of the three parts of the deltoid has a different action. The middle part is thinner than both the anterior and posterior parts.

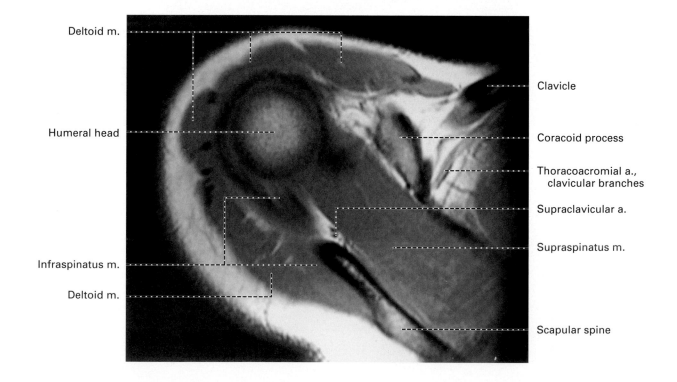

1. This section is through the coracoid process. It is an important site for muscle attachments.

2. The short head of the biceps and the coracobrachialis muscles originate from the tip of the coracoid process.

3. The pectoralis minor muscle inserts on the coracoid process.

4. Coracoacromial and coracoclavicular ligaments also attach to the coracoid process.

5. The supraglenoid tuberosity and superior labrum of the scapula are the sites of origin of the long head of the biceps.

6. Note the course of the long head of the biceps tendon as it passes over the humeral head after originating from the superior labrum and supraglenoid tuberosity of the scapula.

Figure 5.2.8

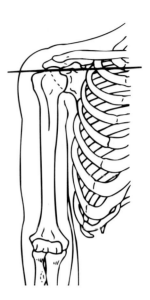

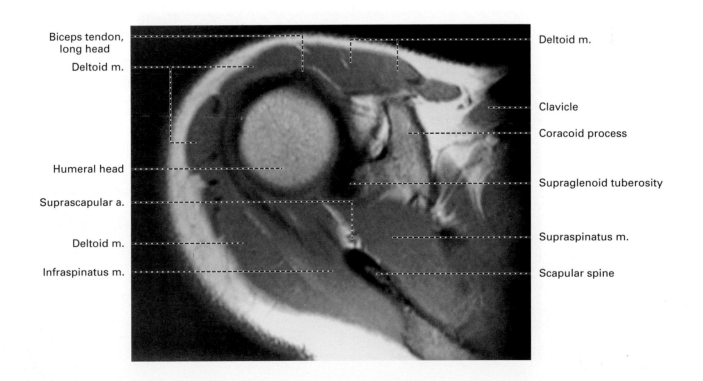

Biceps tendon, long head

Deltoid m.

Humeral head

Suprascapular a.

Deltoid m.

Infraspinatus m.

Deltoid m.

Clavicle

Coracoid process

Supraglenoid tuberosity

Supraspinatus m.

Scapular spine

Figure 5.2.9

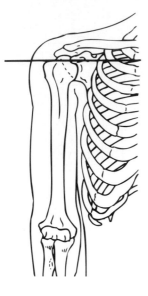

1. Observe the suprascapular artery crossing the supraspinous fossa and coursing toward the infraspinous fossa.

2. Note that the suprascapular artery usually courses above the scapular notch and traverses the scapular ligament whereas the suprascapular nerve usually passes through the scapular notch and beneath the transverse scapular ligament

3. The long head of the biceps tendon is intra-articular at this level.

4. The infraspinatus, teres minor, and posterior fibers of the deltoid are lateral rotators of the arm.

5. The deltopectoral triangle is formed by the clavicle superiorly, the deltoid muscle laterally, and pectoralis major medially.

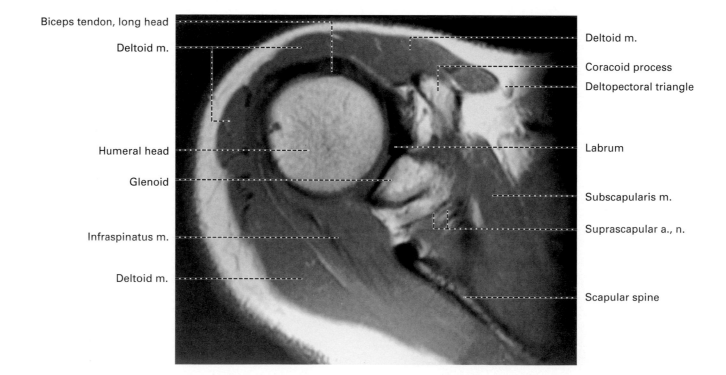

1. The scapular spine separates the supraspinous and infraspinous fossae.

2. Note the insertion of the infraspinatus muscle on the middle facet of the greater tuberosity of the humerus.

3. The anterior and posterior portions of the labrum of the scapula are clearly depicted as small black triangular structures in this section.

4. The suprascapular artery is usually a branch of the thyrocervical trunk.

Figure 5.2.10

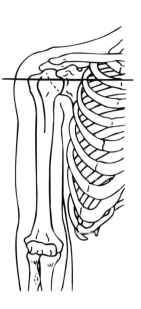

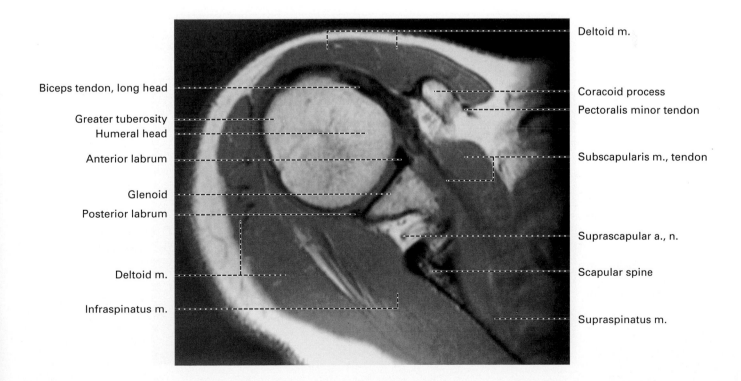

Biceps tendon, long head

Greater tuberosity
Humeral head

Anterior labrum

Glenoid
Posterior labrum

Deltoid m.

Infraspinatus m.

Deltoid m.

Coracoid process
Pectoralis minor tendon

Subscapularis m., tendon

Suprascapular a., n.

Scapular spine

Supraspinatus m.

Figure 5.2.11

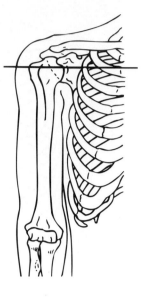

1. Note the origin of the subscapularis muscle from the subscapularis fossa.

2. The glenoid labrum forms a dense fibrous rim around the bony glenoid of the scapula. It deepens the glenoid and increases the articulating surface between the glenoid and the humeral head.

3. This section depicts the short head of biceps, coracobrachialis, and pectoralis minor, all converging toward the coracoid process where they attach.

4. Note that the attachment of the scapula to the thoracic wall is totally muscular. The only joint connecting the upper limb to the trunk is the sternoclavicular joint.

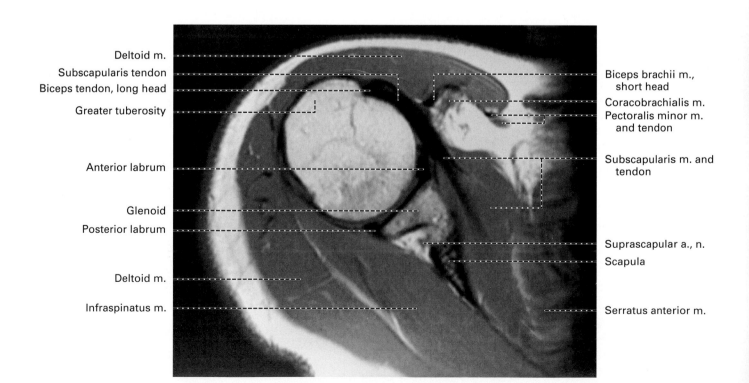

Deltoid m.
Subscapularis tendon
Biceps tendon, long head
Greater tuberosity
Anterior labrum
Glenoid
Posterior labrum
Deltoid m.
Infraspinatus m.

Biceps brachii m., short head
Coracobrachialis m.
Pectoralis minor m. and tendon
Subscapularis m. and tendon
Suprascapular a., n.
Scapula
Serratus anterior m.

1. Note the concave anterior surface of the scapula.

2. The subscapularis muscle, which originates on the dorsal surface of the scapula, courses laterally to insert on the lesser tuberosity of the humerus.

3. The subscapularis muscle is separated from the glenoid cavity of the scapula by the subscapularis bursa, which is an extension of the shoulder joint capsule.

4. The bicipital groove is situated between the greater and lesser tuberosities of the humerus. The long head of the biceps tendon lies within the bicipital groove.

5. The long head of the biceps tendon is surrounded by a synovial sheath while in the bicipital groove.

Figure 5.2.12

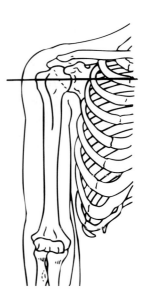

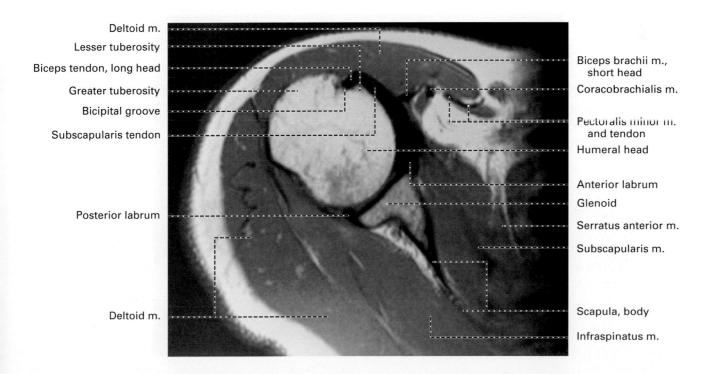

Deltoid m.
Lesser tuberosity
Biceps tendon, long head
Greater tuberosity
Bicipital groove
Subscapularis tendon

Posterior labrum

Deltoid m.

Biceps brachii m., short head
Coracobrachialis m.

Pectoralis minor m. and tendon
Humeral head

Anterior labrum
Glenoid
Serratus anterior m.
Subscapularis m.

Scapula, body
Infraspinatus m.

Figure 5.2.13

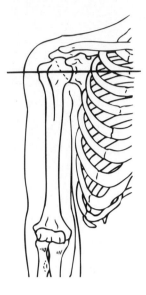

1. The subscapularis muscle and tendon are clearly depicted in this section. The subscapularis, latissimus dorsi, and teres major muscles form the posterior wall of the axilla.

2. The subscapularis inserts on the lesser tuberosity and functions as a medial rotator of the arm.

3. Note the serratus anterior muscle coursing posteriorly to insert on the medial border of the scapula.

4. The serratus anterior muscle forms the medial wall of the axilla.

5. The serratus anterior usually arises from the upper eight ribs.

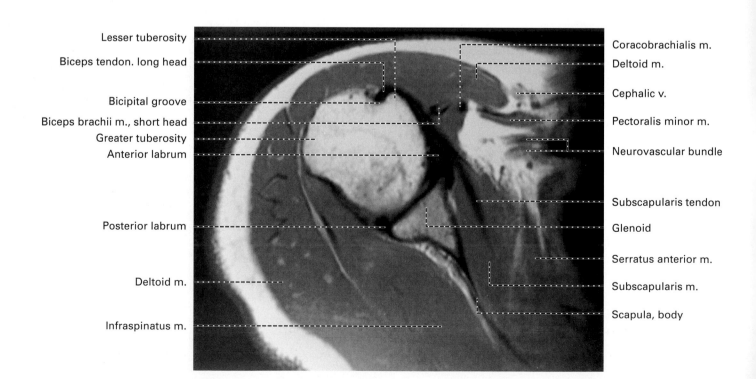

Lesser tuberosity
Biceps tendon. long head
Bicipital groove
Biceps brachii m., short head
Greater tuberosity
Anterior labrum
Posterior labrum
Deltoid m.
Infraspinatus m.

Coracobrachialis m.
Deltoid m.
Cephalic v.
Pectoralis minor m.
Neurovascular bundle
Subscapularis tendon
Glenoid
Serratus anterior m.
Subscapularis m.
Scapula, body

Figure 5.2.14

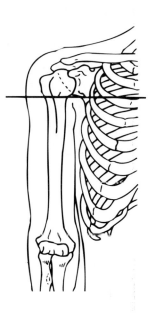

1. Note the neurovascular bundle coursing behind the pectoralis minor muscle.

2. The subclavian artery becomes the axillary artery after it crosses the first rib below the clavicle.

3. The subscapular artery, the largest branch of the axillary artery, is seen on the anterior surface of the subscapularis muscle.

4. The long head of the biceps proceeds distally within the bicipital groove.

5. The transverse cervical and suprascapular arteries are usually branches of the thyrocervical trunk. Branches of these arteries form anastomoses on the dorsum of the scapula.

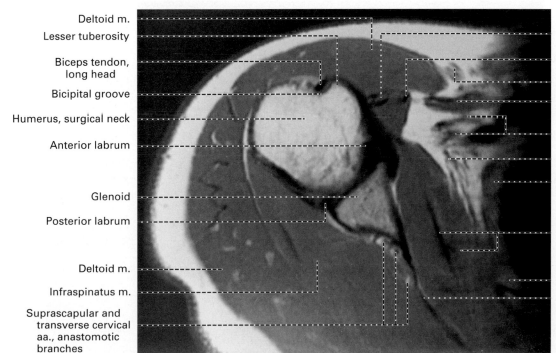

Figure 5.2.15

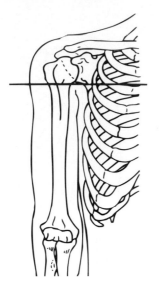

1. Note the cephalic vein coursing proximally in the deltopectoral groove. It usually joins the axillary vein.

2. The bellies of the coracobrachialis and short head of biceps are evident on this section.

3. Teres minor is inseparable from the infraspinatus muscle. The teres minor originates at the superolateral border of the scapula and inserts on the inferior facet of the greater tuberosity of the humerus.

4. The boundaries of the axilla are (1) subscapularis, teres major, and latissimus dorsi muscles, which form the posterior wall of the axilla; (2) pectoralis major and minor, which form the anterior wall; and (3) the serratus anterior, which forms the medial wall.

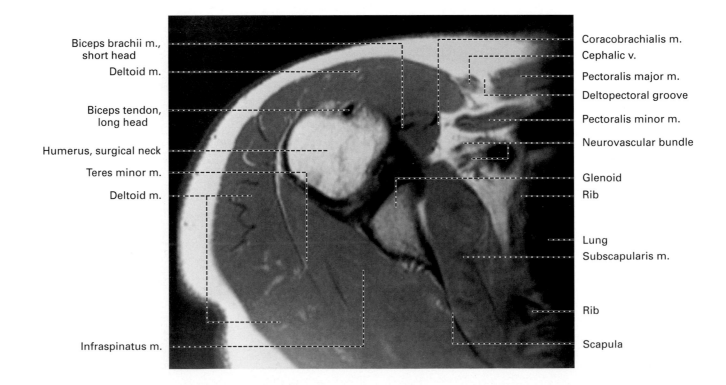

1. This section is at the level of the surgical neck of the humerus.

2. Note that the origin of the long head of triceps is from the infraglenoid tuberosity of the scapula, which is depicted on this section.

3. The neurovascular bundle continues to course distally along with the coracobrachialis muscle.

4. The pectoralis major usually originates from the medial half of the clavicle, sternum, and fifth and sixth costal cartilages.

Figure 5.2.16

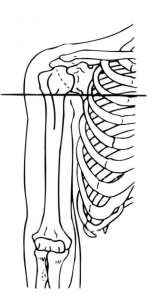

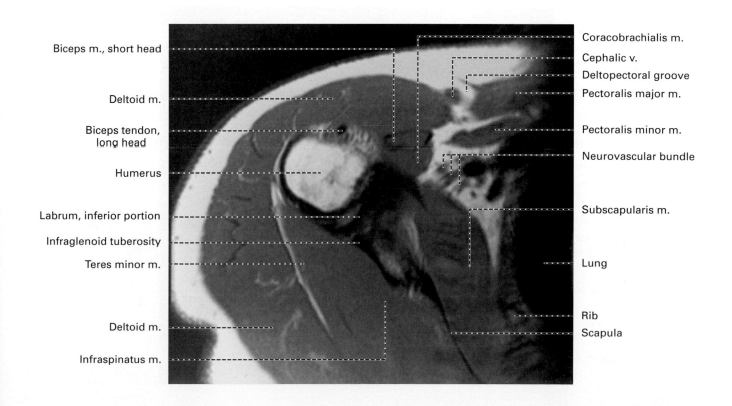

Figure 5.2.17

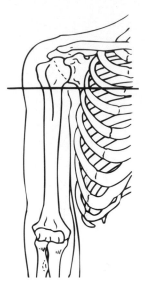

1. The long head of the triceps is clearly demonstrated as it descends from its origin at the infraglenoid tuberosity of the scapula.

2. The short head of the biceps and coracobrachialis descend together along the anteromedial aspect of the humerus.

3. The quadrangular space allows passage of the posterior circumflex humeral artery and axillary nerve.

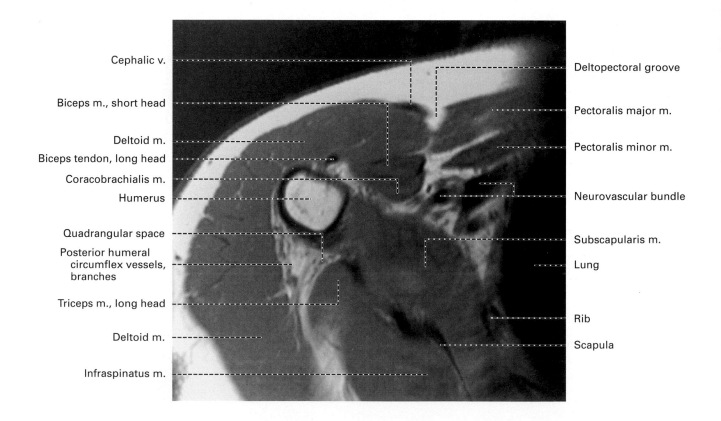

Cephalic v.
Biceps m., short head
Deltoid m.
Biceps tendon, long head
Coracobrachialis m.
Humerus
Quadrangular space
Posterior humeral circumflex vessels, branches
Triceps m., long head
Deltoid m.
Infraspinatus m.

Deltopectoral groove
Pectoralis major m.
Pectoralis minor m.
Neurovascular bundle
Subscapularis m.
Lung
Rib
Scapula

1. Note the origin of the lateral head of the triceps from the posterior surface of the humeral shaft.

2. The individual components of the neurovascular bundle are difficult to identify individually. The axillary vein normally travels anterior to the axillary artery.

3. The posterior circumflex humeral artery supplies the deltoid and triceps muscles.

Figure 5.2.18

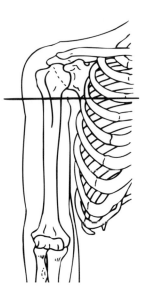

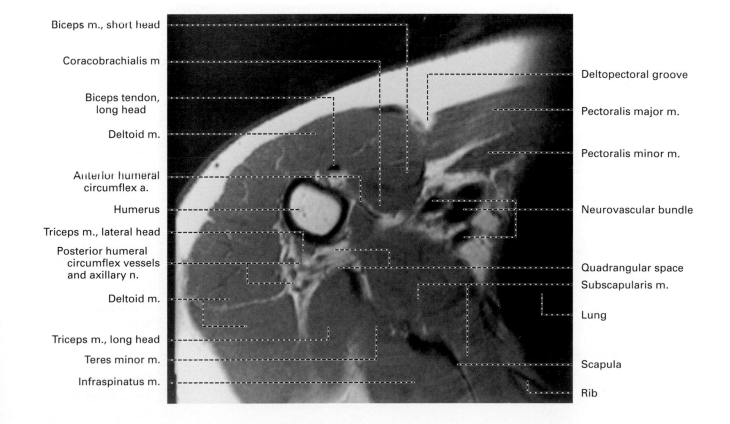

Biceps m., short head

Coracobrachialis m

Biceps tendon, long head

Deltoid m.

Anterior humeral circumflex a.

Humerus

Triceps m., lateral head

Posterior humeral circumflex vessels and axillary n.

Deltoid m.

Triceps m., long head

Teres minor m.

Infraspinatus m.

Deltopectoral groove

Pectoralis major m.

Pectoralis minor m.

Neurovascular bundle

Quadrangular space

Subscapularis m.

Lung

Scapula

Rib

Figure 5.2.19

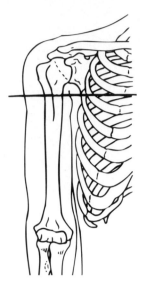

1. In this section, the posterior humeral circumflex vessels and axillary nerve are seen traversing the quadrangular space.

2. The axillary nerve innervates the deltoid and teres minor muscles.

3. The anterior and posterior circumflex humeral vessels anastomose around the surgical neck.

4. The long head of the triceps intersects a space between teres minor and teres major, forming a quadrangular space laterally and a triangular space medially.

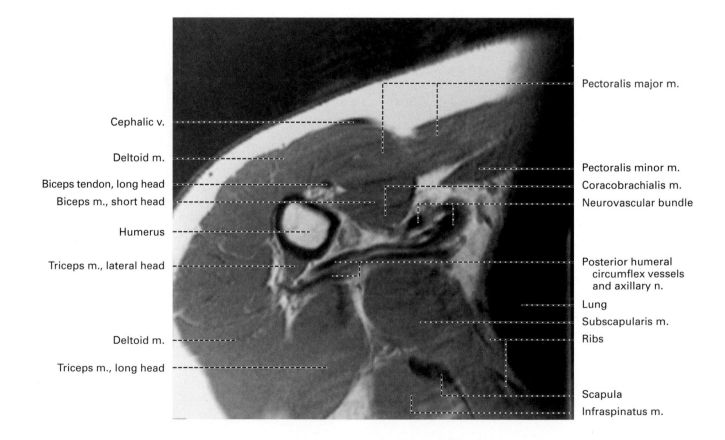

Cephalic v.

Deltoid m.

Biceps tendon, long head

Biceps m., short head

Humerus

Triceps m., lateral head

Deltoid m.

Triceps m., long head

Pectoralis major m.

Pectoralis minor m.

Coracobrachialis m.

Neurovascular bundle

Posterior humeral circumflex vessels and axillary n.

Lung

Subscapularis m.

Ribs

Scapula

Infraspinatus m.

1. The teres major and latissimus dorsi muscles converge to insert on the medial lip and floor of the bicipital groove of the humerus.

2. Pectoralis major is noted approaching its insertion on the lateral lip of the bicipital groove of the humerus.

3. Subscapularis continues to cover the entire anterior surface of the scapula.

4. The axillary nerve, which is in close proximity to the surgical neck of the humerus, innervates the deltoid and teres minor muscles.

Figure 5.2.20

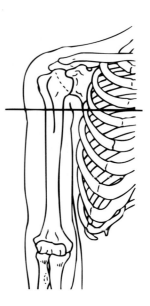

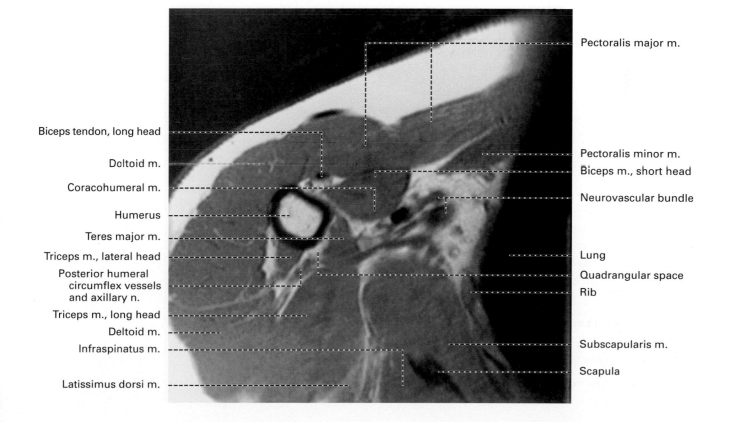

Figure 5.2.21

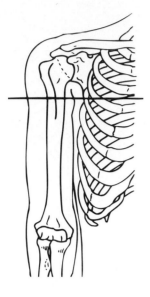

1. The insertion of the pectoralis major muscle on the humerus is covered by the deltoid.

2. In this section, the long head of the biceps is still mainly tendinous.

3. The radial nerve is a continuation of the posterior cord of the brachial plexus. The posterior cord is formed by union of the three posterior divisions of spinal nerves C5 to T1.

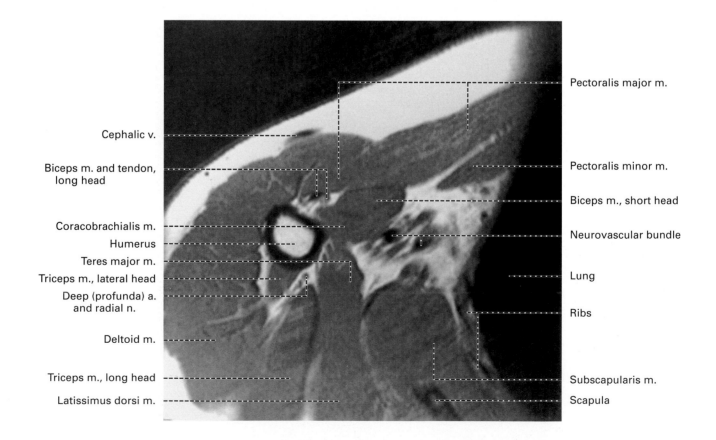

1. As the sections move distally, the deltoid muscle becomes smaller as it converges to insert on the deltoid tuberosity of the humerus.

2. Note that the anterior wall of the axilla is formed by pectoralis major and minor muscles.

3. The cephalic vein ascends laterally in the arm before it drains into the axillary vein.

Figure 5.2.22

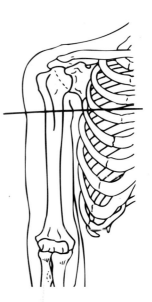

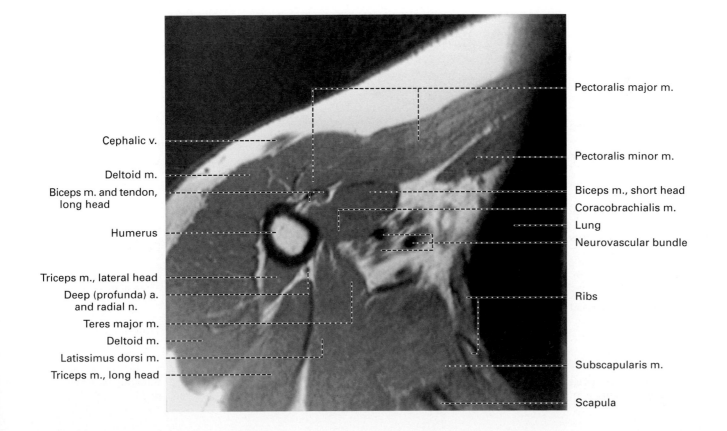

Figure 5.2.23

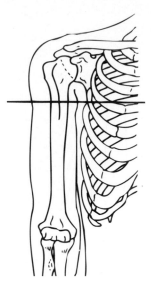

1. The anterolateral thickening in the cortex of the humerus is associated with the formation of the deltoid tuberosity.

2. In the arm, the radial nerve innervates the triceps muscle and all other extensor muscles of the upper limb.

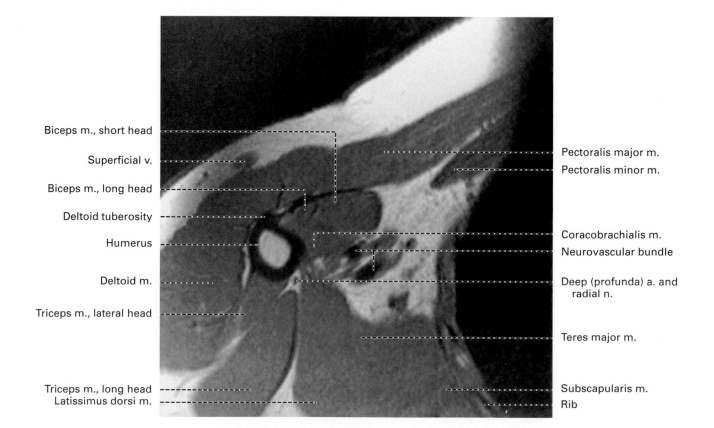

Biceps m., short head

Superficial v.

Biceps m., long head

Deltoid tuberosity

Humerus

Deltoid m.

Triceps m., lateral head

Triceps m., long head
Latissimus dorsi m.

Pectoralis major m.

Pectoralis minor m.

Coracobrachialis m.

Neurovascular bundle

Deep (profunda) a. and radial n.

Teres major m.

Subscapularis m.

Rib

1. The neurovascular bundle courses distally along the posteromedial surface of the coracobrachialis.

2. The long and short heads of biceps are seen separately before they merge into one muscle.

Figure 5.2.24

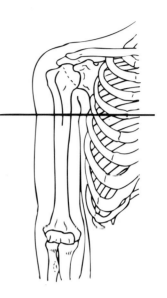

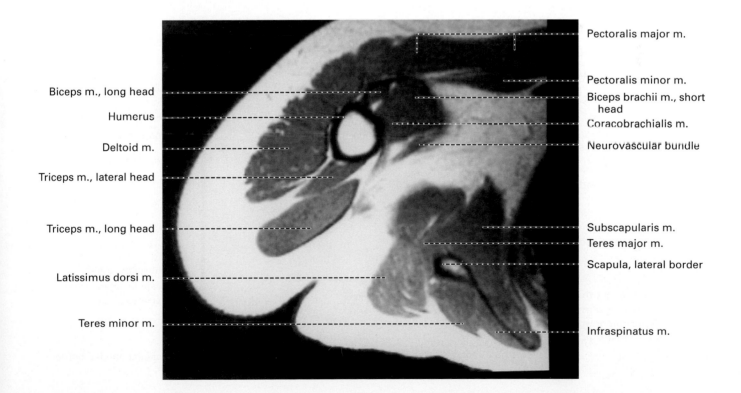

Pectoralis major m.

Pectoralis minor m.

Biceps brachii m., short head

Coracobrachialis m.

Neurovascular bundle

Subscapularis m.

Teres major m.

Scapula, lateral border

Infraspinatus m.

Biceps m., long head

Humerus

Deltoid m.

Triceps m., lateral head

Triceps m., long head

Latissimus dorsi m.

Teres minor m.

Figure 5.2.25

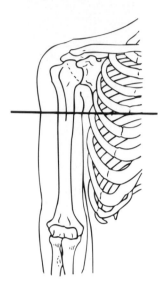

1. This section is at the inferior limit of the axilla.

2. Pectoralis major forms the anterior boundary of the axilla.

3. The lateral and long heads of triceps merge together into one muscle mass.

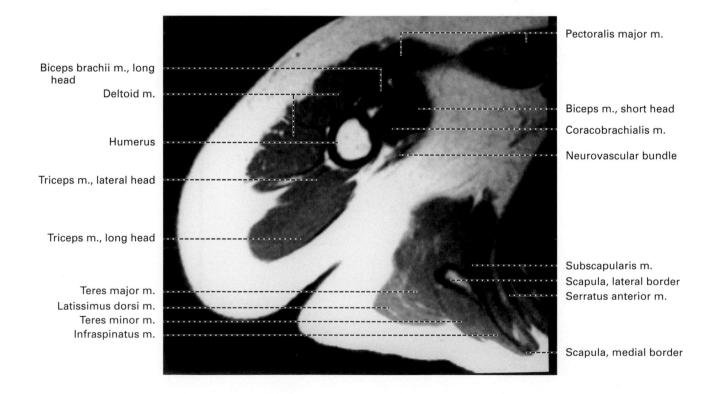

1. The radial nerve separates from the neurovascular bundle; it courses behind the humerus in the radial nerve groove accompanied by the deep (profunda) brachial artery.

2. Deltoid diminishes in size as it approaches its insertion on the deltoid tuberosity.

Figure 5.2.26

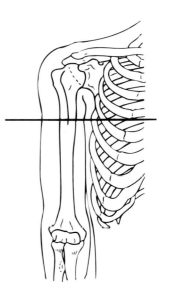

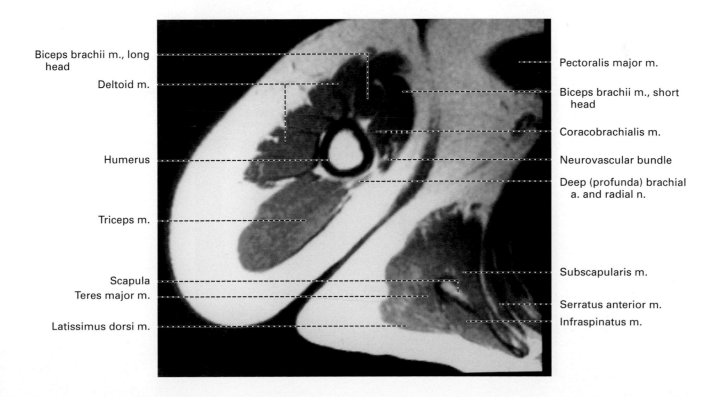

Figure 5.3.1

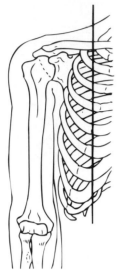

1. The first four images in this series are straight sagittal sections obtained with a large field of view. They are intended to illustrate the relationship between the shoulder girdle and the thorax.

2. This straight section is through the midclavicle.

3. Note that the trapezius muscle inserts on the lateral head of the clavicle.

4. Note the size and extent of pectoralis major and latissimus dorsi muscles.

5. The fibers of the serratus anterior muscle originate at the first and second ribs and converge to insert on the superior angle of the scapula.

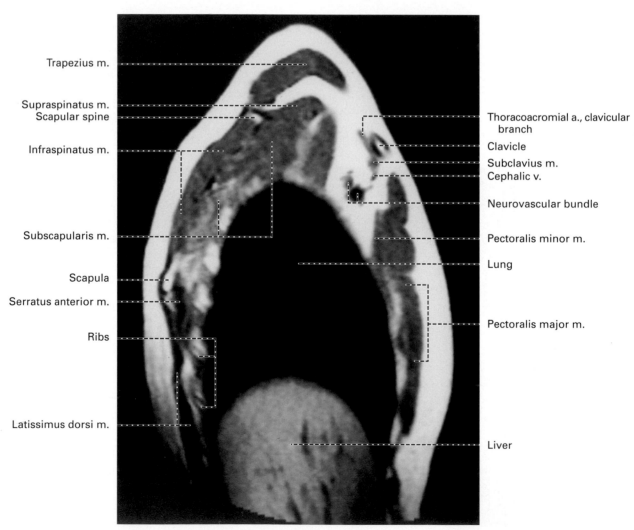

1. This straight sagittal section is through the junction of the middle and lateral thirds of the clavicle.

2. The scapula is heavily invested with muscular attachments.

3. Note the course of the neurovascular bundle posterior to pectoralis major.

4. The cephalic vein is seen in the deltopectoral triangle. More medially, it drains into the axillary vein.

Figure 5.3.2

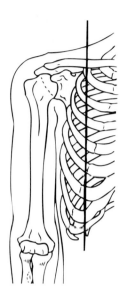

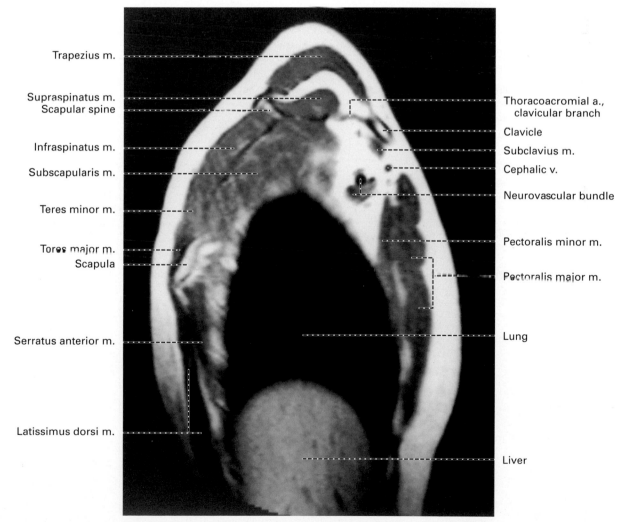

Trapezius m.

Supraspinatus m.
Scapular spine

Infraspinatus m.

Subscapularis m.

Teres minor m.

Teres major m.
Scapula

Serratus anterior m.

Latissimus dorsi m.

Thoracoacromial a.,
clavicular branch

Clavicle

Subclavius m.

Cephalic v.

Neurovascular bundle

Pectoralis minor m.

Pectoralis major m.

Lung

Liver

Figure 5.3.3

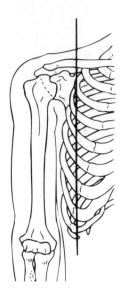

1. Note that portions of the scapula are extremely thin.

2. Note the extent of the serratus anterior muscle. It is a large flat muscle arising from the upper eight ribs and inserts on the medial border of the scapula.

3. Pectoralis minor is seen covered by pectoralis major. Pectoralis minor originates from the third, fourth, and fifth ribs and inserts on the coracoid process.

4. Note that the bulk of the serratus anterior muscle inserts on the inferior angle of the scapula.

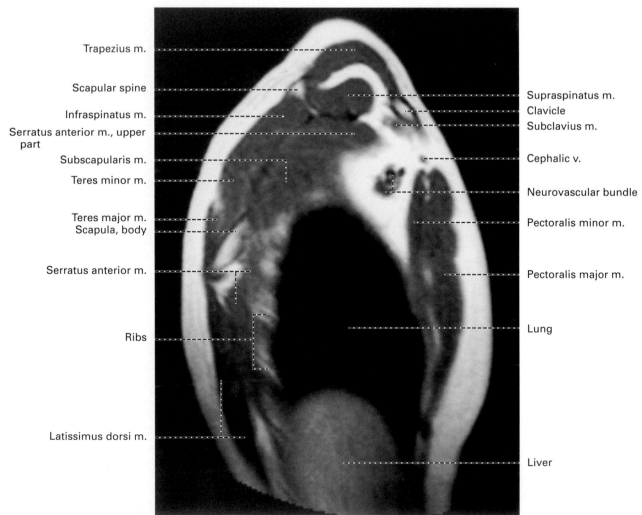

Trapezius m.

Scapular spine

Infraspinatus m.

Serratus anterior m., upper part

Subscapularis m.

Teres minor m.

Teres major m.
Scapula, body

Serratus anterior m.

Ribs

Latissimus dorsi m.

Supraspinatus m.
Clavicle
Subclavius m.

Cephalic v.

Neurovascular bundle

Pectoralis minor m.

Pectoralis major m.

Lung

Liver

1. The cephalic vein courses in the deltopectoral groove before draining into the axillary vein.

2. The subclavian artery is renamed the axillary artery after it crosses the first rib. The axillary artery is renamed the brachial artery after it crosses the teres major muscle.

3. Note the origin of the teres major muscle from the dorsal surface of the inferior angle of the scapula.

Figure 5.3.4

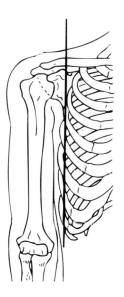

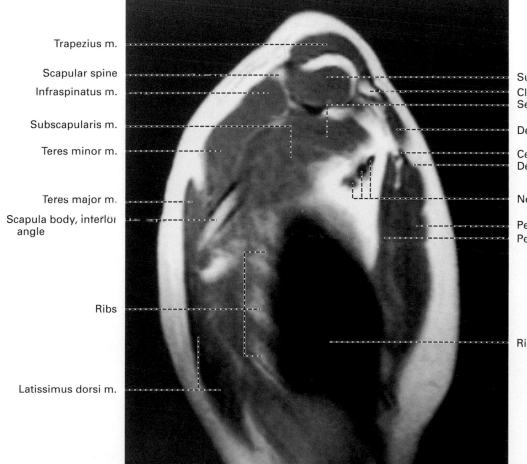

Trapezius m.

Scapular spine

Infraspinatus m.

Subscapularis m.

Teres minor m.

Teres major m.

Scapula body, inferior angle

Ribs

Latissimus dorsi m.

Supraspinatus m.

Clavicle

Serratus anterior m., upper part

Deltoid m.

Cephalic v.

Deltopectoral groove

Neurovascular bundle

Pectoralis major m.

Pectoralis minor m.

Right lung

Figure 5.3.5

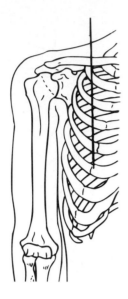

1. The subsequent sections are oblique sagittal images, obtained with small field of view. These sections are intended to demonstrate the musculoskeletal structures surrounding the glenohumeral joint.

2. The supraspinous, infraspinous, and subscapularis fossae are clearly depicted in this section.

3. The upper portion of the serratus anterior is typically thicker than its other parts.

4. The scapula is heavily invested with muscular attachments.

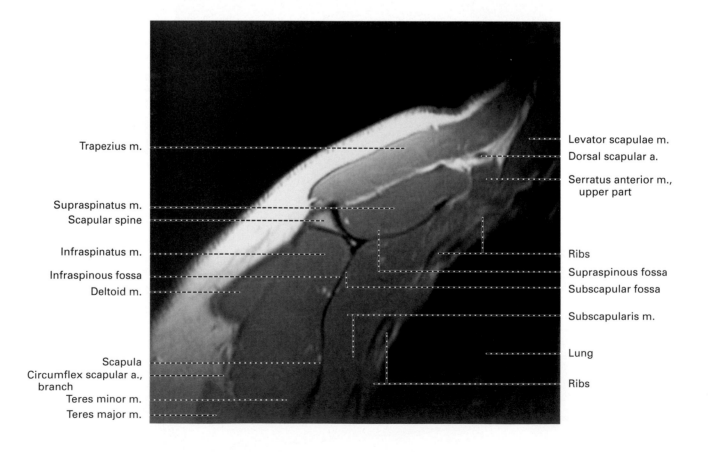

1. Note the origin of the teres major arising from the dorsal surface of the inferior angle of the scapula.

2. The rotator cuff muscles all originate on the scapula, course laterally, and converge to insert on the greater and lesser tuberosities of the humerus.

3. Note that portions of the scapula are extremely thin.

Figure 5.3.6

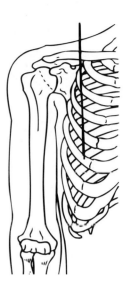

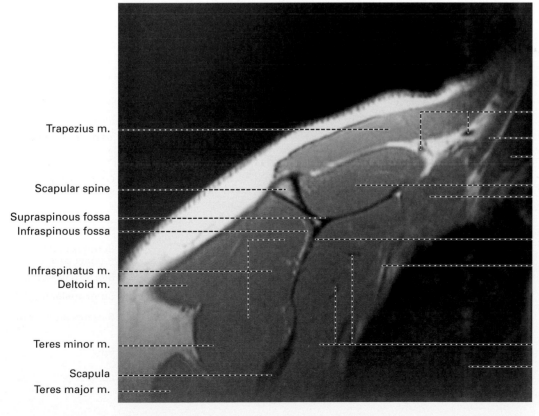

Trapezius m.

Scapular spine

Supraspinous fossa
Infraspinous fossa

Infraspinatus m.
Deltoid m.

Teres minor m.

Scapula
Teres major m.

Transverse cervical a.

Levator scapulae m.
Scalenus medius m.

Supraspinatus m.
Serratus anterior m.,
    upper part

Subscapular fossa

Rib

Subscapularis m.

Lung

Figure 5.3.7

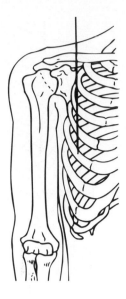

1. As the sections move laterally, the scapula becomes smaller.

2. Note that the upper portion of serratus anterior is thicker than its mid-portion.

3. Note that the subclavian artery courses between scalenus medius and scalenus anterior.

4. The subclavian vein courses anterior to scalenus anterior.

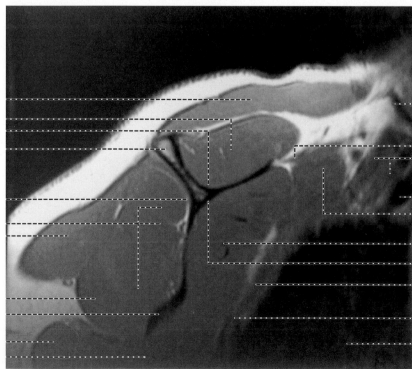

Trapezius m.

Supraspinatus m.
Supraspinous fossa

Scapular spine

Infraspinous fossa

Infraspinatus m.
Deltoid m.

Teres minor m.
Scapula

Teres major m.
Latissimus dorsi m.

Transverse cervical a.

Omohyoid m.
Scalenus medius m.

Subclavian a.
Serratus anterior m.,
    upper part
Subscapularis m.
Subscapular fossa
Serratus anterior m.

Rib

Lung

1. In the axilla, the axillary vein travels anterior to the axillary artery.

2. The supraspinatus and subscapularis muscles continue to occupy the entire supraspinous and subscapularis fossae, respectively.

3. The subscapularis, latissimus dorsi, and teres major muscles form the posterior wall of the axilla.

Figure 5.3.8

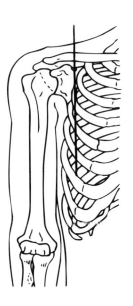

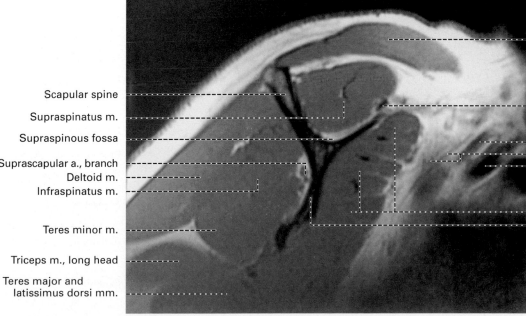

Trapezius m.

Scapular spine

Suprascapular a.

Supraspinatus m.

Supraspinous fossa

Axillary a.
Brachial plexus elements
Axillary v.

Suprascapular a., branch
Deltoid m.
Infraspinatus m.

Teres minor m.

Subscapularis m.
Scapula

Triceps m., long head

Teres major and
latissimus dorsi mm.

Figure 5.3.9

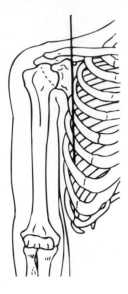

1. Note that the scapular spine has ended and that it has given rise to the acromion process.

2. The coracoid process and clavicle are also depicted in this section.

3. On the superior aspect of the shoulder, the trapezius is demonstrated; it has insertions on the clavicle, acromion process, and scapular spine.

4. The subclavius muscle is seen in this section inserting on the inferior surface of the clavicle.

5. The subclavian artery becomes the axillary artery after it crosses the first rib beneath the clavicle.

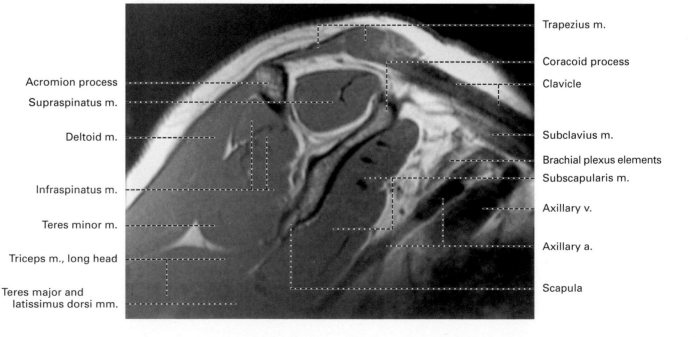

1. This section is through the neck of the scapula.

2. Note the long head of the triceps muscle as it originates from the infraglenoid tubercle.

3. Note that the neurovascular bundle courses on the anterior surface of the subscapularis muscle.

4. The subscapularis, teres major, and latissimus dorsi form the posterior wall of the axilla.

Figure 5.3.10

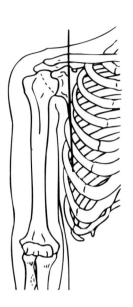

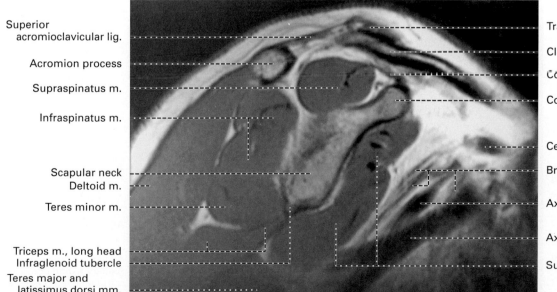

Superior acromioclavicular lig.

Acromion process

Supraspinatus m.

Infraspinatus m.

Scapular neck
Deltoid m.

Teres minor m.

Triceps m., long head
Infraglenoid tubercle

Teres major and latissimus dorsi mm.

Trapezius m.

Clavicle

Coracoclavicular (trapezoid) lig.
Coracoid process

Cephalic v.

Brachial plexus elements

Axillary a.

Axillary v.

Subscapularis m.

Figure 5.3.11

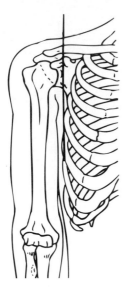

1. This section is through the quadrangular space, which admits the axillary nerve and posterior humeral circumflex artery.

2. The pectoralis minor muscle is seen crossing anterior to the axillary artery.

3. The axillary nerve innervates the deltoid and teres minor muscles.

4. The deltoid takes its origin from the clavicle, acromion process, and also from the spine of the scapula.

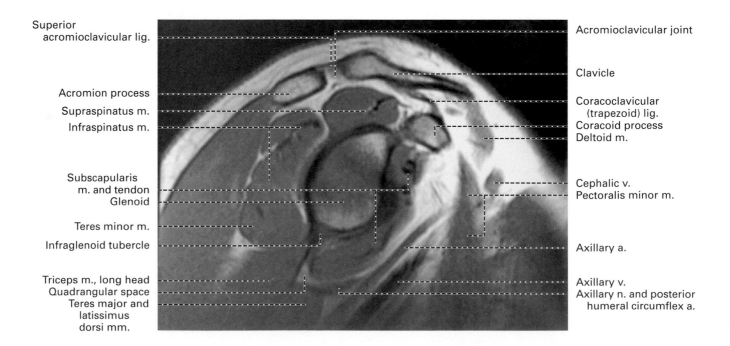

Superior acromioclavicular lig.

Acromion process
Supraspinatus m.
Infraspinatus m.

Subscapularis m. and tendon
Glenoid

Teres minor m.

Infraglenoid tubercle

Triceps m., long head
Quadrangular space
Teres major and latissimus dorsi mm.

Acromioclavicular joint

Clavicle

Coracoclavicular (trapezoid) lig.
Coracoid process
Deltoid m.

Cephalic v.
Pectoralis minor m.

Axillary a.

Axillary v.
Axillary n. and posterior humeral circumflex a.

1. Note the tendon of the long head of the biceps as it originates from the superior aspect of the labrum and supraglenoid tuberosity.

2. The pectoralis minor muscle is seen inserting on the coracoid process.

3. The anterior part of the deltoid muscle originates from the lateral third of the clavicle.

4. The cephalic vein is demonstrated within the deltopectoral triangle.

5. Note the posterior circumflex humeral artery and axillary nerve coursing posteriorly through the quadrangular space.

Figure 5.3.12

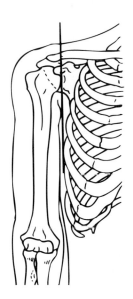

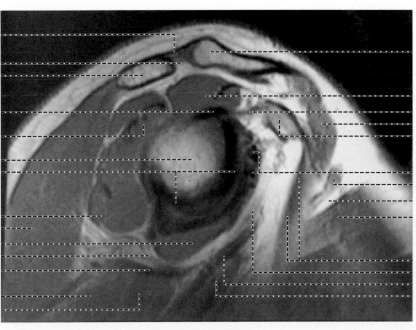

Superior acromioclavicular lig.

Acromioclavicular joint
Acromion process

Biceps tendon, long head
Infraspinatus m.

Humeral head
Glenoid labrum

Teres minor m.
Deltoid m.

Subscapularis m.
Axillary n.

Posterior circumflex humeral a.

Triceps m., long head
Latissimus dorsi and teres major mm.

Clavicle

Supraspinatus m.
Coracohumeral lig.
Deltoid m.
Coracoid process

Subscapularis tendon
Cephalic v.
Deltopectoral triangle
Pectoralis major m.

Pectoralis minor m.
Brachial plexus
Axillary a.
Coracobrachialis and biceps mm., short head

Figure 5.3.13

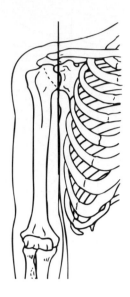

1. This section is just lateral to the axilla.

2. Between the supraspinatus muscle and humeral head, the tendon of the long head of the biceps is seen coursing toward its origin on the labrum and supraglenoid tuberosity.

3. Note the coracobrachialis and the short head of the biceps coursing distally along the anteromedial aspect of the arm.

4. The tendon of the subscapularis is well demonstrated on this section as it courses laterally to insert on the lesser tuberosity of the humerus.

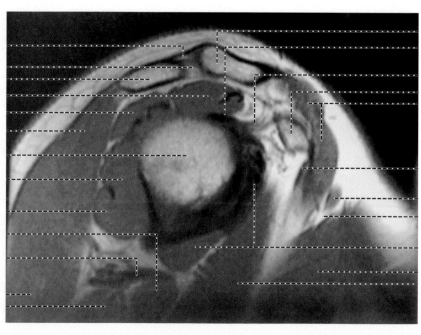

Superior acromioclavicular lig.

Acromioclavicular joint
Acromion process

Supraspinatus m.

Infraspinatus m.

Deltoid m.

Humeral head

Infraspinatus m.

Teres minor m.

Latissimus dorsi and teres major mm.
Posterior circumflex humeral a. and axillary n.
Deltoid m.
Triceps m., long head

Clavicle

Biceps tendon, long head

Coracohumeral lig.

Coracoid process
Deltoid m.

Pectoralis minor tendon

Cephalic v.

Deltopectoral triangle

Subscapularis tendon and m.
Pectoralis major m.
Coracobrachialis and biceps mm., short head

1. Note the latissimus dorsi and teres major muscles as they approach their insertion site on the crest of the lesser tuberosity (also called medial lip of bicipital groove).

2. The subscapularis muscle is almost completely tendinous just prior to its insertion on the lesser tuberosity of the humerus.

3. The four rotator cuff muscles surround the shoulder joint; they retain the head of the humerus within the glenoid cavity.

Figure 5.3.14

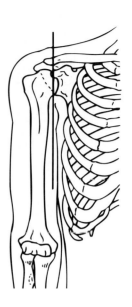

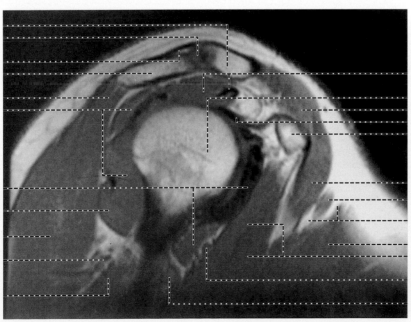

Clavicle
Acromioclavicular joint
Superior
   acromioclavicular lig.
Acromion process

Deltoid m.
Infraspinatus m.

Subscapularis
   tendon and m.

Teres minor m.

Deltoid m.

Posterior circumflex
   humeral a. and
   axillary n.
Triceps m., long head

Supraspinatus m.
   and tendon
Humeral head
Deltoid m.
Biceps tendon, long head
Coracoid process

Deltoid m.

Cephalic v.

Deltopectoral triangle

Pectoralis major m.
Coracobrachialis and
   biceps mm., short head
Anterior circumflex
   humeral a.
Latissimus dorsi and
   teres major mm.

Figure 5.3.15

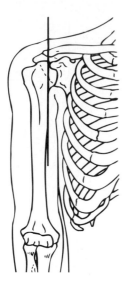

1. Note the origin of coracobrachialis and short head of biceps from the tip of the coracoid process.

2. Note the relationship of the acromion process to the supraspinatus muscle and tendon, which is immediately beneath the acromion. The space between the humeral head and acromion is called the coracoacromial arch.

3. Anteriorly, the deltoid muscle covers both coracobrachialis and short head of biceps as well as the tendons of pectoralis major, subscapularis, and long head of biceps.

4. The space between the supraspinatus and subscapularis tendons is referred to as the rotator cuff interval; this interval should not be misinterpreted as a tear in the rotator cuff.

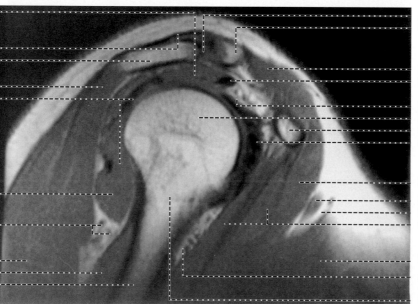

1. Note that the subscapularis is totally tendinous as it inserts onto the lesser tuberosity of the humerus.

2. The other rotator cuff muscles are becoming progressively tendinous as they approach their insertion on the greater tuberosity of the humerus.

3. The tendons of the four rotator cuff muscles blend with the shoulder joint capsule.

4. Note the relationship of the posterior circumflex humeral artery and axillary nerve to the surgical neck. The axillary nerve innervates the deltoid and teres minor muscles.

5. Note that the long head of the biceps tendon can be found consistently within the rotator cuff interval between the supraspinatus and subscapularis tendons.

Figure 5.3.16

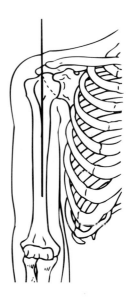

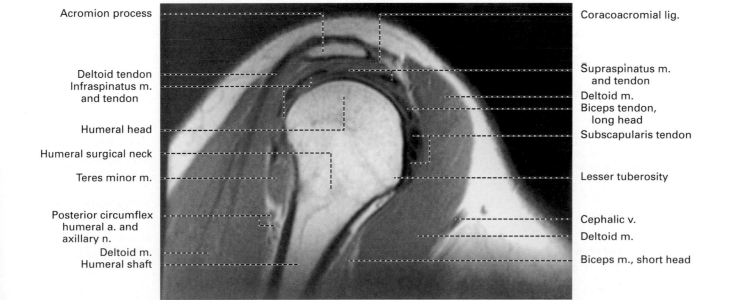

Acromion process

Deltoid tendon
Infraspinatus m. and tendon

Humeral head

Humeral surgical neck

Teres minor m.

Posterior circumflex humeral a. and axillary n.

Deltoid m.
Humeral shaft

Coracoacromial lig.

Supraspinatus m. and tendon

Deltoid m.
Biceps tendon, long head

Subscapularis tendon

Lesser tuberosity

Cephalic v.

Deltoid m.

Biceps m., short head

Figure 5.3.17

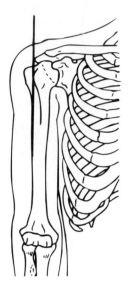

1. This section shows the insertions of the subscapularis tendon onto the lesser tuberosity of the humerus.

2. The other rotator cuff tendons are also depicted in this section.

3. Note the long head of the biceps tendon coursing distally within the bicipital groove.

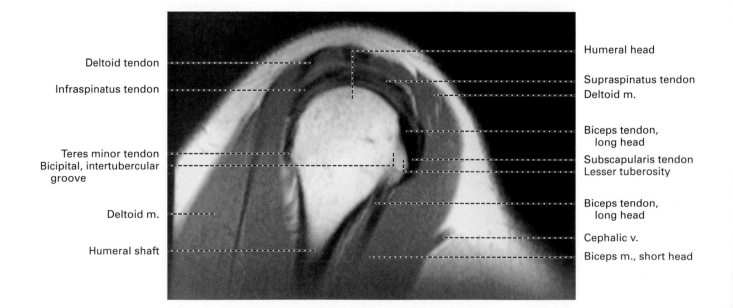

Deltoid tendon

Infraspinatus tendon

Teres minor tendon
Bicipital, intertubercular groove

Deltoid m.

Humeral shaft

Humeral head

Supraspinatus tendon
Deltoid m.

Biceps tendon,
long head

Subscapularis tendon
Lesser tuberosity

Biceps tendon,
long head

Cephalic v.

Biceps m., short head

1. The insertions of the infraspinatus and teres minor tendons on the greater tuberosity of the humerus are depicted on this section.

2. In the vicinity of the shoulder joint, the long head of the biceps tendon is intracapsular.

3. The tendon of the long head of biceps is located in the bicipital groove and is covered by a synovial sheath for a short distance. The synovial sheath is an extension of the shoulder joint capsule.

Figure 5.3.18

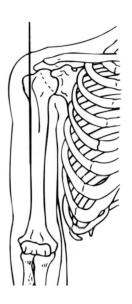

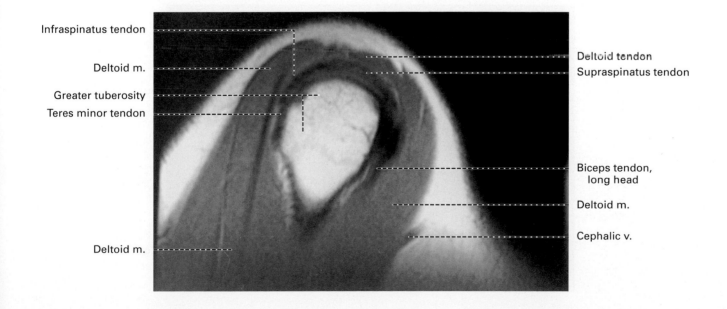

Infraspinatus tendon

Deltoid m.

Greater tuberosity
Teres minor tendon

Deltoid m.

Deltoid tendon
Supraspinatus tendon

Biceps tendon,
long head

Deltoid m.

Cephalic v.

Figure 5.3.19

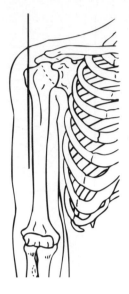

1. This sagittal section passes through the lateral aspect of the shoulder, demonstrating the insertion of the supraspinatus tendon onto the greater tuberosity of the humerus.

2. The deltoid muscle surrounds the shoulder joint from three sides: anterior, lateral, and posterior.

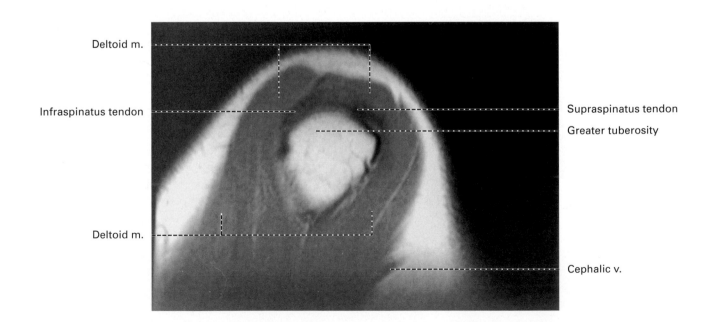

1. This is a straight sagittal section through the lateral musculature of the shoulder.

2. Note the multipennate configuration of the deltoid muscle.

3. The fascicles of the deltoid converge to insert on the deltoid tuberosity.

4. The biceps and triceps are demonstrated on the anterior and posterior aspects of the arm, respectively.

Figure 5.3.20

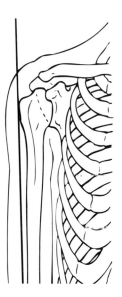

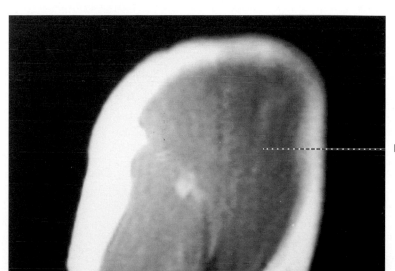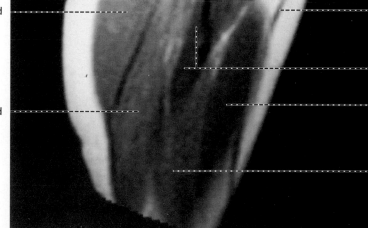

Deltoid m.

Triceps m., long head

Cephalic v.

Deltoid tuberosity

Biceps brachii m.

Triceps m., lateral head

Brachialis m.

Chapter 6

ARM

Musculature of the Arm

The musculature of the arm includes coracobrachialis, biceps brachii, brachialis, triceps brachii, and anconeus.

Coracobrachialis, biceps, and brachialis extend along the front of the arm. Triceps is found on the dorsum of the arm and extend from the scapula and humerus to the olecranon process of the ulna.

The ventral or flexor group of muscles includes coracobrachialis, biceps brachii, and brachialis. Coracobrachialis is a round but untapered muscle that arises from the coracoid process of the scapula and inserts onto the humerus at its middle third. Biceps brachii arises from two heads. The short head is closely associated with coracobrachialis and arises from the coracoid process. The long head arises by a tendon from the supraglenoid tuberosity of the scapula. The fusiform bellies formed from these two origins become fused and insert onto the radial tuberosity and into the fascia of the forearm.

Brachialis, located beneath the biceps muscle, arises from the lower three-fifths of the humerus and inserts onto the coronoid process of the ulna.

The muscles of the ventral group are innervated by the musculocutaneous nerve.

There are two muscles in the dorsal or extensor group: triceps brachii and anconeus. Triceps is a complex muscle with three heads: long scapular, lateral humeral, and medial humeral. These heads fuse distally and insert by a common tendon onto the olecranon process of the ulna. Anconeus is located primarily in the forearm but belongs morphologically and physiologically with the triceps.

Both muscles are supplied by branches of the radial nerve and extend the forearm. In addition, the long head of triceps extends and adducts the arm at the shoulder.

Table 6-1. Anatomy of the Arm

Muscle	Origin	Insertion	Nerve Supply	Arterial
Coracobrachialis	Coracoid process	Shaft of humerus above the middle of the bone	Musculocutaneous n. (C5, C6, C7)	Muscular branches of the axillary and brachial
Biceps brachii	Short head, coracoid process; long head, supraglenoid tubercle and superior part of glenoid labrum	Tuberosity of the radius and by an aponeurotic expansion to the fascia on the ulnar side of the forearm	Musculocutaneous n. (C5, C6)	Muscular branches of the brachial
Brachialis	Anterior surface, lateral and medial sides of the lower three fifths of the humerus, medial intermuscular septum above origin of coracobrachialis and brachialis	Capsule of elbow joint and ulnar tuberosity	Musculocutaneous n. (C5, C6)	Muscular branches of the brachial
Triceps	Long head, infraglenoid tuberosity of the scapula, the lateral part of the posterior surface of the humerus; medial head, from the posterior surface of the humerus below the radial groove and dorsal surfaces of the medial and lateral intermuscular septa	Primary tendon inserts onto the olecranon process of the ulna and laterally, by an expansion over anconeus, into the dorsal fascia of the forearm	Radial n. (C6, C7, C8)	Muscular branches of the axillary via posterior circumflex humeral, anterior circumflex humeral, and deep brachial
Anconeus	Posterior surface of the lateral epicondyle, and the adjacent part of the elbow joint capsular ligament	Onto the radial side of the olecranon and adjacent part onto the shaft of the ulna	Nerve to anconeus (C7, C8, T1)	Interosseus recurrent branch of the posterior interosseus and/or common interosseus, and from the deep brachial via middle collateral

1. This section is through the inferior portion of the axilla.

2. The pectoralis major is completing its insertion on the lateral lip of the bicipital groove.

3. The deltoid is beginning to insert on the deltoid tubercle of the humerus.

4. Observe the cephalic vein coursing superiorly within the deltopectoral groove.

Figure 6.1.1

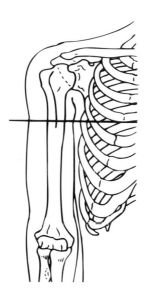

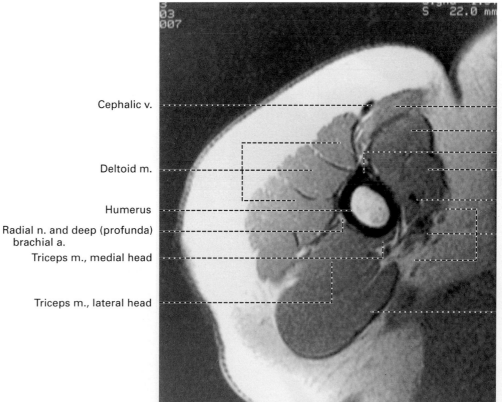

Cephalic v.

Deltoid m.

Humerus

Radial n. and deep (profunda) brachial a.

Triceps m., medial head

Triceps m., lateral head

Pectoralis major m.

Biceps brachii m., long head

Deltoid tuberosity

Biceps brachii m., short head

Coracobrachialis m.

Neurovascular bundle (brachial a. and v.; median and ulnar nn.)

Triceps m., long head

Figure 6.1.4

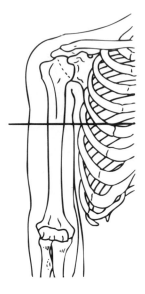

1. The brachialis takes its origin from the distal half of the anterior surface of the humerus.

2. All three heads of the triceps and the triceps tendon are depicted in this section.

3. In the arm, the radial nerve innervates all three heads of the triceps.

4. All the muscles of the anterior compartment of the arm are innervated by the musculocutaneous nerve.

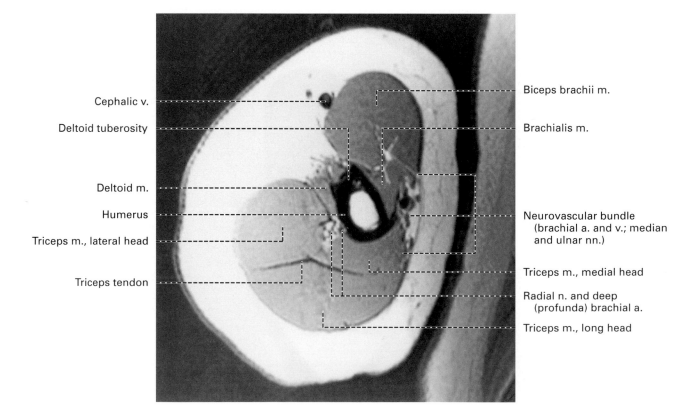

Cephalic v.

Deltoid tuberosity

Deltoid m.

Humerus

Triceps m., lateral head

Triceps tendon

Biceps brachii m.

Brachialis m.

Neurovascular bundle (brachial a. and v.; median and ulnar nn.)

Triceps m., medial head

Radial n. and deep (profunda) brachial a.

Triceps m., long head

1. The brachialis continues to enlarge as sections move distally in the arm.

2. Note the location of the medial and lateral intermuscular septa.

3. The neurovascular bundle is situated within the medial intermuscular septum.

4. The lateral head of the triceps originates from the posterior aspect of the humeral shaft proximally.

5. The medial head of the triceps originates from the posterior aspect of the distal two-thirds of the humeral shaft.

Figure 6.1.5

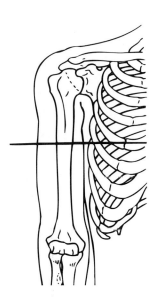

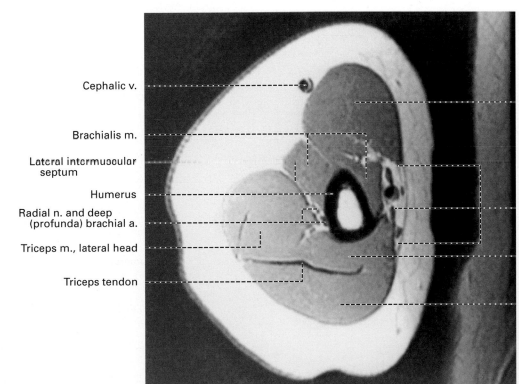

Cephalic v.

Brachialis m.

Lateral intermuscular septum

Humerus

Radial n. and deep (profunda) brachial a.

Triceps m., lateral head

Triceps tendon

Biceps brachii m.

Neurovascular bundle (brachial a. and v.; median and ulnar nn.)

Triceps m., medial head

Triceps m., long head

Figure 6.1.6

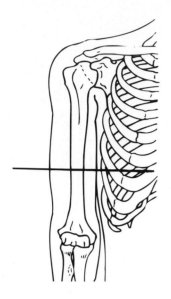

1. A thick tendon separates the medial and long heads of triceps.

2. All three heads of triceps are well developed in this level.

3. At this level, the neurovascular bundle consists of the brachial artery, the basilic vein, and the median and ulnar nerves.

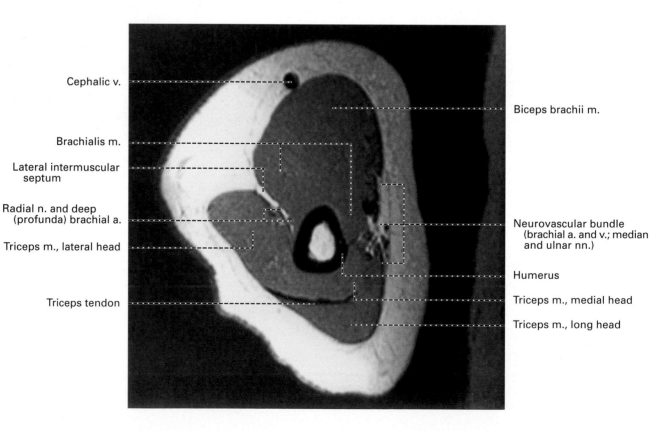

Cephalic v.

Brachialis m.

Lateral intermuscular septum

Radial n. and deep (profunda) brachial a.

Triceps m., lateral head

Triceps tendon

Biceps brachii m.

Neurovascular bundle (brachial a. and v.; median and ulnar nn.)

Humerus

Triceps m., medial head

Triceps m., long head

1. The image shows the origin of the brachioradialis from the proximal part of the lateral supracondylar ridge.

2. Note that the distal humerus is just starting to flatten and the lateral supracondylar ridge appears at this level.

3. Note the course of the radial nerve just above the elbow. It courses distally between the brachioradialis and brachialis muscles.

4. The ulnar nerve now courses some distance posterior to the neurovascular bundle and on the medial surface of the triceps muscle.

Figure 6.1.7

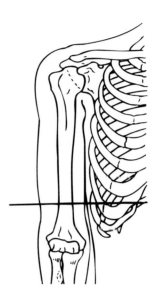

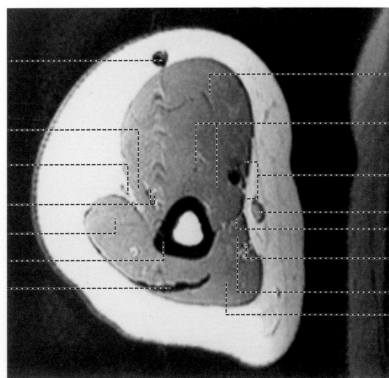

Cephalic v.

Brachioradialis m.

Lateral intermuscular septum

Radial n. and deep (profunda) brachial a.

Triceps m., lateral head

Humerus, lateral supracondylar ridge

Triceps tendon

Biceps brachii m.

Brachialis m.

Neurovascular bundle (brachial a. and v.; median n.)

Basilic v.

Medial intermuscular septum

Ulnar n.

Triceps m., medial head

Triceps m., long head

Figure 6.1.8

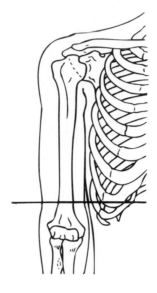

1. The ulnar nerve continues its course posterior to the neurovascular bundle on the medial surface of the triceps muscle.

2. The median nerve continues in the distal arm as part of the neurovascular bundle in close proximity to the brachial artery.

3. Note the extensor Carpi radialis longus as it originates from the distal part of the lateral supracondylar ridge.

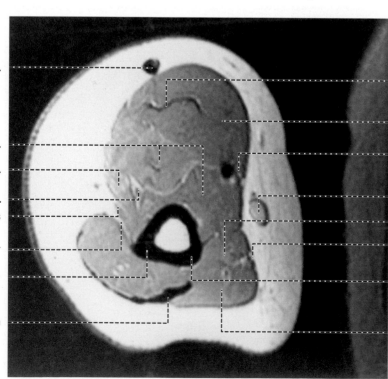

Cephalic v.

Brachialis m.

Brachioradialis m.

Radial n. and deep (profunda) brachial a.

Extensor carpi radialis longus m.

Lateral intermuscular septum

Lateral supracondylar ridge

Triceps tendon

Biceps brachii tendon

Biceps brachii m.

Neurovascular bundle (brachial a. and v.; median n.)

Basilic v.

Triceps m., medial head

Ulnar n.

Humerus, medial supracondylar ridge

Triceps m., long head

1. The distal humerus continues to flatten; both the medial and lateral supra-condylar ridges are quite prominent in this section.

2. The biceps tapers in the distal arm and the brachialis becomes the largest muscle of the anterior compartment.

3. In the distal arm, the radial nerve courses distally in the anterior compart-ment between brachialis and brachioradialis, supplying brachioradialis and occasionally the lateral edge of the brachialis muscle.

4. The triceps tapers distally and its tendinous part becomes more prominent just prior to its insertion on the olecramon process.

Figure 6.1.9

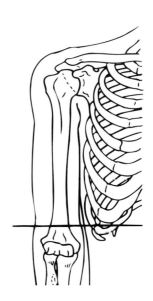

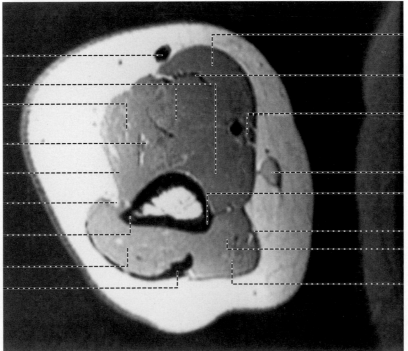

Cephalic v.

Brachialis m.

Brachioradialis m.

Radial n. and deep (profunda) brachial a.

Extensor carpi radialis longus m.

Lateral intermuscular septum

Lateral supracondylar ridge

Triceps m., lateral head

Triceps tendon

Biceps brachii m.

Biceps brachii tendon

Neurovascular bundle (brachial a. and v.; median n.)

Basilic v.

Humerus, medial supracondylar ridge

Ulnar n.

Triceps m., medial head

Triceps m., long head

Figure 6.2.1

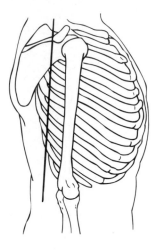

1. This section passes through the most posterior aspect of the arm.

2. The triceps (long head) is partially demonstrated.

3. Some shoulder muscles are depicted in this section, but they are demonstrated to better advantage in the section of the shoulder (see Ch. 5).

4. The serratus anterior arises from the upper eight or nine ribs; it courses superiorly and posteriorly to insert on the medial border of the scapula.

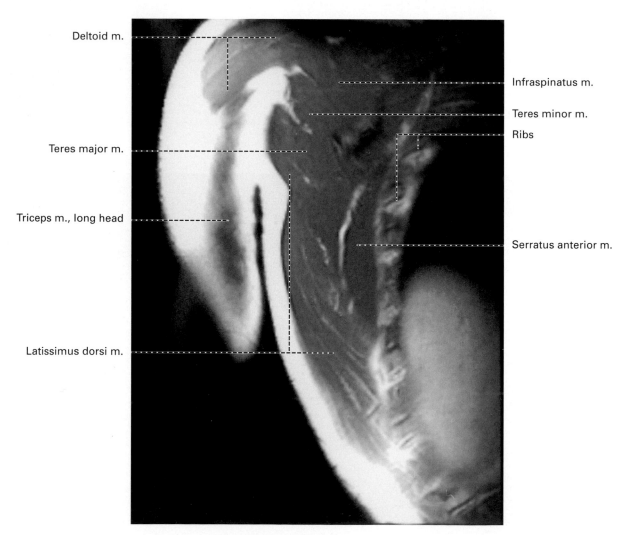

Deltoid m.

Infraspinatus m.

Teres minor m.

Ribs

Teres major m.

Triceps m., long head

Serratus anterior m.

Latissimus dorsi m.

1. The long head of the triceps courses distally, posterior to teres major and latissimus dorsi and anterior to teres minor.

2. The posterior portion of the deltoid originates from the spine of the scapula.

3. Latissimus dorsi, teres major, and subscapularis form the posterior wall of the axilla.

Figure 6.2.2

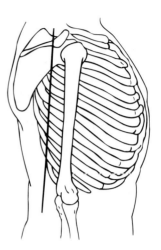

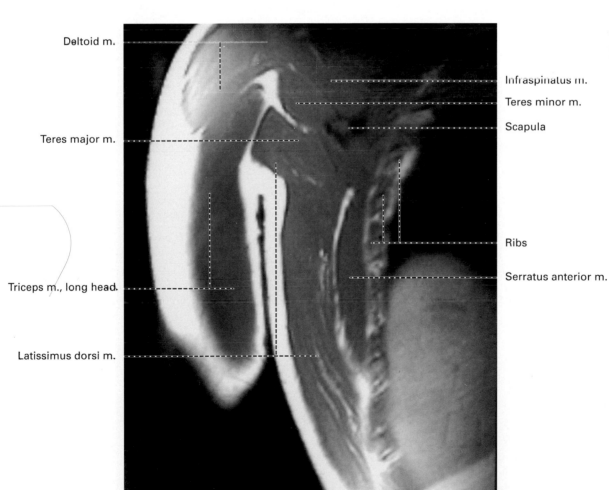

Figure 6.2.3

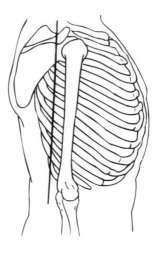

1. The only muscle of the posterior compartment of the arm is triceps, which receives its innervation from the radial nerve.

2. Triceps is separated from the anterior compartment muscles by the medial and lateral intermuscular septa.

3. The origin of the long head of triceps, from the infraglenoid tuberosity, is covered by the deltoid posteriorly.

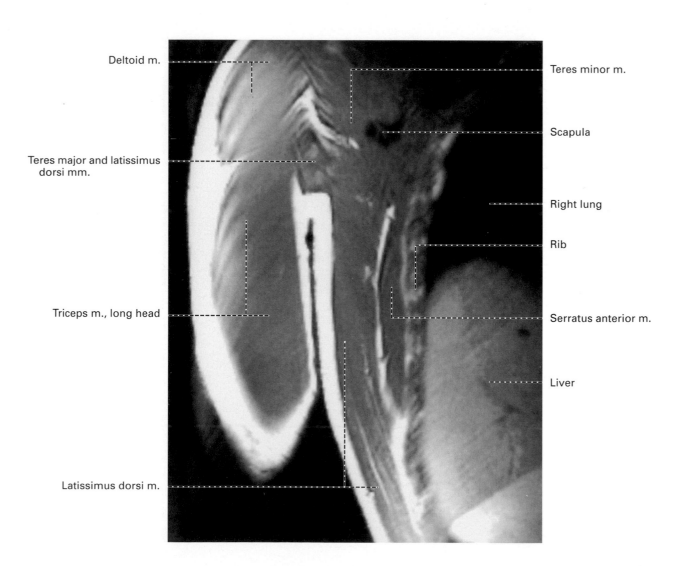

Deltoid m.

Teres major and latissimus dorsi mm.

Triceps m., long head

Latissimus dorsi m.

Teres minor m.

Scapula

Right lung

Rib

Serratus anterior m.

Liver

1. Note the extent of latissimus dorsi and serratus anterior muscles.

2. Latissimus dorsi originates from the lower six thoracic spinous processes, lumbar and sacral spinous processes, crest of the ilium, and lower four ribs. It inserts along with teres major on the crest of the lesser tuberosity.

3. The lateral head of the triceps is partially outlined.

4. The quadrangular space admits the posterior circumflex humeral artery and axillary nerve.

Figure 6.2.4

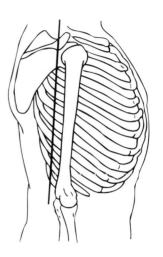

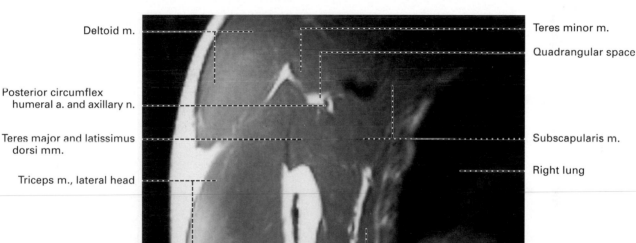

Deltoid m.

Posterior circumflex
humeral a. and axillary n.

Teres major and latissimus
dorsi mm.

Triceps m., lateral head

Triceps m., long head

Latissimus dorsi m.

Teres minor m.

Quadrangular space

Subscapularis m.

Right lung

Liver

Serratus anterior m.

Figure 6.2.5

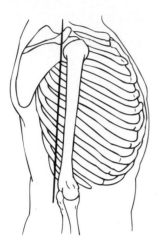

1. All three heads of triceps are demonstrated in this section.

2. The posterior circumflex humeral artery and axillary nerve exist through the quadrangular space.

3. The long and lateral heads of triceps cover the posterior surface of its medial head.

4. The axillary nerve innervates the deltoid and teres minor muscles.

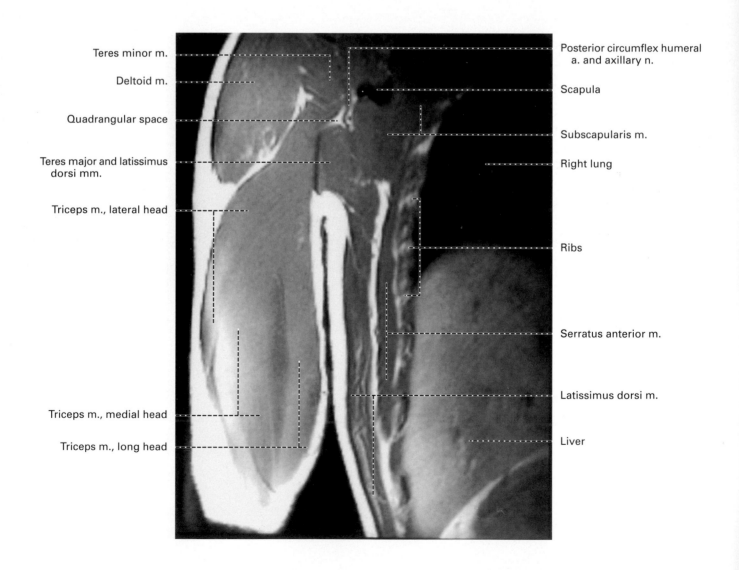

Teres minor m.

Deltoid m.

Quadrangular space

Teres major and latissimus dorsi mm.

Triceps m., lateral head

Triceps m., medial head

Triceps m., long head

Posterior circumflex humeral a. and axillary n.

Scapula

Subscapularis m.

Right lung

Ribs

Serratus anterior m.

Latissimus dorsi m.

Liver

1. The course of the radial nerve and deep (profunda) brachial artery is partially outlined in this section.

2. The radial nerve and deep (profunda) brachial artery have a spiral posterior course close to the surface of the bone in the radial groove.

3. All three heads of the triceps muscle receive their nerve supply from the radial nerve.

4. Note that the scapular attachment to the thoracic wall is entirely muscular.

Figure 6.2.6

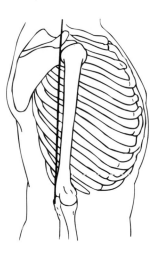

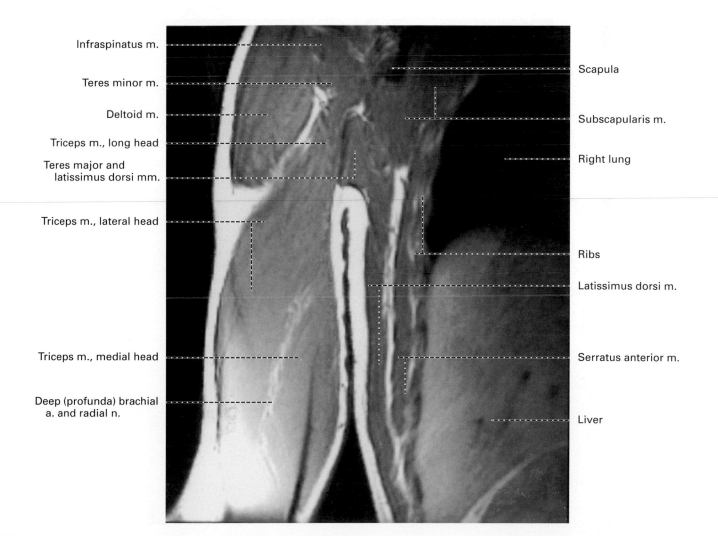

Infraspinatus m.

Teres minor m.

Deltoid m.

Triceps m., long head

Teres major and latissimus dorsi mm.

Triceps m., lateral head

Triceps m., medial head

Deep (profunda) brachial a. and radial n.

Scapula

Subscapularis m.

Right lung

Ribs

Latissimus dorsi m.

Serratus anterior m.

Liver

Figure 6.2.7

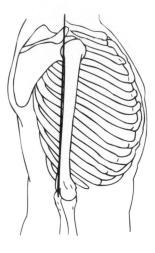

1. Note the relationship of teres minor to the long head of triceps. The long head of triceps passes between teres minor and teres major.

2. The long head of triceps originates from the infraglenoid tuberosity.

3. Note the posterior humeral circumflex artery in this section just posterior to the humeral neck.

4. The subscapularis, latissimus dorsi, and teres major muscles form the posterior wall of the axilla.

Teres minor m.

Deltoid m.

Posterior circumflex humeral a. and axillary n.

Triceps m., long head

Teres major and latissimus dorsi mm.

Deep (profunda) brachial a. and radial n.

Triceps m., lateral head

Triceps m., medial head

Scapula, infraglenoid tuberosity

Subscapularis m.

Right lung

Serratus anterior m.

Liver

Latissimus dorsi m.

1. This section is through the posterior shaft of the humerus.

2. The origin of brachialis is partially demonstrated. It originates from the anterior half of the anterior surface of the humerus.

3. Note the radial collateral artery (a terminal branch of the deep brachial) and the radial nerve posterior to the brachialis muscle.

4. The posterior circumflex humeral artery supplies the deltoid and triceps muscles; it also anastomoses with the anterior circumflex humeral artery around the surgical neck of the humerus.

Figure 6.2.8

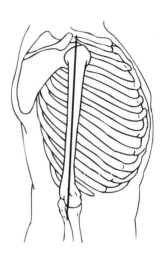

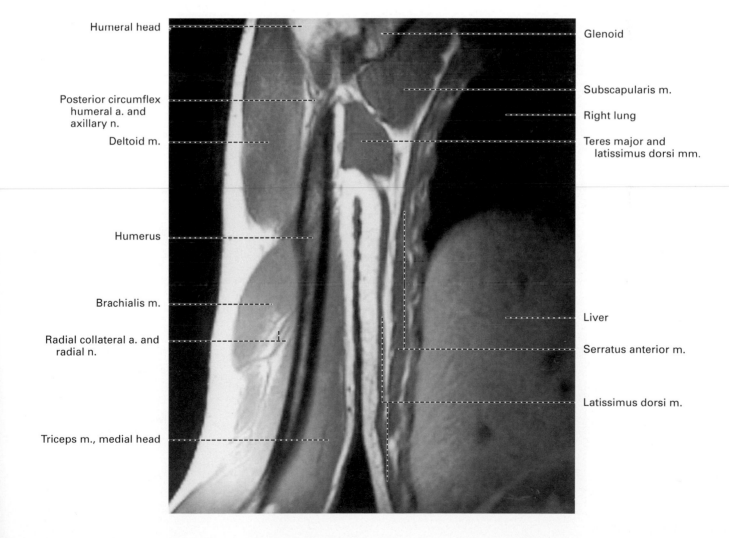

Humeral head

Posterior circumflex humeral a. and axillary n.

Deltoid m.

Humerus

Brachialis m.

Radial collateral a. and radial n.

Triceps m., medial head

Glenoid

Subscapularis m.

Right lung

Teres major and latissimus dorsi mm.

Liver

Serratus anterior m.

Latissimus dorsi m.

Figure 6.2.9

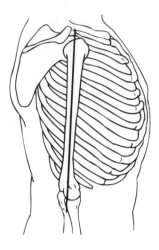

1. Note the deltoid insertion on the deltoid tuberosity.

2. Teres major and latissimus dorsi are seen approaching their insertion on the crest of the lesser tuberosity just inferior to the insertion of the subscapularis muscle.

3. The anterior margin of latissimus dorsi is demonstrated in this section.

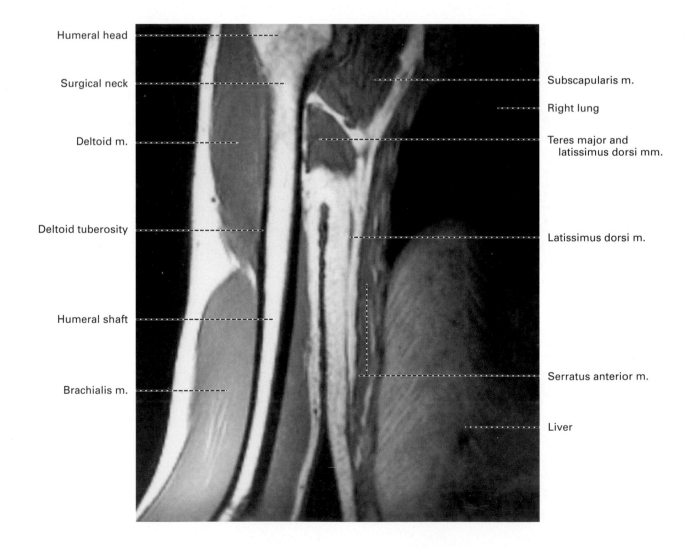

1. This section passes through the anterior shaft of the humerus.

2. Teres major and latissimus dorsi are seen inserting on the crest of the lesser tuberosity.

3. Note serratus anterior covering the lateral aspects of the rib cage. It originates from the upper eight ribs.

4. Serratus anterior forms the medial wall of the axilla.

Figure 6.2.10

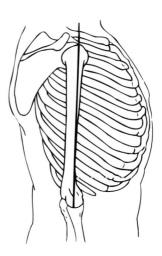

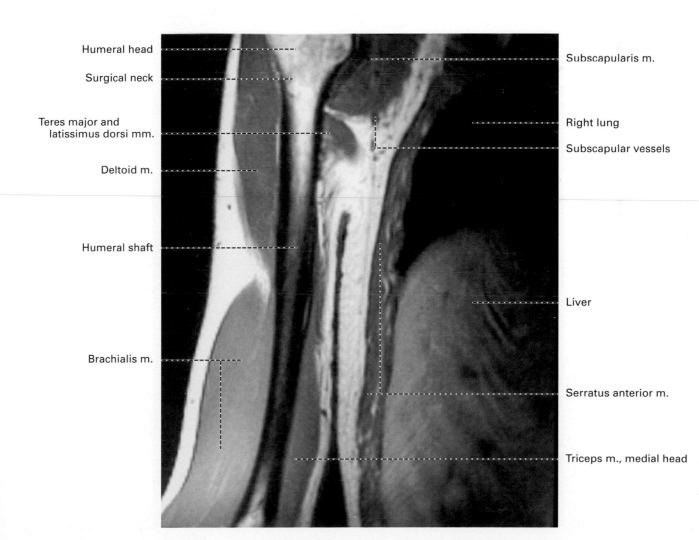

Humeral head

Surgical neck

Teres major and
latissimus dorsi mm.

Deltoid m.

Humeral shaft

Brachialis m.

Subscapularis m.

Right lung

Subscapular vessels

Liver

Serratus anterior m.

Triceps m., medial head

Figure 6.2.11

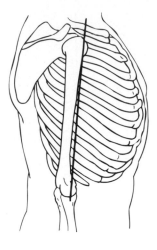

1. Note the insertion of pectoralis major on the crest of the greater tuberosity.

2. The neurovascular bundle is seen coursing distally on the anterior surface of subscapularis and medial surface of coracobrachialis.

3. The long head of the biceps tendon is demonstrated in this section. It is situated just lateral to the short head of biceps. Proximally, the long head of the biceps tendon travels in the bicipital groove.

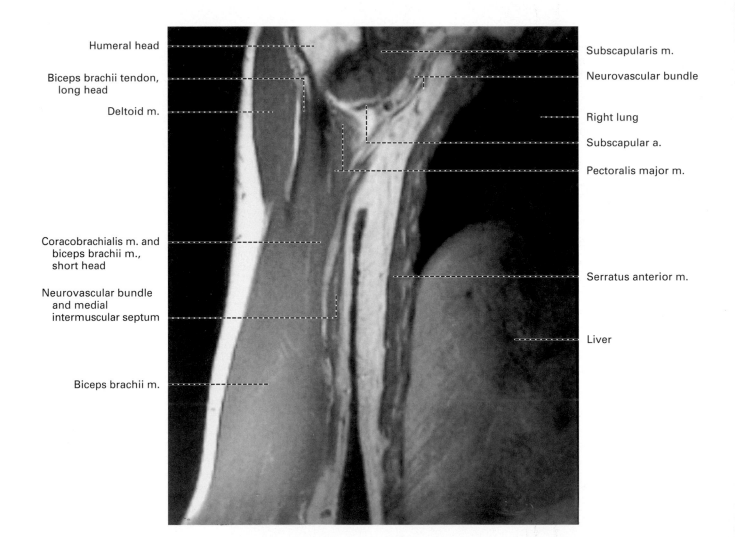

Humeral head

Biceps brachii tendon, long head

Deltoid m.

Coracobrachialis m. and biceps brachii m., short head

Neurovascular bundle and medial intermuscular septum

Biceps brachii m.

Subscapularis m.

Neurovascular bundle

Right lung

Subscapular a.

Pectoralis major m.

Serratus anterior m.

Liver

1. Note the insertion of the subscapularis muscle on the lesser tuberosity.

2. The deltoid muscle covers all the other muscle insertions at the humeral head and neck.

3. The anterior humeral circumflex artery is clearly depicted in this section as it originates from the axillary artery.

Figure 6.2.12

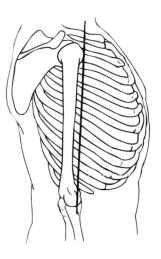

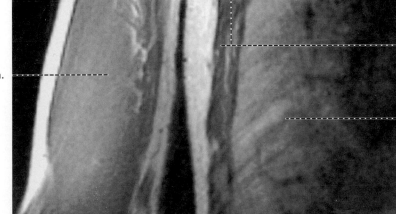

Humeral head

Subscapularis m.

Deltoid m.

Biceps brachii tendon, long head

Coracobrachialis m. and biceps brachii m., short head

Biceps brachii m.

Neurovascular bundle

Anterior humeral circumflex a.

Right lung

Serratus anterior m.

Liver

Figure 6.2.13

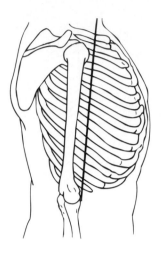

1. The neurovascular bundle courses posterior to the pectoralis minor 1 to 2 cm inferior to the tip of the coracoid process.

2. The axillary vein courses anterior to the axillary artery.

3. The anterior portion of the deltoid originates on the distal third of the clavicle and acromion process.

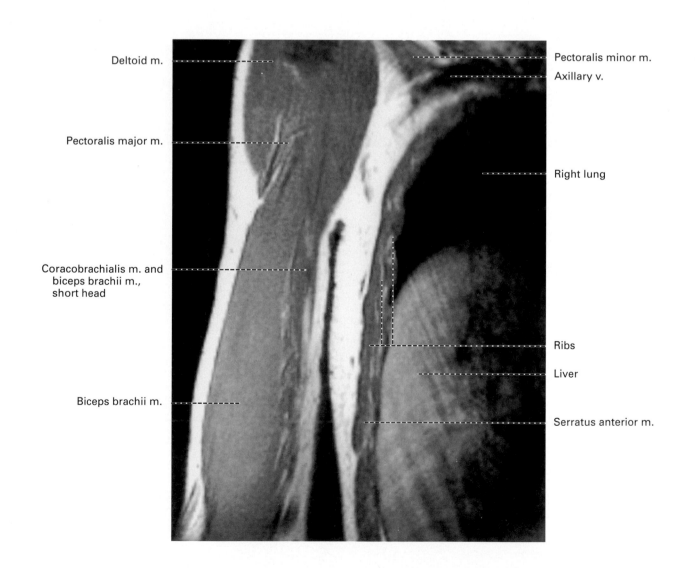

Deltoid m.

Pectoralis minor m.

Axillary v.

Pectoralis major m.

Right lung

Coracobrachialis m. and biceps brachii m., short head

Biceps brachii m.

Ribs

Liver

Serratus anterior m.

1. This section passes superficially through the anterior aspect of arm and shoulder.

2. The cephalic vein is apparent in the subcutaneous tissues on the antero-lateral aspect of the arm prior to entering the deltopectoral groove.

3. Pectoralis minor lies anterior to the microvascular bundle.

Figure 6.2.14

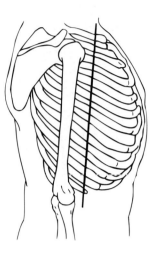

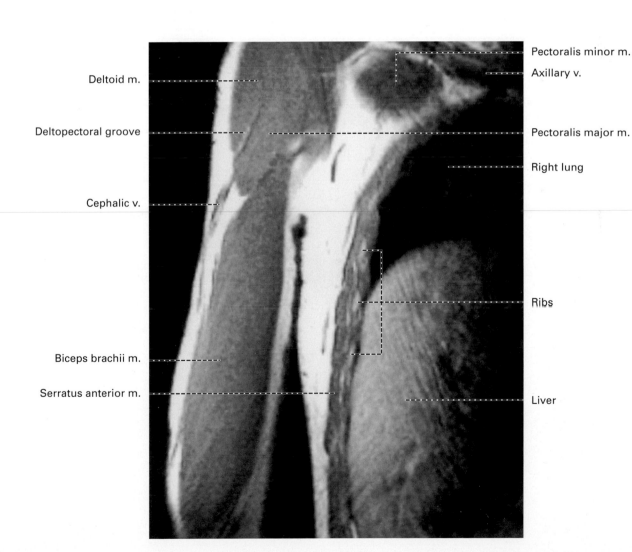

Figure 6.2.15

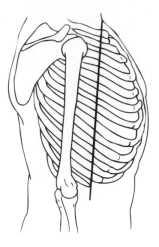

1. This section passes through the most anterior portion of biceps brachii.

2. The clavicular head of pectoralis major is demonstrated in this section.

3. Pectoralis major forms the anterior wall of the axilla. Its insertion on the humerus is covered by the deltoid.

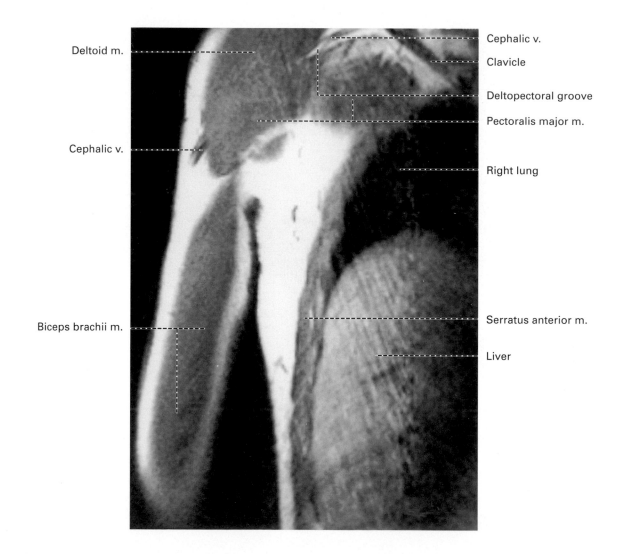

Deltoid m.

Cephalic v.

Biceps brachii m.

Cephalic v.

Clavicle

Deltopectoral groove

Pectoralis major m.

Right lung

Serratus anterior m.

Liver

Figure 6.3.1

1. This is the most medial section.

2. The brachial artery and median nerve are seen coursing distally into the cubital fossa.

3. The brachial artery lies between the biceps tendon and median nerve.

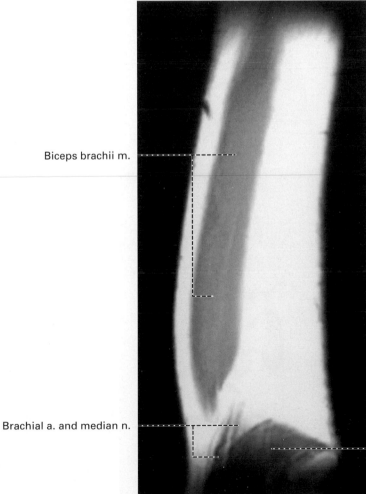

Biceps brachii m.

Brachial a. and median n.

Superficial flexor mm.

Figure 6.3.2

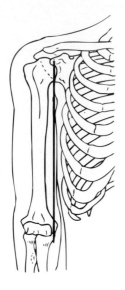

1. Note the neurovascular bundle coursing distally on the medial surface of coracobrachialis in the proximal arm and on the medial surface of brachialis in the distal arm.

2. Note the length of the biceps muscle. It traverses two joints, the shoulder and the elbow.

3. The ulnar nerve courses distally, posterior to the intermuscular septum and on the surface of the medial head of the triceps.

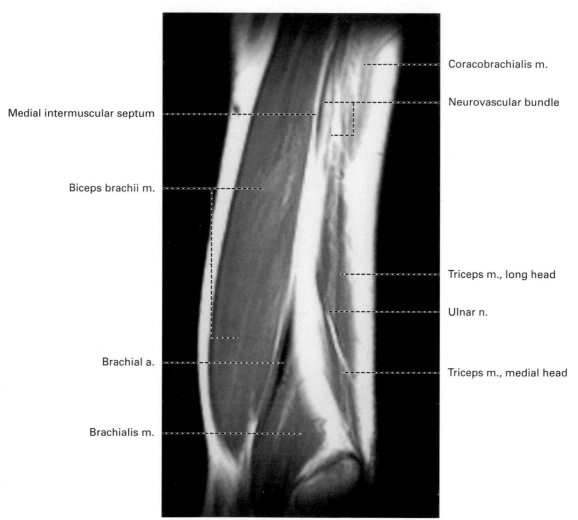

Coracobrachialis m.

Neurovascular bundle

Medial intermuscular septum

Biceps brachii m.

Triceps m., long head

Ulnar n.

Brachial a.

Triceps m., medial head

Brachialis m.

1. Note the medial intermuscular septum separating triceps from the muscles in the anterior compartment.

2. All the muscles of the anterior compartment, including coracobrachialis, are innervated by the musculocutaneous nerve.

3. Coracobrachialis is demonstrated approaching its insertion on the shaft of the proximal humerus.

Figure 6.3.3

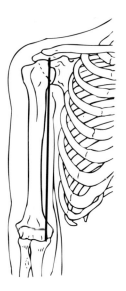

Cephalic v.	Coracobrachialis m.
	Triceps m., long head
Neurovascular bundle	
Biceps brachii m.	
	Medial intermuscular septum
Brachialis m.	
	Humerus, medial epicondyle

Figure 6.3.4

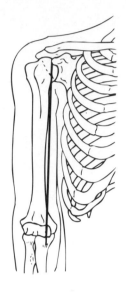

1. The olecranon fossa and posterior fat pad are well depicted in this section.

2. The coronoid fossa and anterior fat pad are also seen.

3. In the posterior compartment of the arm there is only one muscle, the triceps.

4. The triceps has three heads: long, medial, and lateral. The triceps is innervated by the radial nerve.

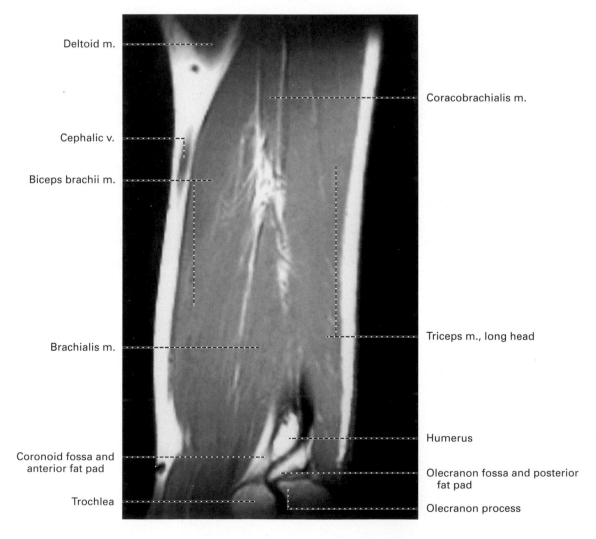

1. The medial head of triceps is covered by the long and lateral heads.

2. Note the origin of brachialis from the anterior surface of the humerus.

3. The musculocutaneous nerve is seen distally between biceps and brachialis, both of which it innervates.

Figure 6.3.5

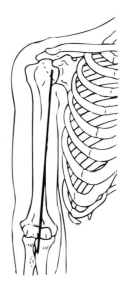

Deltoid m.

Coracobrachialis m.

Biceps brachii m.

Triceps m., medial head

Triceps m., long head

Brachialis m.

Humerus

Triceps tendon

Olecranon fossa and posterior fat pad

Trochlea

Olecranon process

Figure 6.3.6

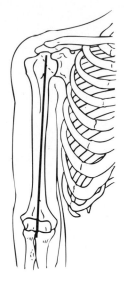

1. As the sections proceed laterally, some of the extensor muscles become evident as they originate from the lateral supracondylar ridge.

2. The brachialis muscle is the main flexor of the forearm.

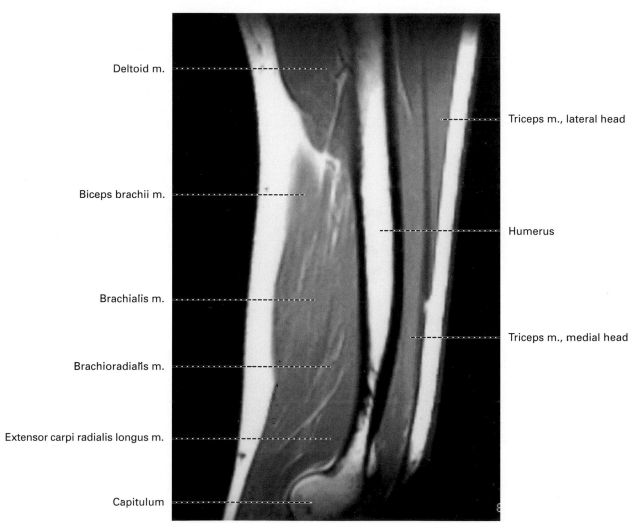

Deltoid m.

Triceps m., lateral head

Biceps brachii m.

Humerus

Brachialis m.

Triceps m., medial head

Brachioradialis m.

Extensor carpi radialis longus m.

Capitulum

1. Brachioradialis and extensor carpi radialis longus originate from the lateral supracondylar crest (ridge).

2. The remainder of the extensor originates from the lateral epicondyle.

Figure 6.3.7

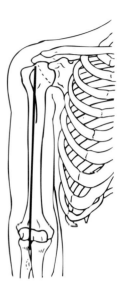

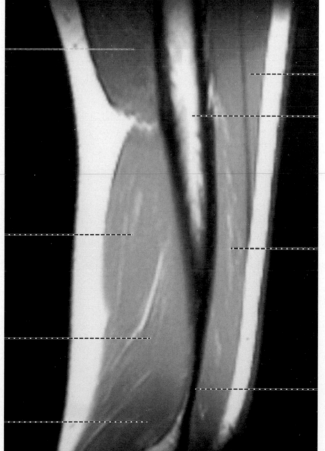

Deltoid m.

Triceps m., lateral head

Humerus

Brachialis m.

Triceps m., medial head

Brachioradialis m.

Lateral supracondylar crest

Extensor carpi radialis longus m.

Lateral epicondyle

Figure 6.3.8

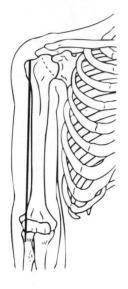

1. The radial nerve and deep (profunda) brachial artery course distally and posteriorly, adjacent to the humerus, in the radial sulcus.

2. Note the lateral intermuscular septum, which separates the anterior and posterior compartments of the arm.

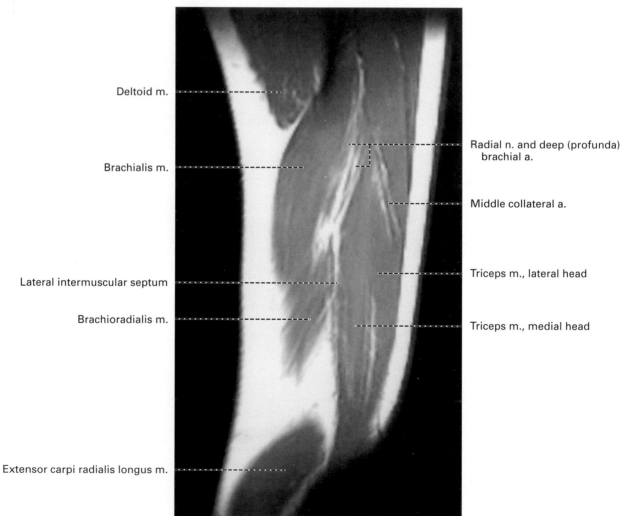

Deltoid m.

Brachialis m.

Radial n. and deep (profunda) brachial a.

Middle collateral a.

Lateral intermuscular septum

Triceps m., lateral head

Brachioradialis m.

Triceps m., medial head

Extensor carpi radialis longus m.

1. In this lateral section, the only prominent muscle is the lateral head of the triceps. Brachialis and deltoid are only partially demonstrated.

Figure 6.3.9

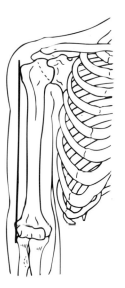

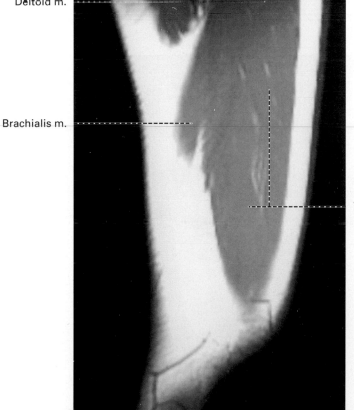

Deltoid m.

Brachialis m.

Triceps m., lateral head

Figure 6.3.10

1. The lateral head of the triceps originates from the posterior and lateral surfaces of the humerus, superior and lateral tot he radial (nerve) groove.

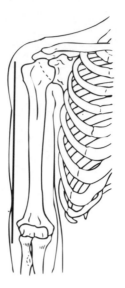

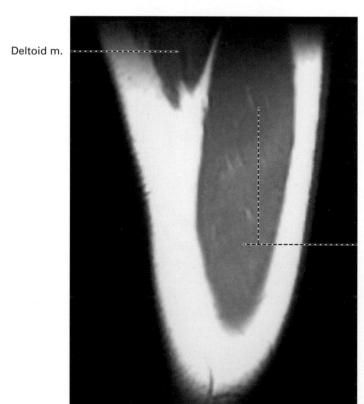

Deltoid m.

Triceps m., lateral head

1. This is the most lateral section. Only the lateral aspect of triceps and deltoid is seen in this section.

Figure 6.3.11

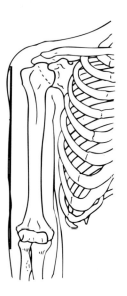

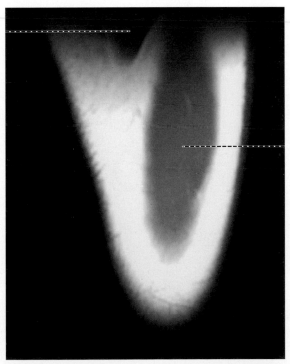

Deltoid m.

Triceps m., lateral head

Chapter 7

ELBOW

Figure 7.1.1

1. This section is through the medial and lateral supracondylar ridges of the humerus.

2. The brachioradialis and extensor carpi radialis longus muscles take their origin from the lateral supracondylar ridge.

3. Just proximal to the elbow joint, the radial nerve courses distally between the brachioradialis and brachialis muscles.

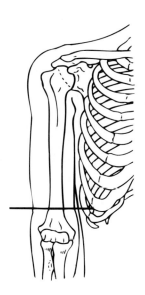

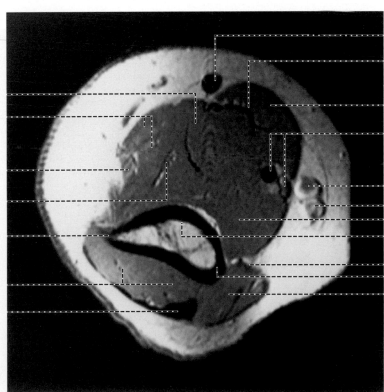

Brachialis m.

Brachioradialis m.

Extensor carpi radialis longus m.

Radial n.

Lateral supracondylar ridge

Triceps m., lateral and medial heads

Triceps tendon

Cephalic v.

Biceps brachii tendon

Biceps brachii m.

Neurovascular bundle (brachial a. and v.; median n.)

Median cubital v.

Basilic v.

Brachialis m.

Humerus

Ulnar n.

Medial supracondylar ridge

Triceps m., long head

Figure 7.1.2

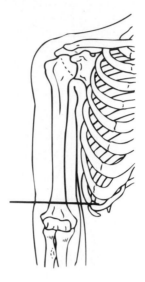

1. The median cubital vein is a major superficial vein in the elbow connecting the basilic and cephalic veins.

2. The ulnar nerve continues to take a more posterior course before it passes behind the medial epicondyle.

3. At the elbow, the median nerve travels medial to the brachial artery.

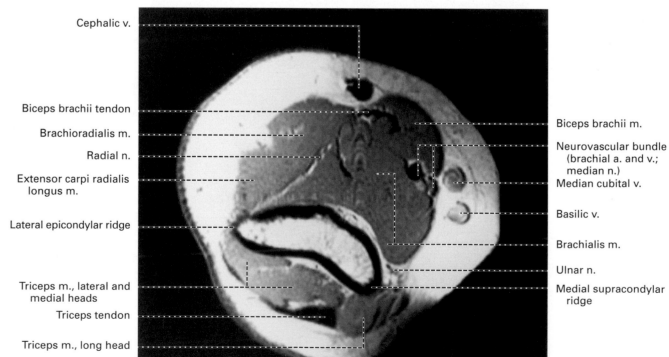

Cephalic v.

Biceps brachii tendon

Brachioradialis m.

Radial n.

Extensor carpi radialis longus m.

Lateral epicondylar ridge

Triceps m., lateral and medial heads

Triceps tendon

Triceps m., long head

Biceps brachii m.

Neurovascular bundle (brachial a. and v.; median n.)

Median cubital v.

Basilic v.

Brachialis m.

Ulnar n.

Medial supracondylar ridge

1. This section is through the olecranon fossa, which accommodates the olecranon process of the ulna when the forearm is in extension.

2. The belly of biceps brachii becomes smaller and its tendon more prominent as the sections move distally.

3. Note the irregularly flat configuration of the distal humerus.

Figure 7.1.3

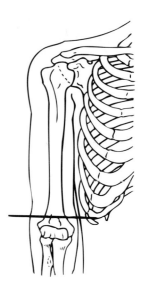

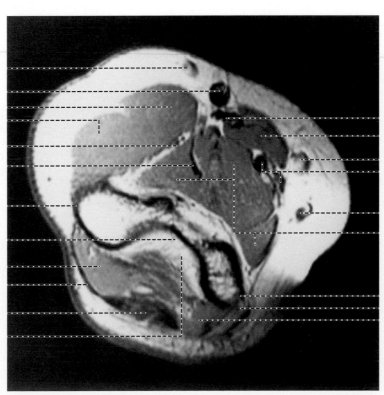

Superficial v.

Cephalic v.

Brachioradialis m.

Extensor carpi radialis longus m.

Radial n.

Brachialis tendon

Lateral supracondylar ridge

Olecranon fossa

Triceps m.

Tricipital aponeurosis

Triceps tendon

Posterior fat pad

Biceps brachii tendon

Biceps brachii m.

Median cubital v.

Neurovascular bundle (brachial a. and v.; median n.)

Basilic v.

Brachialis m.

Medial supracondylar ridge

Ulnar n.

Triceps m., long head

Figure 7.1.4

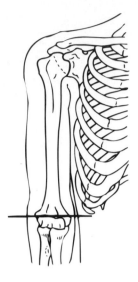

1. As the belly of biceps brachii diminishes in size, it gives rise to the biceps tendon and to the bicipital aponeurosis.

2. Note the origin of the common flexor tendon from the medial epicondyle. The common extensor tendon originates from the lateral epicondyle.

3. Note the ulnar nerve posterior to the medial epicondyle.

4. The brachial artery and median nerve continue to move from a medial to an anterior position.

5. The triceps muscle inserts on the superior surface of the olecranon and the deep fascia over the anconeus via the tricipital aponeurosis.

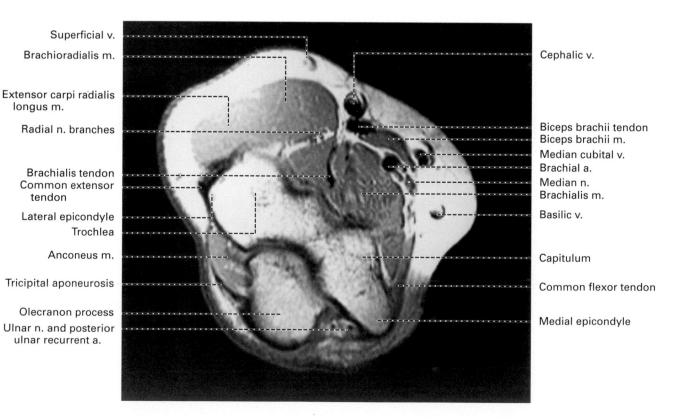

1. This section passes through the trochlea and capitulum.

2. The anconeus muscle originates with the common extensor tendon from the lateral epicondyle and inserts on the posterolateral aspect of the proximal ulna.

3. Note the bicipital aponeurosis arising from the biceps tendon.

4. Note that the ulnar nerve is accompanied by the posterior ulnar recurrent artery, a branch of the ulnar artery.

Figure 7.1.5

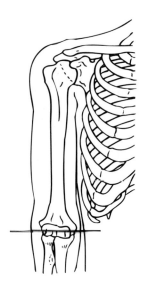

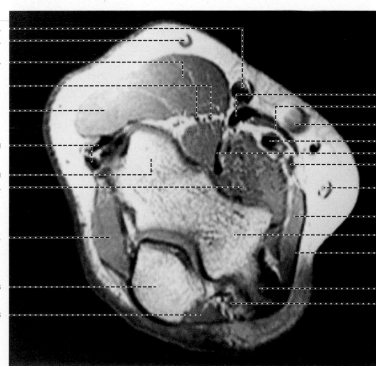

Cephalic v.
Superficial v.

Brachioradialis m.
Radial n., deep and
superficial branches

Extensor carpi radialis
longus m.

Common extensor tendon

Trochlea
Brachialis m.

Anconeus m.

Olecranon process

Flexor carpi ulnaris

Biceps brachii tendon
Bicipital aponeurosis

Medial cubital v.

Brachial a.
Brachialis tendon
Median n.

Basilic v.

Pronator teres m.

Capitulum

Common flexor tendon

Medial epicondyle

Ulnar n. and posterior ulnar
recurrent a.

Figure 7.1.6

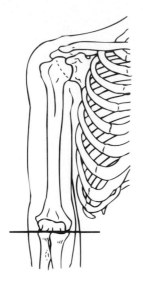

1. The lateral and medial boundaries of the cubital fossa are depicted in this section. The lateral boundary is formed by the brachioradialis muscle and medial boundary by pronator teres muscle.

2. In the cubital fossa, the brachial artery is surrounded by the medial nerve on its medial side, the biceps tendon on its lateral side, and the bicipital aponeurosis anteriorly.

3. The radial nerve lies directly on the joint capsule.

4. The ulnar nerve in this section is covered by the flexor carpi ulnaris muscle.

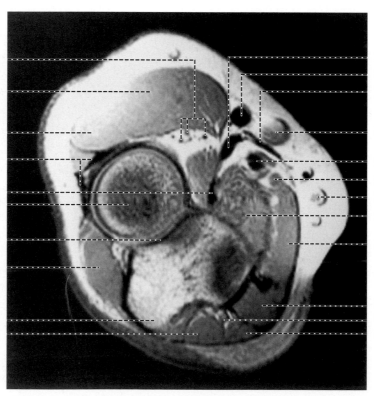

Radial n. branches
Brachioradialis m.
Extensor carpi radialis longus m.
Common extensor tendon
Brachialis tendon
Radial head
Radial notch
Anconeus m.
Ulna, posterior border
Flexor carpi ulnaris m.

Biceps brachii tendon
Cephalic v.
Bicipital aponeurosis
Median cubital v.
Brachial a.
Median n.
Basilic v.
Brachialis m.
Pronator teres m.
Flexor carpi radialis m.
Ulnar n.
Palmaris longus m.

1. The flexor carpi ulnaris muscle has two heads; one originates as part of the common flexor tendon, from the medial epicondyle; the other originates from the medial border of the olecranon and posterior aspect of the ulnar shaft.

2. Note the proximal radioulnar joint with the radial head articulating with the proximal ulna at the radial notch.

3. Note the origin of the supinator muscle mainly from the supinator crest and fossa of the ulna. The other origins include the lateral epicondyle, radial collateral ligament, and the annular ligament.

4. The brachialis muscle diminishes in size and becomes partially tendinous as it approaches its insertion on the coronoid process.

Figure 7.1.7

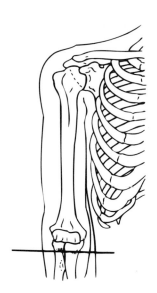

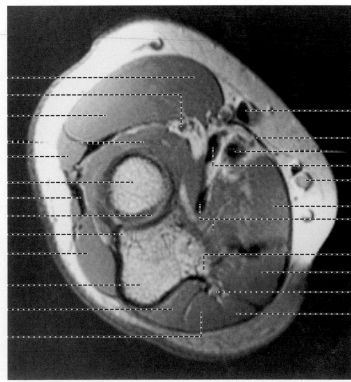

Brachioradialis m.
Radial n.
Extensor carpi radialis longus and brevis mm.
Supinator m.
Extensor digitorum m.
Radial head
Extensor carpi ulnaris tendon
Radial notch
Supinator crest
Anconeus m.
Ulna
Flexor carpi ulnaris m., ulnar head
Flexor digitorum superficialis m.

Cephalic v.
Bicipital aponeurosis
Brachial a.
Biceps brachii tendon
Basilic v.
Pronator teres m.
Brachialis tendon and m.
Coronoid process
Flexor carpi radialis m.
Ulnar n.
Palmaris longus m.

Figure 7.1.8

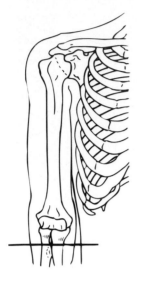

1. The bicipital aponeurosis inserts into the deep fascia on the anterior surface of pronator teres.

2. Note how the supinator muscle wraps around the proximal radius and inserts onto its lateral surface.

3. In this section, the brachialis tendon is seen inserting on the coronoid process.

4. In this section, the brachial artery is seen dividing into the radial and ulnar arteries.

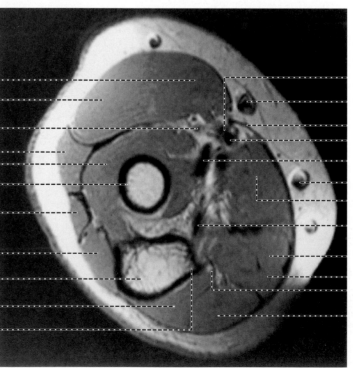

Brachioradialis m.

Flexor carpi radialis longus and brevis mm.

Radial n.

Extensor digitorum m.
Supinator m.

Radial neck

Extensor carpi ulnaris m.

Anconeus m.

Ulna

Flexor carpi ulnaris m.

Coronoid process

Radial a.

Cephalic v.

Bicipital aponeurosis
Ulnar a.

Biceps brachii tendon

Basilic v.
Pronator teres m.

Brachialis tendon

Flexor carpi radialis m.

Palmaris longus m.
Ulnar nerve

Flexor digitorum superficialis m.

1. Note the location of the ulnar nerve coursing distally between the flexor digitorum profundus and superficialis muscles.

2. The ulnar nerve innervates flexor carpi ulnaris and half of flexor digitorum profundus. The rest of the flexors in the forearm are supplied by the median nerve.

3. The median nerve continues to move deeper in the forearm. In this section, it is covered by the pronator teres muscle.

4. The brachialis tendon is completing its insertion onto the coronoid process of the ulna and the biceps tendon is completing its insertion onto the radial tuberosity.

Figure 7.1.9

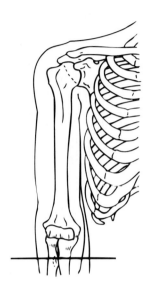

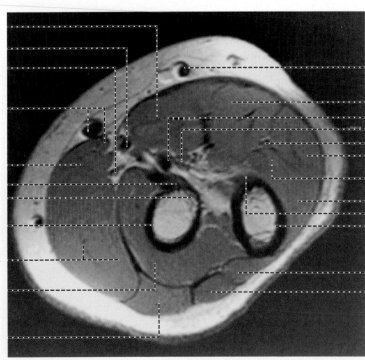

Pronator teres m.

Radial a.

Radial n., superficial branch

Cephalic and median cubital vv.

Brachioradialis m.

Biceps brachii tendon

Radial tuberosity

Radius

Extensor carpi radialis longus and brevis mm.

Supinator m.

Extensor digitorum m.

Basilic v.

Flexor carpi radialis m.
Ulnar a.
Median n.
Ulnar n.
Flexor digitorum superficialis m.
Flexor digitorum profundus m.
Flexor carpi ulnaris m.
Brachialis tendon
Ulna

Anconeus m.

Extensor carpi ulnaris m.

Figure 7.1.10

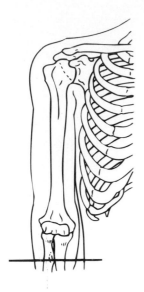

1. This section is at the apex of the cubital fossa, where the pronator teres and brachioradialis muscles meet.

2. Most individual flexor and extensor muscles in the distal elbow and forearm can be distinguished.

3. In the forearm, the ulnar nerve travels between the flexor digitorum profundus and flexor carpi ulnaris muscles.

4. The radial nerve (superficial branch) in the elbow and proximal forearm can be found covered by the brachioradialis muscle.

5. The supinator muscle is innervated by the deep branch of the radial nerve.

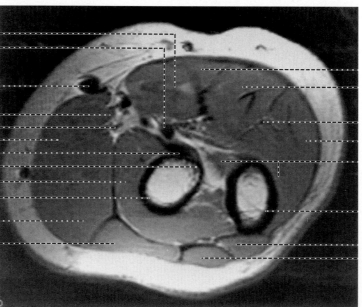

Left side labels:
- Pronator teres m.
- Ulnar a.
- Cephalic v.
- Radial a.
- Radial n.
- Brachioradialis m.
- Biceps brachii tendon
- Radial tuberosity
- Supinator m.
- Radius
- Extensor carpi radialis longus m.
- Extensor digitorum

Right side labels:
- Flexor carpi radialis m.
- Flexor digitorum superficialis m.
- Ulnar n.
- Flexor carpi ulnaris m.
- Flexor digitorum profundus m.
- Flexor digitorum superficialis m.
- Ulna
- Anconeus m.
- Extensor carpi ulnaris m.

1. This is the most posterior section of the elbow.

2. Note the origin of the ulnar head of flexor carpi ulnaris from the olecranon process.

3. Note the insertions of the triceps and anconeus onto the olecranon.

Figure 7.2.1

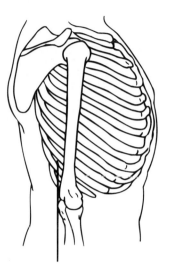

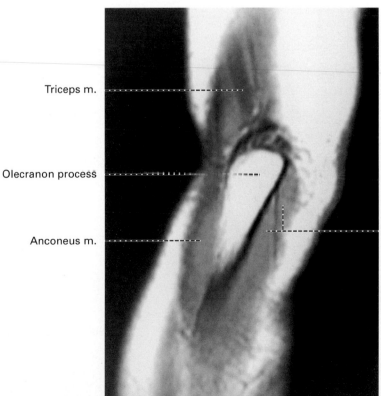

Triceps m.

Olecranon process

Anconeus m.

Flexor carpi ulnaris m.

229

Figure 7.2.2

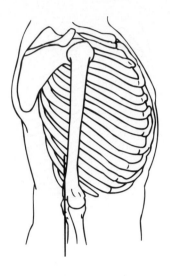

1. Note the insertion of the triceps tendon on the olecranon process.

2. The anconeus muscle is clearly depicted in this section. It originates from the posterior surface of the lateral epicondyle and inserts on the olecranon process and proximal ulna posteriorly.

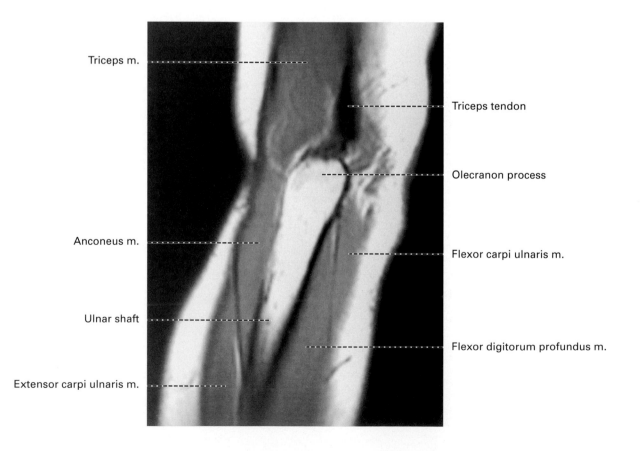

Triceps m.

Triceps tendon

Olecranon process

Anconeus m.

Flexor carpi ulnaris m.

Ulnar shaft

Flexor digitorum profundus m.

Extensor carpi ulnaris m.

1. Note the course of the ulnar nerve as it crosses behind the medial epicondyle and enters the forearm between the two heads of the flexor carpi
ulnaris.

2. The ulnar nerve innervates the flexor carpi ulnaris and the medial half of
the flexor digitorum profundus.

3. Note the supinator crest of the ulna, which serves as a major origin for the
supinator muscle.

4. The triceps and its tendon are clearly depicted in this section.

Figure 7.2.3

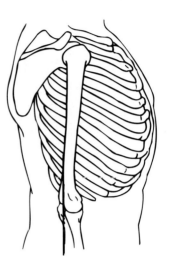

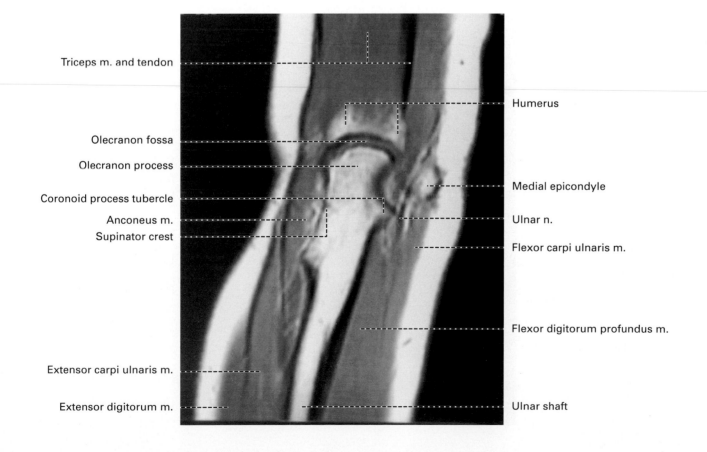

Triceps m. and tendon

Olecranon fossa

Olecranon process

Coronoid process tubercle

Anconeus m.

Supinator crest

Extensor carpi ulnaris m.

Extensor digitorum m.

Humerus

Medial epicondyle

Ulnar n.

Flexor carpi ulnaris m.

Flexor digitorum profundus m.

Ulnar shaft

Figure 7.2.4

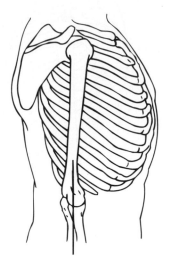

1. Note that the ulnar nerve in the elbow region is covered by the flexor carpi ulnaris. The ulnar nerve enters the forearm between the humeral and ulnar heads of flexor carpi ulnaris.

2. The olecranon fossa and the olecranon process are depicted in this section. The olecranon fossa houses the olecranon process when the elbow is in full extension.

3. Note the origin of the extensor carpi radialis brevis and extensor digitorum muscles from the lateral epicondyle.

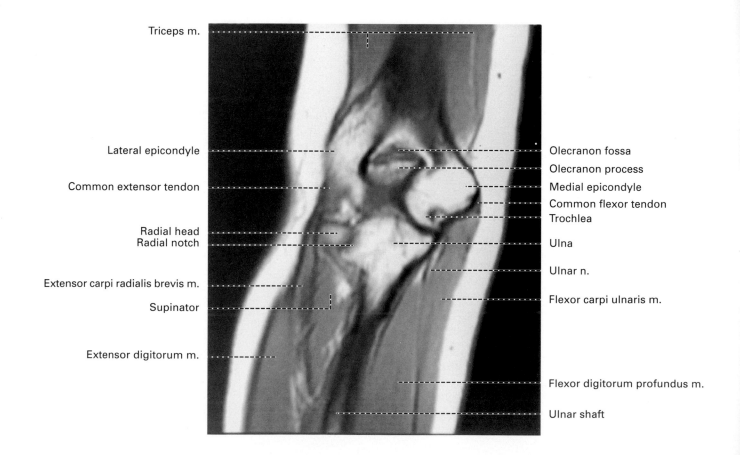

1. The common flexor tendon, originating from the medial epicondyle, is clearly depicted in this section.

2. The most medial flexor muscle is the flexor carpi ulnaris, which covers the flexor digitorum profundus.

3. The flexor carpi ulnaris and the medial half of the flexor digitorum profundus are innervated by the ulnar nerve. All the other flexors are innervated by the median nerve.

Figure 7.2.5

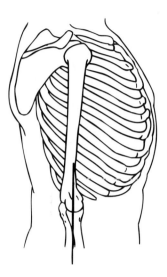

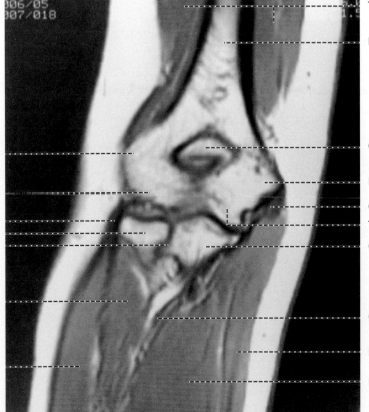

Triceps m.

Humeral shaft

Olecranon fossa

Medial epicondyle

Common flexor tendon

Trochlea

Coronoid process

Common interosseous a.

Flexor carpi ulnaris m.

Flexor digitorum profundus m.

Lateral epicondyle

Capitulum

Common extensor tendon
Radial head
Radial notch

Supinator m.

Extensor carpi radialis brevis m.

Figure 7.2.6

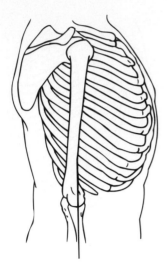

1. In this section, the pronator teres is seen originating from the proximal aspect of the medial epicondyle. It has another small head that originates from the medial side of the coronoid process.

2. Note how the supinator muscle wraps around the proximal radius.

3. The supinator muscle originates from the lateral epicondyle, radial collateral and annular ligaments, and supinator crest of the ulna. It inserts onto the posterior, lateral, and anterior surfaces of the proximal radius.

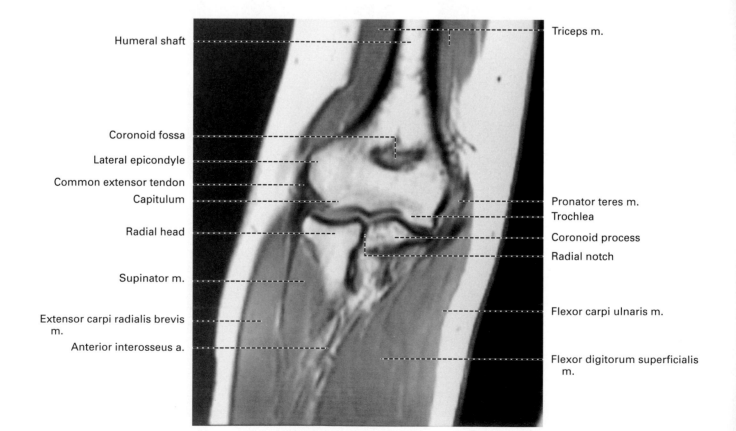

Figure 7.2.7

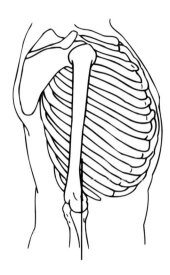

1. Note that tl
section.

2. The ulnar a
itorum pro

3. Distal to tl
tinue toget

4. Note the te
tuberosity.

5. The floor c
by the sup

1. The radiocapitular articulation is clearly depicted in this section.

2. The radial and coronoid fossae house the radial head and coronoid process when the elbow is in full flexion.

3. Note the large size of the flexor digitorum profundus. It originates from three sites: medial epicondyle, coronoid process, and anterior surface of the radial shaft proximally.

4. All the flexor muscles are innervated by the median nerve except the flexor carpi ulnaris and medial half of the flexor digitorum profundus, which are innervated by the ulnar nerve.

Brachio

R

Su

Brachio
Radial

Extensor ca
brevis m.

Extensor ca
longus m.

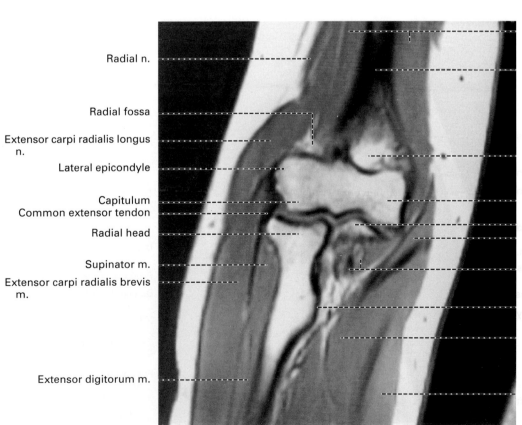

Radial n.

Radial fossa

Extensor carpi radialis longus n.

Lateral epicondyle

Capitulum
Common extensor tendon

Radial head

Supinator m.

Extensor carpi radialis brevis m.

Extensor digitorum m.

Brachialis m.

Humeral shaft, anterior cortex

Coronoid fossa

Trochlea

Coronoid process
Pronator teres m.

Brachialis m. and tendon

Radial tuberosity

Flexor digitorum superficialis m.

Flexor carpi ulnaris m.

Figu

Figure 7.2.10

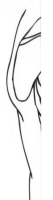
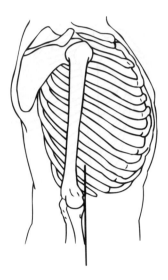

1. The brachioradialis and extensor carpi radialis longus muscles originate proximal to the elbow joint, from the lateral supracondylar ridge of the humerus.

2. In the cubital fossa, the median nerve lies medial to the brachial artery and the biceps tendon lies lateral to the brachial artery.

3. The biceps tendon is seen coursing toward its insertion on the radial tuberosity.

Extens

Cor

Extens
m.

Extens
m.

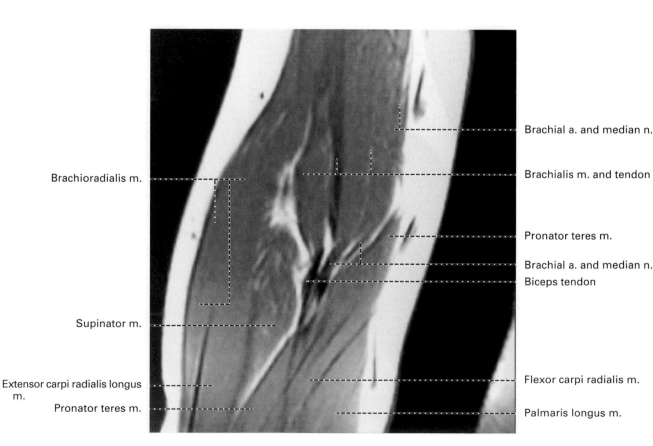

1. The cubital fossa and its boundaries are clearly depicted in this section.

2. Brachioradialis forms the lateral boundary and pronator teres forms the medial boundary.

3. The floor of the cubital fossa is formed by the brachialis and supinator muscles.

4. The supinator is innervated by the deep branch of the radial nerve.

Figure 7.2.11

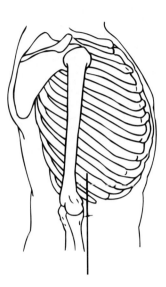

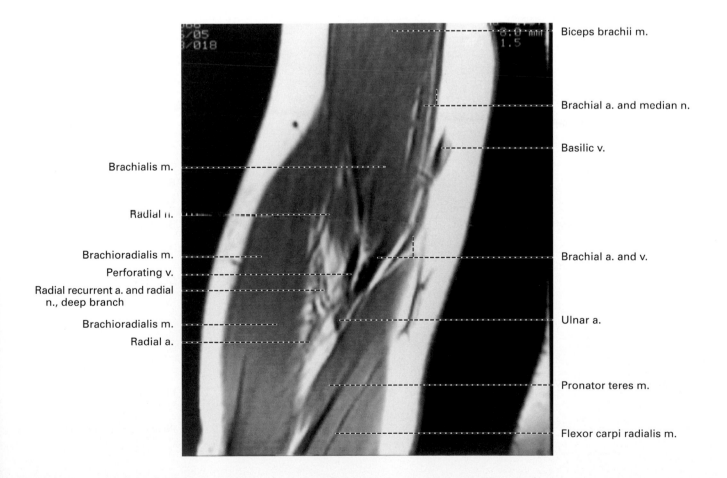

Biceps brachii m.

Brachial a. and median n.

Basilic v.

Brachialis m.

Radial n.

Brachioradialis m.

Perforating v.

Radial recurrent a. and radial n., deep branch

Brachioradialis m.

Radial a.

Brachial a. and v.

Ulnar a.

Pronator teres m.

Flexor carpi radialis m.

Figure 7.2.12

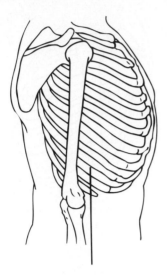

1. The median nerve, brachial artery, and biceps tendon are seen entering the cubital fossa.

2. Pronator teres and flexor carpi radialis muscles are also depicted in this section. These muscles are superficial flexors of the arm and wrist.

3. The median nerve in the cubital fossa courses medial to the brachial artery.

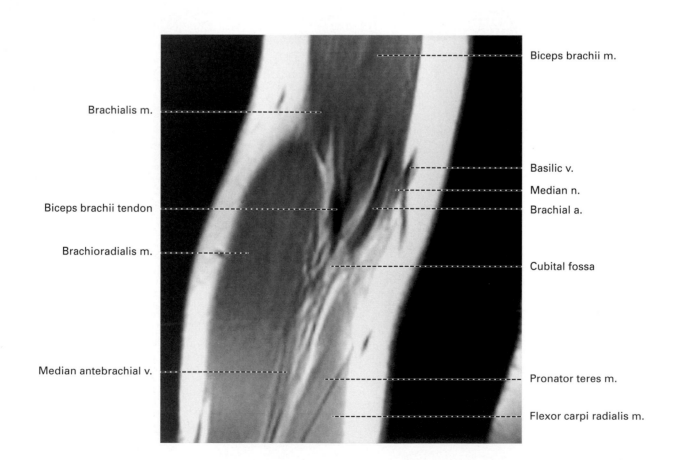

Biceps brachii m.

Brachialis m.

Basilic v.

Median n.

Biceps brachii tendon

Brachial a.

Brachioradialis m.

Cubital fossa

Median antebrachial v.

Pronator teres m.

Flexor carpi radialis m.

1. The most prominent muscle proximally on the anterior surface of the fore-arm is brachioradialis.

2. Brachioradialis arises from the upper two-thirds of the supracondylar ridge of the humerus and inserts on the lateral side of the styloid process of the radius at its base.

3. The radial nerve crosses the elbow into the forearm beneath brachioradialis.

Figure 7.2.13

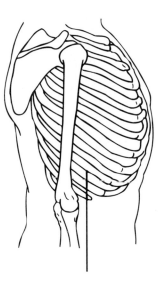

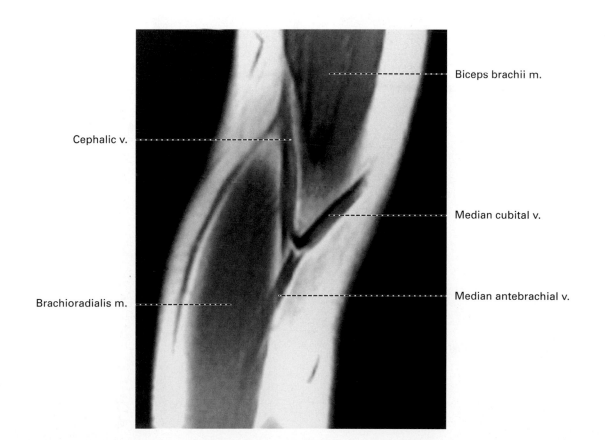

Figure 7.2.14

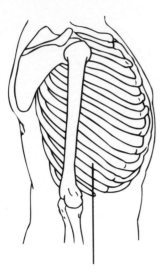

1. This section is through the anterior aspect of the elbow.

2. The biceps and some of the superficial veins are depicted in this section.

3. The cephalic vein continues to course proximally on the anterolateral surface of the arm.

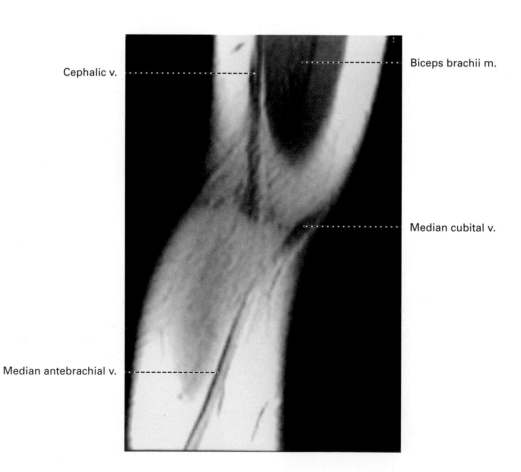

Cephalic v.

Biceps brachii m.

Median cubital v.

Median antebrachial v.

1. This is the most medial section of the elbow. It passes through the medial epicondyle of the humerus.

2. The medial epicondyle serves as the origin for the common flexor tendon.

3. Muscles that totally or partially originate from the medial epicondyle function as flexor-pronators; they include pronator teres, flexor carpi radialis, palmaris longus, flexor carpi ulnaris, and flexor digitorum superficialis.

Figure 7.3.1

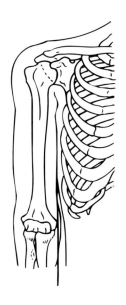

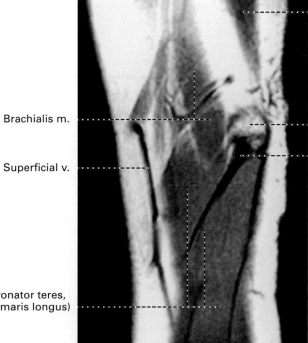

Triceps m.

Brachialis m.

Superficial v.

Medial epicondyle

Common flexor tendon

Superficial flexor mm. (pronator teres, flexor carpi radialis, palmaris longus)

Figure 7.3.10

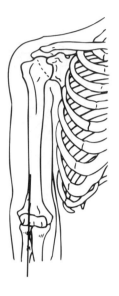

1. The supinator is demonstrated in this section. It is seen wrapping around the radius where it inserts on its lateral surface.

2. The supinator muscle originates from the lateral epicondyle, radial collateral and annular ligaments, the supinator fossa, and the crest of the ulna. It inserts on the posterior, lateral, and anterior surfaces of the proximal radius.

3. The supinator is innervated by the deep branch of the radial nerve.

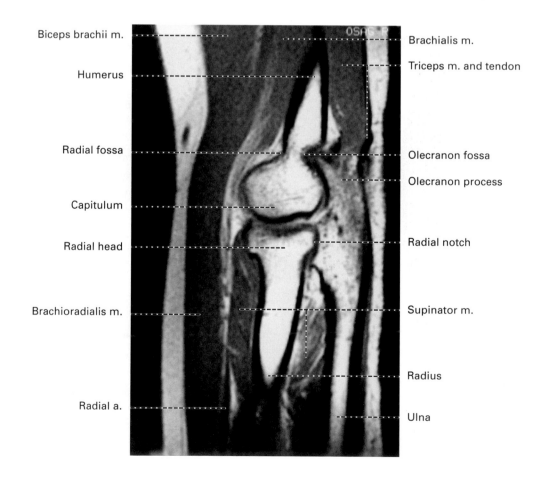

1. Anconeus is seen posterior to the elbow joint. It arises from the lateral epicondyle and inserts on the lateral aspect of the olecranon.

2. The extensor carpi radialis longus and brachioradialis both originate from the lateral supracondylar crest. The remainder of the extensor muscles originate from the lateral epicondyle.

3. Note the relationship of the supinator muscle to the proximal radius.

Figure 7.3.11

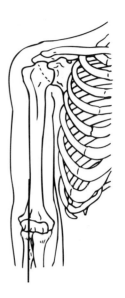

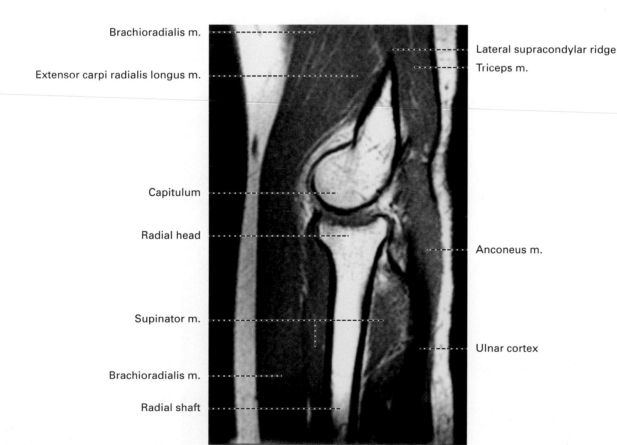

Brachioradialis m.

Extensor carpi radialis longus m.

Lateral supracondylar ridge

Triceps m.

Capitulum

Radial head

Anconeus m.

Supinator m.

Ulnar cortex

Brachioradialis m.

Radial shaft

Figure 7.3.12

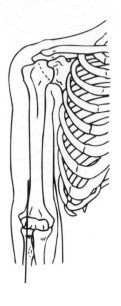

1. This section passes lateral to the humeral shaft, where the lateral intermuscular septum is demonstrated. It separates the triceps in the posterior compartment from muscles in the anterior compartment.

2. Note the articulation between the capitulum and the radial head.

3. Note the relationship of the anconeus muscle to the elbow joint. It covers the posterolateral aspect of the joint.

4. Extensor carpi ulnaris is depicted in this section. It originates from the lateral epicondyle.

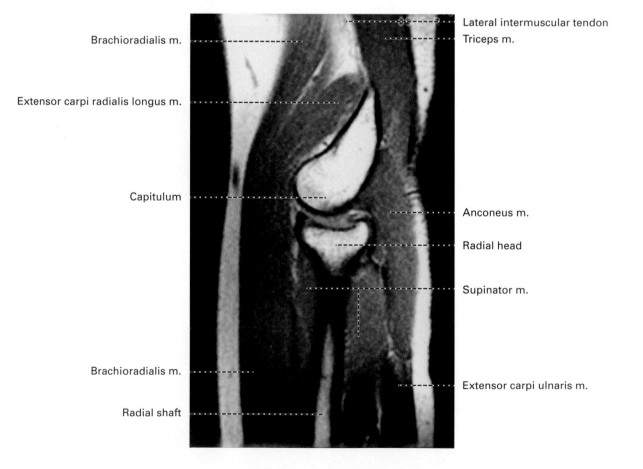

Brachioradialis m.

Extensor carpi radialis longus m.

Capitulum

Brachioradialis m.

Radial shaft

Lateral intermuscular tendon

Triceps m.

Anconeus m.

Radial head

Supinator m.

Extensor carpi ulnaris m.

1. This section is through the lateral epicondyle, which serves as the origin for the common extensor tendon.

2. The extensor digitorum muscle originates from the lateral epicondyle.

3. All the extensors in the forearm are innervated by the radial nerve.

Figure 7.3.13

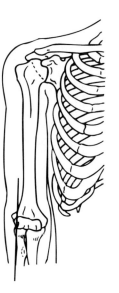

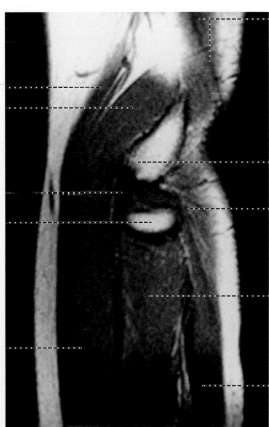

Triceps m.

Brachioradialis m.

Extensor carpi radialis longus m.

Lateral epicondyle

Common extensor tendon

Anconeus m.

Radial head

Supinator m.

Brachioradialis and extensor carpi radialis longus mm.

Extensor digitorum m.

Figure 7.3.14

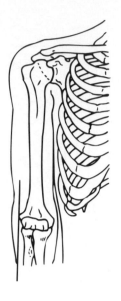

1. The brachioradialis and extensor carpi radialis longus muscles originate from the lateral supracondylar ridge proximal to the lateral epicondyle.

2. The common extensor tendon is demonstrated in this section.

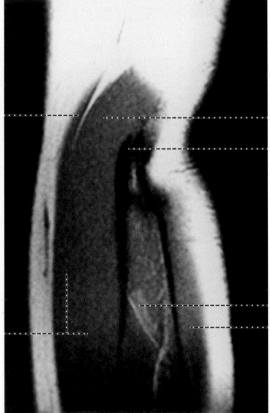

Brachioradialis m.

Extensor carpi radialis longus m.

Common extensor tendon

Extensor carpi radialis brevis m.

Extensor digitorum m.

Brachioradialis and extensor carpi radialis longus mm.

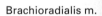

1. The prominent mass of muscles on the anterolateral aspect of the forearm consists of brachioradialis and extensor carpi radialis longus and brevis.

2. Because brachioradialis is innervated by the radial nerve, it is classified as an extensor. It lies on the anterior or flexor surface of the forearm and functions as a flexor of the elbow.

Figure 7.3.15

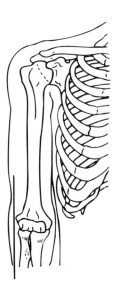

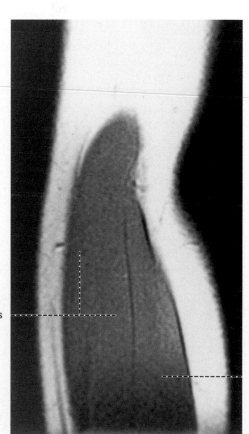

Brachioradialis and extensor carpi radialis longus mm.

Extensor carpi radialis brevis m.

Figure 7.3.16

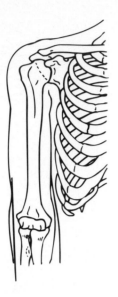

1. This is the most lateral section of the elbow. It mainly demonstrates the extensor carpi radialis longus and brevis muscles.

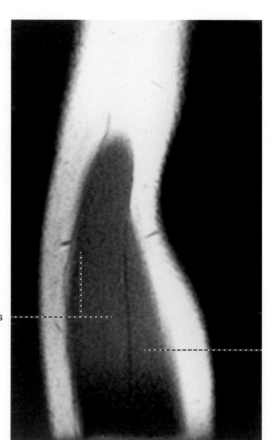

Brachioradialis and extensor carpi radialis longus mm.

Extensor carpi radialis brevis m.

Chapter 8

FOREARM

Table 8-1. (*Continued*)

Muscle	Origin	Insertion	Nerve Supply	Arterial Supply
Extensor pollicis longus	Middle third of the dorsal surface of the ulna, adjacent interosseus membrane	Base of the distal phalanx of the thumb	Deep radial (posterior interosseus) n. (C7, C8)	Posterior interosseous
Extensor indicis	Proximal part of distal third of posterior surface of the ulna, interosseus membrane	Dorsal aponeurosis on the ulnar side of the index finger, adjacent to the base of proximal phalanx	Deep radial (posterior interosseus) n. (C7, C8)	Posterior interosseous
Pronator teres	Two heads: (1) humeral head (superior half of ventral surface of medial epicondyle) and (2) ulnar head (medial border of the coronoid process)	Onto middle third of lateral surface of the radius	Median n. (C6, C7)	Anterior ulnar recurrent and posterior ulnar recurrent
Flexor carpi radialis	Medial epicondyle of humerus	Base of the second metacarpal and, usually, base of the third metacarpal	Median n. (C6, C7)	Anterior interosseous
Palmaris longus	Medial epicondyle	Flexor retinaculum and palmar aponeurosis	Median n. (C7, C8)	Anterior interosseus
Flexor carpi ulnaris	Two heads: (1) medial epicondyle and (2) medial side of the olecranon, upper two-thirds of the dorsal border of ulna	Primarily onto the pisiform	Ulnar n. (C7, C8)	Muscular branches of ulnar and anterior interosseus and posterior ulnar recurrent
Flexor digitorum superficialis	Two heads: (1) ulnar (medial epicondyle, ventral surface of the epicondyle, ulnar collateral ligament, ulnar tuberosity, medial border of coronoid process) and (2) radial (anterior oblique line and ventral border below the radial oblique line)	Ventral surface of the shaft of the middle phalanx of each finger	Median n. (C7, C8, T1)	Ulnar recurrent posterior branch and muscular branches of anterior interosseus
Flexor digitorum profundus	Proximal three-fourths of medial and anterior surface of ulna and interosseus membrane	Bases of the distal phalanges of the second to fifth digits	Median, anterior interosseous branch (C8, T1)	Ulnar recurrent posterior branch, common and anterior interosseus muscular branches
Flexor pollicis longus	Ventral surface of radius, oblique line, and adjacent interosseus membrane	Base of the distal phalanx of the thumb	Median, anterior interosseus branch (C8, T1)	Muscular branches of the anterior interosseus
Pronator quadratus	Medial side, ventral surface of distal fourth of the ulna	Distal quarter of ventral surface of the radius	Median, anterior interosseous (C8, T1)	Anterior interosseus artery, anterior and posterior terminal branches

1. This section passes through the apex of the cubital fossa.

2. The radial artery travels distally in the forearm beneath the brachioradialis muscle.

3. The median nerve travels distally between the flexor digitorum superficialis and flexor digitorum profundus muscles.

4. The median nerve innervates most of the flexors in the forearm except the carpi ulnaris and the medial half of the flexor digitorum profundus.

Figure 8.1.1

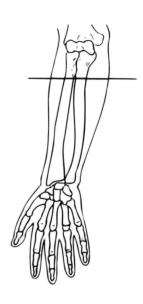

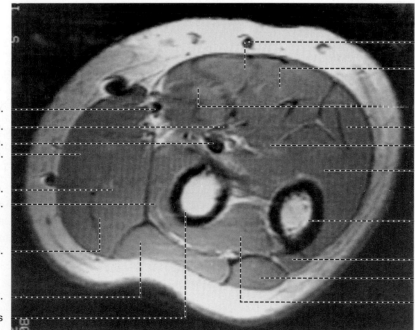

Flexor carpi radialis m.

Flexor digitorum superficialis m.

Pronator teres m

Flexor carpi ulnaris m.

Ulnar n.

Flexor digitorum profundus m.

Ulna

Anconeus m.

Extensor carpi ulnaris m.

Supinator m.

Radial a.

Median n.

Ulnar a.

Brachioradialis m.

Extensor carpi radialis brevis m.

Supinator m.

Extensor carpi radialis brevis m.

Extensor digitorum m.

Radius

Figure 8.1.2

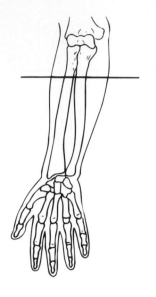

1. The ulnar nerve is seen between the flexor carpi ulnaris and flexor digitorum profundus muscles. It maintains this relation throughout most of its course in the forearm.

2. In the forearm, the ulnar nerve innervates flexor carpi ulnaris and the medial half of the flexor digitorum profundus.

3. The insertion of the supinator muscle on the anterolateral aspect of the proximal radius is depicted in this section.

4. The anterior interosseous artery, depicted in this section, is a branch of the ulnar artery.

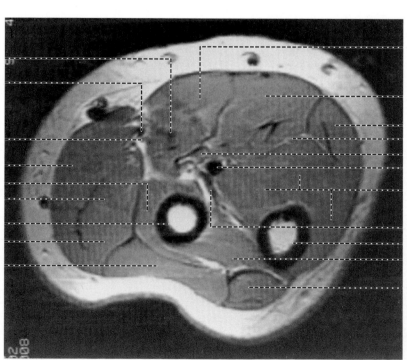

Pronator teres m.

Radial a.

Radial n., superficial branch

Brachioradialis m.

Supinator m.

Extensor carpi radialis longus m.

Radius

Extensor carpi radialis brevis m.

Extensor digitorum m.

Flexor carpi radialis m.

Flexor digitorum superficialis m.

Flexor carpi ulnaris m.

Ulnar n.

Median n.

Ulnar a.

Flexor digitorum profundus m.

Anterior interosseus a.

Ulna

Supinator m.

Extensor carpi ulnaris m.

Figure 8.1.3

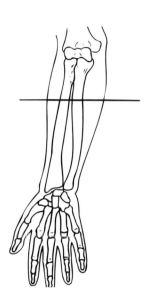

1. The pronator teres muscle is noted deep in the forearm as it courses toward its insertion on the anterolateral surface of the radius at about its midshaft. The distal part of pronator teres is covered by brachioradialis and extensor carpi radialis longus muscles.

2. The radial nerve innervates all the extensors in the forearm. The nerve's superficial branch is seen in this section covered by the brachioradialis. Brachioradialis is supplied by this nerve. The deep branch supplies the supinator, then passes through the supinator muscle; it supplies all the extensor muscles posterior to it.

3. Several superficial veins are depicted in this section. These veins merge together at the elbow to form the basilic and cephalic veins.

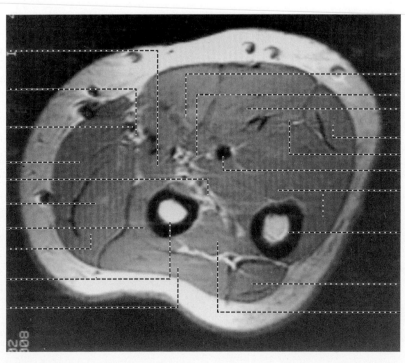

Pronator teres m.

Radial n., superficial branch

Radial a.

Brachioradialis m.

Anterior interosseous artery

Extensor carpi radialis longus m.

Supinator m.

Extensor carpi radialis brevis m.

Radius

Extensor digitorum m.

Flexor carpi radialis m.

Median n.

Flexor digitorum superficialis m

Flexor carpi ulnaris m.

Ulnar n.

Ulnar a.

Flexor digitorum profundus m.

Ulna

Extensor carpi ulnaris m.

Supinator m.

Figure 8.1.4

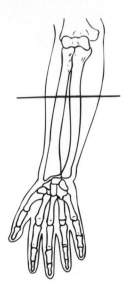

1. The belly of the brachioradialis muscle diminishes in size as the sections move distally.

2. The pronotor teres is shown close to its insertion on the anterolateral surface of the radius.

3. Note that the shaft of the ulna is more superficial than the shaft of the radius. The ulna, in the forearm, can be easily palpated under the skin.

4. The extensor muscles originate from the lateral epicondyle. The only exceptions are the brachioradialis and extensor carpi radialis longus muscles, which originate from the lateral supracondylar ridge.

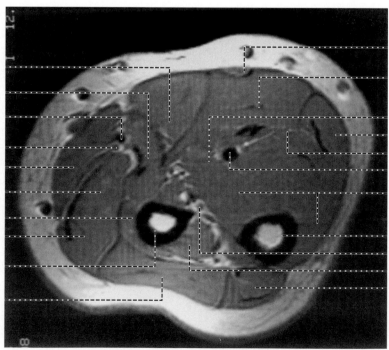

Flexor carpi radialis m.

Pronator teres m.

Radial a.

Radial n., superficial branch

Brachioradialis m.

Extensor carpi radialis longus m.

Supinator m.

Extensor carpi radialis brevis m.

Radius

Extensor digitorum m.

Palmaris longus m.

Flexor digitorum superficialis m.

Median n.

Flexor carpi ulnaris m.

Ulnar n.

Ulnar a.

Flexor digitorum profundus m.

Ulna

Anterior interosseus a.

Supinator m.

Flexor carpi ulnaris m.

1. Note that the shafts of the radius and ulna have now assumed a triangular configuration.

2. The interosseous membrane, which provides a site of origin for two deep flexors and four extensor muscles, is depicted in this section.

3. Note that the extensor pollicis longus, abductor pollicis longus, and flexor digitorum profundus muscles originate, in part, from the interosseous membrane.

4. Note the origin of the flexor pollicis longus muscle from the anterior surface of the radius at its middle third.

Figure 8.1.5

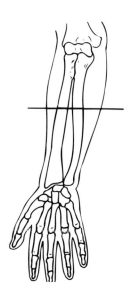

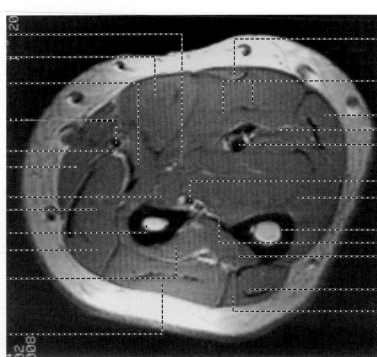

Median n.

Flexor carpi radialis m.

Pronator teres m.

Radial a.

Radial n., superficial branch

Brachioradialis m.

Flexor pollicis longus m.
Extensor carpi radialis longus m.

Radius

Extensor carpi radialis brevis m.

Abductor pollicis longus m.

Extensor digitorum m.

Palmaris longus m.

Flexor carpi digitorum superficialis m.

Flexor carpi ulnaris m.
Ulnar n.
Ulnar a.

Anterior interosseus a.

Flexor digitorum profundus m.

Ulna
Interosseus membrane
Extensor pollicis longus m.

Extensor carpi ulnaris m.

Extensor digiti minimi m.

Figure 8.1.6

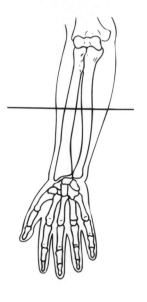

1. The posterior interosseous as well as the anterior interosseous artery are branches of the common interosseous artery, which is a tributary of the ulnar artery.

2. Note that at this level the extensor muscles occupy the posterior and lateral aspects of the forearm.

3. The abductor pollicis longus originates from the posterior surface of the radius at its middle third and from the adjacent interosseous membrane.

4. Note the origin of the flexor pollicis longus from the anterior surface of the radius at its middle third.

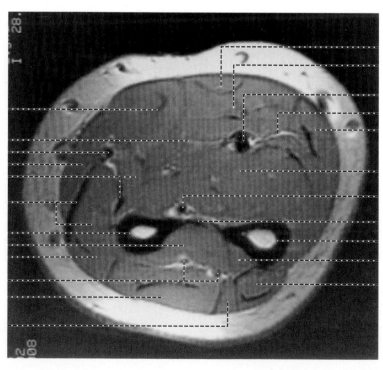

Flexor carpi radialis m.

Median n.
Radial a.
Brachioradialis m.
Pronator teres m. and tendon

Extensor carpi radialis longus m.

Radius
Abductor pollicis longus m.
Extensor carpi radialis brevis m.
Posterior interosseus vessels
Extensor digitorum m.

Extensor digiti minimi m. and tendon

Palmaris longus m.
Flexor digitorum superficialis m.
Ulnar a.
Ulnar n.
Flexor carpi ulnaris m.

Flexor digitorum profundus m.
Anterior interosseus a.

Interosseus membrane

Ulna

Extensor pollicis longus m.

Extensor carpi ulnaris m.

1. This section is near the middle of the forearm. At this level, the pronator teres muscle completes its insertion on the radius.

2. Note that most of the forearm muscles have a prominent tendinous component at this level near the middle of the forearm.

3. Note the relationships of the median and ulnar nerves to the surrounding structures. The median nerve continues to course distally between the flexor digitorum profundus and superficialis muscles; the ulnar nerve courses distally between the flexor digitorum profundus and flexor carpi ulnaris muscles.

4. Note that the flexor muscle mass in the forearm is considerably larger than the extensor muscle mass.

Figure 8.1.7

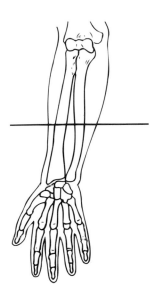

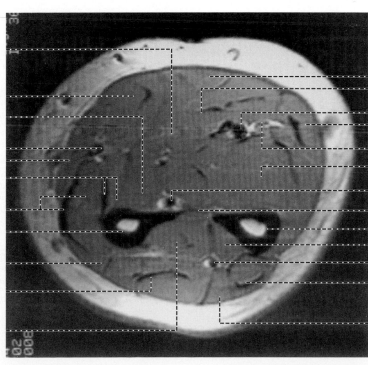

Median n.

Flexor carpi radialis m.

Flexor pollicis longus m.

Radial a.
Brachioradialis m.

Pronator teres m. and tendon

Extensor carpi radialis
longus m. and tendon

Radius

Extensor carpi
radialis brevis m.

Extensor digitorum m.
and tendon

Abductor pollicis longus m.

Palmaris longus m.
Flexor digitorum superficialis
m. and tendon
Ulnar a.
Flexor carpi ulnaris m.
and tendon
Ulnar n.

Flexor digitorum
profundus m.
Anterior interosseous a.

Interosseous membrane

Ulna

Extensor pollicis longus m.

Posterior interosseous a.

Extensor carpi ulnaris m.
and tendon

Extensor digiti minimi m.

Figure 8.1.8

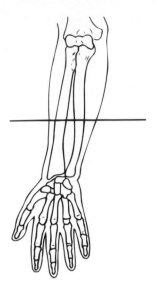

1. The interosseous membrane is well developed and distinctly visualized in this section.

2. Anteriorly, the interosseous membrane is bounded by the flexor digitorum profundus and to a much lesser extent by the flexor pollicis longus. Posteriorly, it is bounded by the abductor pollicis longus and to a lesser extent by the extensor pollicis longus.

3. Note that the ulnar nerve and artery are now coursing distally together. They are covered by the flexor carpi ulnaris muscle.

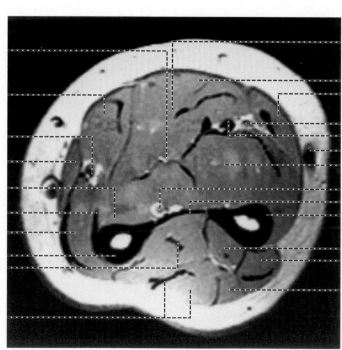

Median n.

Flexor carpi radialis m. and tendon

Radial a. and n., superficial branch

Brachioradialis m.

Flexor pollicis longus m.

Pronator teres tendon

Extensor carpi radialis longus and brevis mm. and tendons
Radius
Abductor pollicis longus m. and tendon

Extensor digitorum m. and tendon

Flexor digitorum superficialis m. and tendons

Palmaris longus m.
Flexor carpi ulnaris m. and tendon

Ulnar n.
Ulnar a.
Basilic v.
Flexor digitorum profundus m. and tendons
Anterior interosseous a. and n.
Interosseous membrane
Ulna

Extensor pollicis longus m.
Extensor carpi ulnaris m. and tendon

Extensor digiti minimi m.

1. Note that in this section, which is just distal to the midforearm, the brachioradialis is completely tendinous and the radial artery is quite superficial.

2. The extensor indicis muscle is seen for the first time as it takes its origin from the posterior aspect of the ulna and interosseous membrane.

3. Note that the extensor pollicis longus muscle is originating from the posterior surface of the ulna.

4. In this section, abductor pollicis longus and extensor pollicis brevis migrate laterally prior to crossing over extensor carpi radialis longus and brevis, as seen in more distal sections.

Figure 8.1.9

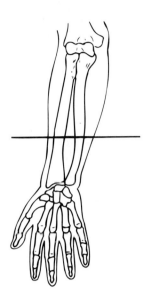

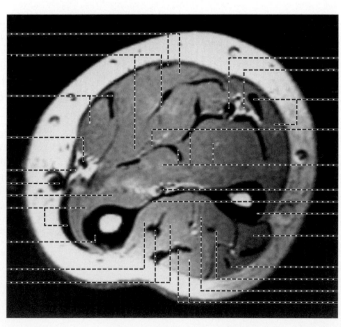

Palmaris longus m. and tendon

Flexor digitorum superficialis m. and tendon

Flexor carpi radialis m. and tendon

Radial a. and radial n., superficial branch

Brachioradialis tendon
Cephalic v.
Flexor pollicis longus m.
Extensor carpi radialis longus and brevis mm. and tendons

Radius

Extensor pollicis brevis m.
Abductor pollicis longus m. and tendon

Ulnar a.
Ulnar n.

Flexor carpi ulnaris m. and tendon

Median n.

Flexor digitorum profundus m. and tendons
Anterior interosseous a. and n.
Anterior interosseous membrane
Ulna

Extensor carpi ulnaris m.

Extensor digiti minimi m.
Extensor pollicis longus m.
Extensor indicis m.
Extensor digitorum m. and tendons

Figure 8.1.10

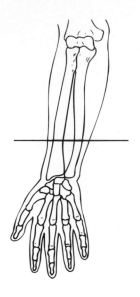

1. The abductor pollicis longus and extensor pollicis brevis muscles continue their migration laterally.

2. The extensor carpi radialis longus and brevis muscles are almost entirely tendinous in the distal third of the forearm.

3. The ulnar nerve and artery continue to course distally between the flexor carpi ulnaris and flexor digitorum profundus muscles.

4. The median nerve, which innervates most of the flexors in the forearm, is still coursing between the flexor digitorum profundus and superficialis muscles.

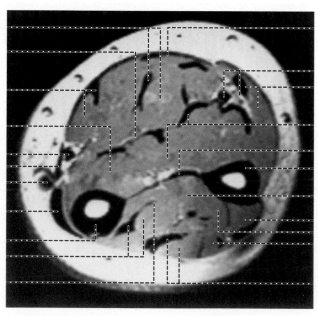

Flexor digitorum superficialis m. and tendon

Median n.

Flexor carpi radialis m. and tendon

Flexor pollicis longus m.

Radial a.
Brachioradialis tendon
Cephalic v.

Extensor carpi radialis longus and brevis mm. and tendons

Radius

Abductor pollicis longus m. and tendon

Extensor pollicis brevis m.

Palmaris longus tendon

Ulnar a. and n.
Flexor carpi ulnaris m. and tendon

Flexor digitorum profundus m. and tendons
Interosseous membrane
Ulna

Extensor indicis m.

Extensor carpi ulnaris m.
Extensor pollicis longus m.
Extensor digiti minimi m.

Extensor digitorum m. and tendons

1. The abductor pollicis longus and extensor pollicis brevis muscles are cropping out from beneath extensor digitorum, just prior to crossing over the extensor carpi radialis longus and brevis muscles.

2. In the distal forearm, the radial artery is quite superficial and is easily palpated.

3. The brachioradialis muscle is represented in the distal forearm by its small tendon.

4. The extensor indicis muscle originates on the posterolateral surface of the distal third of the ulna and the posterolateral surface of the interosseous membrane.

Figure 8.1.11

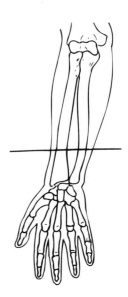

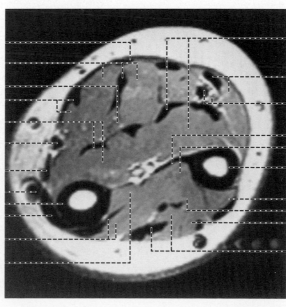

Palmaris longus tendon

Flexor digitorum superficialis m. and tendons

Median n.

Flexor carpi radialis m. and tendon

Flexor pollicis longus m. and tendon

Radial a.

Brachioradialis tendon

Cephalic v.
Radius
Extensor carpi radialis longus and brevis tendons
Abductor pollicis longus m. and tendon
Extensor pollicis brevis m.

Flexor digitorum profundus m. and tendons

Flexor carpi ulnaris n. and tendon

Ulnar a. and n.

Interosseous membrane
Extensor indicis m.

Ulna

Extensor carpi ulnaris m.
Extensor pollicis longus m.
Extensor digiti minimi m.

Extensor digitorum m. and tendons

Figure 8.1.12

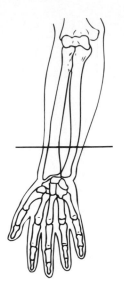

1. The muscle mass of the forearm diminishes in distal sections and tendons of individual muscles become prominent.

2. Note that the distal radius starts to flatten and enlarge as it approaches the wrist.

3. The radial artery continues in its course distally adjacent to the flexor carpi radialis tendon, where it can be palpated under the skin.

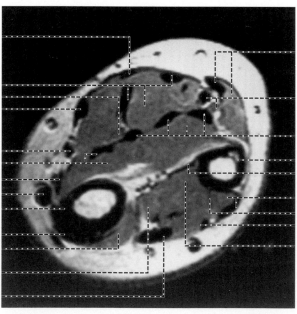

Palmaris longus tendon

Flexor digitorum
superficialis m. and tendons
Median n.
Flexor carpi radialis tendon

Radial a.
Flexor pollicis longus m. and tendon
Brachioradialis tendon
Cephalic v.
Radius
Extensor carpi radialis
longus and brevis tendons
Abductor pollicis longus m.
and tendon
Extensor pollicis brevis m.

Extensor digitorum tendons

Flexor carpi ulnaris m. and tendons

Ulnar a. and n.

Flexor digitorum profundus m.
and tendons
Ulna
Interosseous membrane

Extensor carpi ulnaris m. and tendon
Extensor indicis m.
Extensor digiti quinti m. and tendon

Extensor pollicis longus m.

1. This section passes through the proximal portion of pronator quadratus. This muscle originates from the anterior surface of the distal one-fourth of the ulna and runs transversely to insert on the anterior surface of the radius.

2. The radius continues to enlarge and flatten.

3. The abductor pollicis longus has cropped out from beneath the flexor digitorum. Distally, it will be joined by the extensor pollicis brevis tendon and both will cross over extensor carpi radialis longus and brevis tendons.

4. The brachioradialis tendon courses close to the distal radius as it approaches its insertion on the lateral side of the base of the styloid process of the radius.

Figure 8.1.13

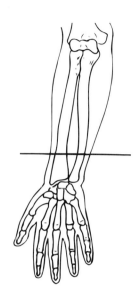

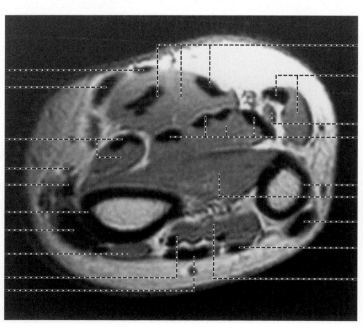

Palmaris longus tendon
Flexor carpi radialis tendon

Flexor pollicis longus m. and tendon

Radial a.
Brachioradialis tendon

Radius
Extensor carpi radialis longus and brevis tendons
Abductor pollicis longus m. and tendon
Extensor pollicis brevis tendon
Extensor digitorum tendons and extensor digiti quinti tendon

Flexor digitorum superficialis m. and tendon
Flexor carpi ulnaris m. and tendon

Ulnar n. and a.
Flexor digitorum profundus m. and tendons

Ulna
Pronator quadratus m.

Extensor carpi ulnaris tendon

Extensor indicis tendon

Extensor pollicis longus m.

Figure 8.3.1

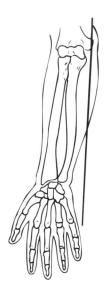

1. This is the most medial sagittal section of the forearm. It passes through the medial epicondyle.

2. Posterior to the medial epicondyle passes the ulnar nerve, which enters the forearm between the two heads of the flexor carpi ulnaris.

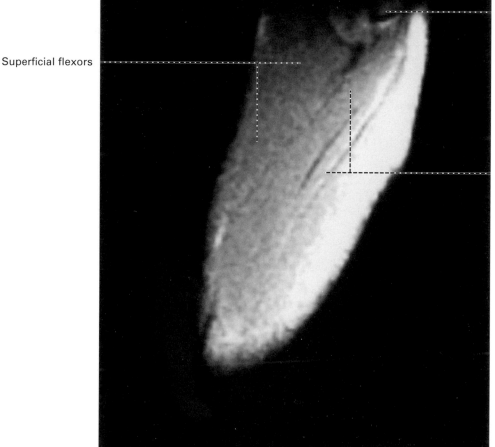

Medial epicondyle

Superficial flexors

Flexor carpi ulnaris and flexor digitorum profundus mm.

1. This section passes through the medial aspect of the trochlea and trochlear notch.

2. The ulnar nerve travels distally between the flexor carpi ulnaris and flexor digitorum profundus muscles.

3. In the forearm, the ulnar nerve supplies the flexor carpi ulnaris and the medial half of the flexor digitorum profundus muscles.

Figure 8.3.2

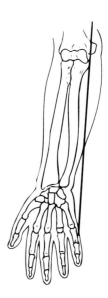

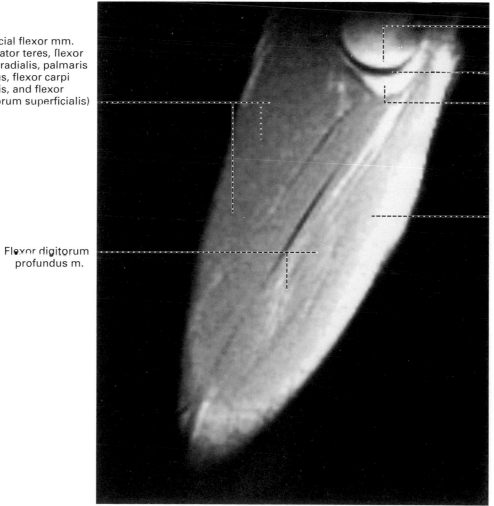

Superficial flexor mm. (pronator teres, flexor carpi radialis, palmaris longus, flexor carpi ulnaris, and flexor digitorum superficialis)

Flexor digitorum profundus m.

Trochlea

Trochlear notch

Coronoid process

Flexor carpi ulnaris m.

Chapter 9

WRIST

1. This section is through pronator quadratus muscle proximal to the radio-carpal joint.

2. Note the origin of pronator quadratus from the anterior surface of the distal ulna. It runs transversely and inserts onto the anterior surface of the radius.

3. Four individual tendons of the flexor digitorum profundus are demonstrated on this section. The flexor digitorum superficialis tendons are not yet completely divided.

4. The brachioradialis tendon is depicted in this section prior to its insertion onto the base of the radial styloid process.

Figure 9.1.1

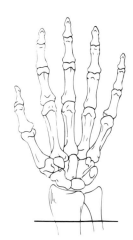

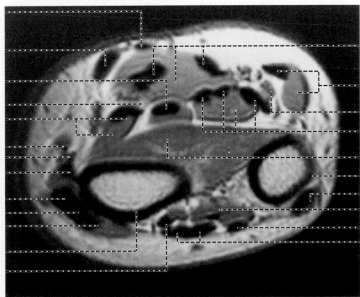

Palmaris longus tendon

Flexor carpi radialis tendon

Flexor digitorum profundus indicis tendon (II)

Median n.

Flexor pollicis longus m. and tendon

Radial a.

Brachioradialis tendon

Abductor pollicis longus

Extensor pollicis brevis tendon

Extensor carpi radialis longus

Extensor carpi radialis brevis tendon

Radius

Extensor pollicis longus tendon

Flexor digitorum superficialis m. and tendon

Flexor carpi ulnaris m. and tendon

Ulnar a., n.

Flexor digitorum profundus m. and tendon

Pronator quadratus m.

Ulna

Extensor carpi ulnaris tendon

Extensor indicis tendon

Extensor digiti minimi tendon

Extensor digitorum tendons

Figure 9.1.2

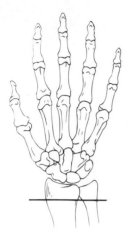

1. Note the extensor carpi ulnaris coursing distally within the ulnar groove.

2. The extensor pollicis longus tendon has exited from beneath the tendons of extensor digitorum.

3. The tendon of palmaris longus flattens before it crosses the wrist superficial to the flexor retinaculum. It proceeds distally to become the palmar aponeurosis.

4. Note the superficial position of the radial artery, where it can be easily palpated.

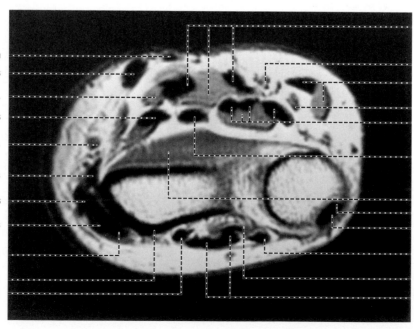

Palmaris longus tendon

Flexor carpi radialis tendon

Median n.

Flexor pollicis longus tendon

Radial a.

Abductor pollicis longus tendon

Extensor pollicis brevis tendon

Extensor carpi radialis longus tendon

Extensor carpi radialis brevis tendon

Radius

Extensor pollicis longus tendon

Flexor digitorum superficialis m. and tendons

Ulnar a., n.

Flexor carpi ulnaris m. and tendon

Ulnar a., n.

Flexor digitorum profundus m. and tendons (III, IV, V)

Flexor digitorum profundus indicis tendon (II)

Pronator quadratus m.

Ulna and ulnar groove

Extensor carpi ulnaris tendon

Extensor digiti minimi tendon

Extensor indicis tendon

Extensor digitorum tendons

1. This section is through the distal radioulnar joint. It is separated from the radiocarpal joint by the triangular fibrocartilage.

2. Note the groove on the dorsal surface of the distal ulna that houses the extensor carpi ulnaris tendon.

3. The extensor carpi ulnaris tendon continues distally to insert onto the base of the fifth metacarpal.

4. The brachioradialis muscle is completing its insertion onto the base of the radial styloid process.

Figure 9.1.3

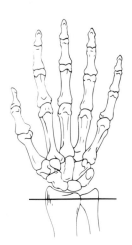

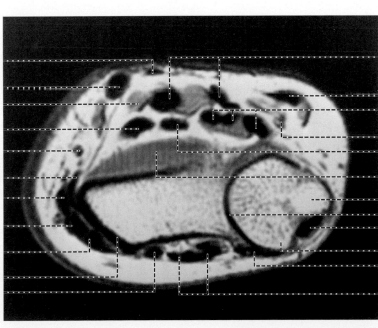

Palmaris longus tendon	Flexor digitorum superficialis tendons
Flexor carpi radialis tendon	Flexor carpi ulnaris tendon
Median n.	Flexor digitorum profundus tendons (III, IV, V)
Flexor pollicis longus tendon	Ulnar a., n.
Radial a.	Flexor digitorum profundus indicis tendon (II)
Brachioradialis tendon	Pronator quadratus m.
Abductor pollicis longus tendon	Ulna, styloid process
Extensor carpi radialis longus tendon	Distal radioulnar joint
Extensor carpi radialis brevis tendon	Extensor carpi ulnaris tendon
Radius	Ulna
Extensor pollicis longus tendon	Extensor digiti minimi tendon
	Extensor digitorum tendons

Figure 9.1.4

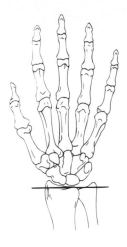

1. This section is through the dorsal radial tubercle (Lister's tubercle) at the level of the triangular fibrocartilage.

2. In the wrist, the radial artery can be found lateral to the tendon of the flexor carpi radialis.

3. The ulnar artery and nerve reach the wrist together and are covered partially by the tendon of flexor carpi ulnaris.

4. The median nerve crosses the wrist by passing through the carpal tunnel, whereas the ulnar nerve crosses the wrist superficial to the flexor retinaculum.

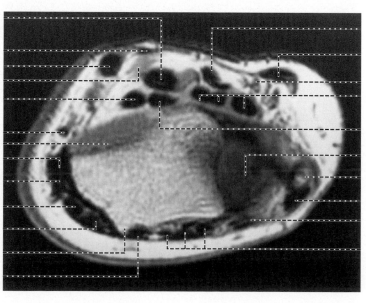

Flexor digitorum superficialis tendons (II, III)
Palmaris longus tendon
Flexor carpi radialis tendon
Median n.
Flexor pollicis longus tendon

Radial a.
Pronator quadratus m.
Abductor pollicis longus tendon
Extensor pollicis brevis tendon
Extensor carpi radialis longus tendon
Extensor carpi radialis brevis tendon
Dorsal radial tubercle (Lister's tubercle)
Extensor pollicis longus tendon

Flexor digitorum superficialis tendons (IV, V)
Flexor carpi ulnaris tendon

Ulnar a., n.
Flexor digitorum profundus tendons (III, IV, V)

Flexor digitorum profundus indicis tendon (II)

Triangular fibrocartilage

Ulnar styloid process

Extensor carpi ulnaris tendon

Extensor digiti minimi tendon

Extensor digitorum and extensor indicis tendons

1. This section is through the radiocarpal joint and proximal to the carpal tunnel.

2. The extensor retinaculum is identified in this section; it is seen anchoring the extensor tendons to bone.

3. Note that the lunate articulates with the radius and triangular fibrocartilage. The triquetrum articulates with the triangular fibrocartilage only when the hand is adducted.

4. Beyond the extensor retinaculum the flexor pollicis longus starts its lateral course in order to reach the thumb.

Figure 9.1.5

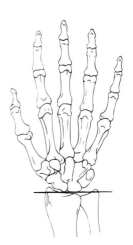

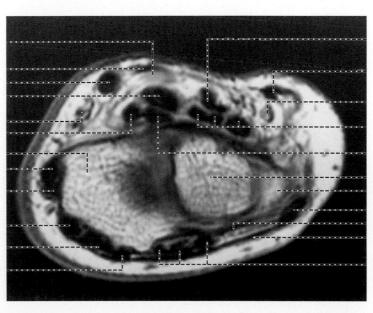

Median n

Palmaris longus tendon
Flexor carpi radialis tendon
Flexor digitorum superficialis
tendons (II, III)
Radial a.
Flexor pollicis longus tendon

Radius
Abductor pollicis longus
tendon
Extensor pollicis brevis
tendon

Extensor carpi radialis longus
tendon
Extensor carpi radialis brevis
tendon
Extensor pollicis longus
tendon

Flexor digitorum superficialis
tendons (IV, V)

Flexor carpi ulnaris tendon

Ulnar a., n.

Flexor digitorum profundus
tendons (III, IV, V)
Flexor digitorum profundus
indicis tendon (II)
Lunate
Triquetrum

Extensor carpi ulnaris tendon
Extensor digiti minimi tendon
Extensor retinaculum

Extensor digitorum and
extensor indicis tendons

Figure 9.1.6

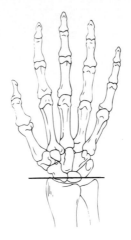

1. This section is through the bones of the proximal carpal row just proximal to the region of the carpal tunnel.

2. Note that the flexor carpi ulnaris tendon is completing its insertion on the pisiform.

3. The palmaris longus tendon continues to flatten prior to becoming the palmar aponeurosis.

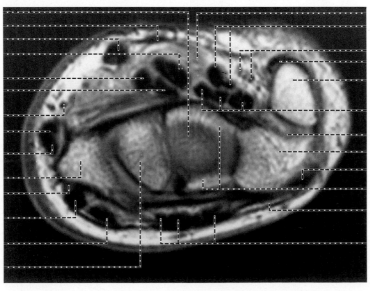

Concavity of lunate
Palmaris longus tendon
Flexor carpi radialis tendon
Flexor digitorum superficialis tendons (II, III)
Flexor pollicis longus tendon
Flexor digitorum profundus indicis tendon (II)
Radial a.
Abductor pollicis longus tendon
Extensor pollicis brevis tendon
Radial styloid process
Extensor carpi radialis longus tendon
Extensor carpi radialis brevis tendon
Extensor pollicis longus tendon
Scaphoid, proximal pole

Median n.
Flexor digitorum superficialis tendons (IV, V)
Ulnar a., n.
Flexor carpi ulnaris tendon
Pisiform
Flexor digitorum profundus tendons (III, IV, V)
Pisotriquetral joint
Triquetrum
Extensor carpi ulnaris tendon
Lunate, distal portion
Extensor retinaculum
Extensor digitorum and extensor indicis tendons

1. This section is through the proximal portion of the carpal tunnel.

2. The proximal portion of the carpal tunnel is bounded medially by the pisiform and laterally by the tuberosity of the scaphoid.

3. Note the position of the median nerve just beneath the flexor retinaculum.

4. The flexor carpi radialis tendon courses distally immediately volar to the tuberosity of the scaphoid.

5. The extensor pollicis longus shifts its course laterally prior to crossing over the extensor carpi radialis longus and brevis tendons.

6. Note the origin of the abductor digiti minimi from the pisiform.

Figure 9.1.7

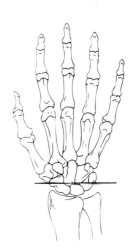

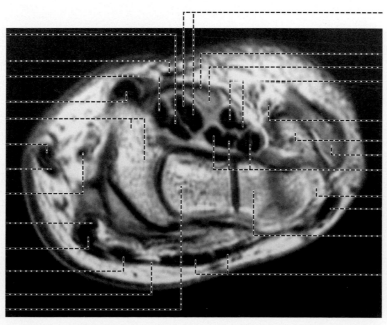

Flexor digitorum profundus indicis tendon (II)
Palmaris longus tendon
Flexor pollicis longus tendon
Flexor carpi radialis tendon
Scaphoid and scaphoid tuberosity
Abductor pollicis longus tendon
Extensor pollicis brevis tendon
Radial a.
Extensor carpi radialis longus tendon
Extensor carpi radialis brevis tendon
Extensor pollicis longus tendon
Extensor retinaculum
Capitate

Flexor digitorum superficialis tendons (II, III)
Flexor retinaculum
Median n.
Flexor digitorum superficialis tendons (IV, V)
Ulnar a., n.
Pisiform
Abductor digiti minimi m.
Flexor digitorum profundus tendons (III, IV, V)
Triquetrum
Extensor carpi ulnaris tendon
Hamate
Extensor digitorum and extensor indicis tendons

Figure 9.1.8

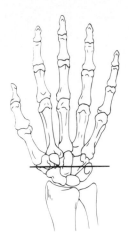

1. This section is partly through the bones of the distal carpal row.

2. The flexor retinaculum and median nerve beneath it are clearly depicted in this section.

3. Note the position of the palmaris longus tendon, which is superficial to the flexor retinaculum.

4. In this section, the extensor pollicis longus tendon is seen crossing over the extensor carpi radialis longus and brevis tendons.

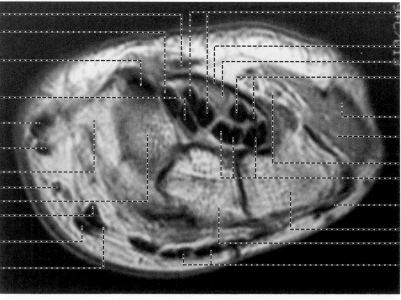

Palmaris longus tendon
Flexor pollicis longus tendon
Flexor carpi radialis tendon
Flexor digitorum profundus indicis tendon (II)
Abductor pollicis longus tendon
Extensor pollicis brevis tendon
Trapezium
Radial a.
Scaphoid tuberosity
Extensor carpi radialis longus tendon
Extensor pollicis longus tendon
Extensor carpi radialis brevis tendon

Flexor digitorum superficialis tendons (II, III)
Flexor retinaculum
Median n.
Flexor digitorum superficialis tendons (IV, V)
Abductor digiti minimi m.
Opponens digiti minimi m.
Ulnar a., n.
Flexor digitorum profundus tendons
Extensor carpi ulnaris tendon
Hamate
Capitate
Extensor digitorum and extensor indicis tendons

1. This section is through the distal carpal row and distal portion of the carpal tunnel.

2. Two bones form the boundaries on each side of the carpal tunnel. These are the pisiform and hamulus of the hamate on the medial side and scaphoid tuberosity and tubercle of the trapezium on the lateral side.

3. Note the origin of the abductor pollicis longus tendon from the flexor retinaculum.

4. Note that the flexor carpi radialis is not included in the content of the carpal tunnel.

Figure 9.1.9

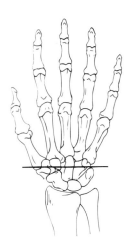

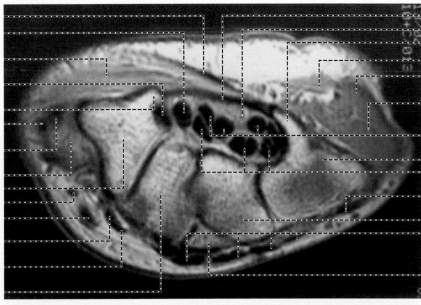

Palmar aponeurosis
Flexor pollicis longus tendon
Abductor pollicis brevis m.
Flexor carpi radialis tendon
Tubercle of trapezium
Extensor pollicis brevis tendon
Abductor pollicis brevis tendon
First metacarpal, base
Trapezium
Radial a.
Extensor pollicis longus tendon
Extensor carpi radialis longus tendon
Extensor carpi radialis brevis tendon
Trapezoid

Flexor retinaculum
Median n.
Hook of hamate
Palmaris brevis m.
Abductor digiti minimi m.
Opponens digiti minimi m.
Flexor digitorum superficialis tendons
Hamate
Flexor digitorum profundus tendons
Extensor carpi ulnaris tendon
Capitate
Extensor digitorum and extensor indicis tendons
Third metacarpal, styloid process

Figure 9.1.10

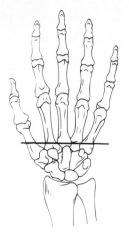

1. The extensor carpi radialis longus and brevis have completed their insertion onto the bases of the second and third metacarpals, respectively.

2. Extensor carpi ulnaris has completed its insertion onto the base of the fifth metacarpal.

3. Flexor carpi radialis has completed its insertion onto the base of the second metacarpal on its volar side.

4. The opponens pollicis and opponens digiti minimi muscles originate from the surface of the flexor retinaculum.

Abductor pollicis brevis m.
Opponens pollicis m.
Flexor retinaculum
Flexor pollicis longus tendon
Base of first metacarpal
Extensor pollicis brevis tendon
Flexor digitorum profundus tendons
Extensor pollicis longus tendon
Second metacarpal, base
Third metacarpal, base

Palmar aponeurosis
Opponens digiti minimi m.
Palmaris brevis m.
Abductor digiti minimi m.
Flexor digitorum superficialis tendons
Median n.
Fifth metacarpal, base
Fourth metacarpal, base
Extensor digitorum and extensor indicis tendons

1. This section is through the dorsum of the wrist. Some of the extensor tendons are demonstrated, as well as the base of the third metacarpal and its styloid process. All these are palpable structures on the dorsum of the wrist.

2. Note the lateral course of the extensor pollicis longus in the direction of the thumb. It takes this course just distal to the radial tubercle (Lister's tubercle).

3. Extensor digiti minimi can be seen just lateral to the head of the ulna. It crosses the wrist posterior to the distal radioulnar joint.

4. Note the extensor carpi radialis brevis as it courses distally to insert on the base of the third metacarpal.

Figure 9.2.1

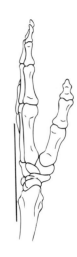

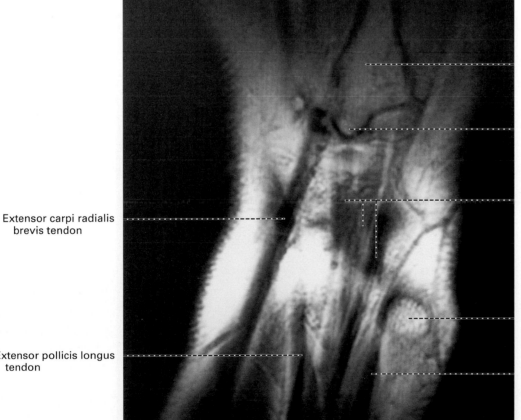

Third metacarpal, base

Third metacarpal, styloid process

Extensor digitorum tendons

Ulnar head

Third metacarpal, base

Extensor carpi radialis brevis tendon

Extensor pollicis longus tendon

Figure 9.2.2

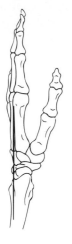

1. The extensor carpi ulnaris is seen in the ulnar groove at the head of the ulna.

2. The extensor carpi radialis longus is seen inserting onto the base of the second metacarpal.

3. The extensor pollicis longus tendon continues its course in the direction of the thumb and the extensor digiti minimi also continues its course toward the little finger.

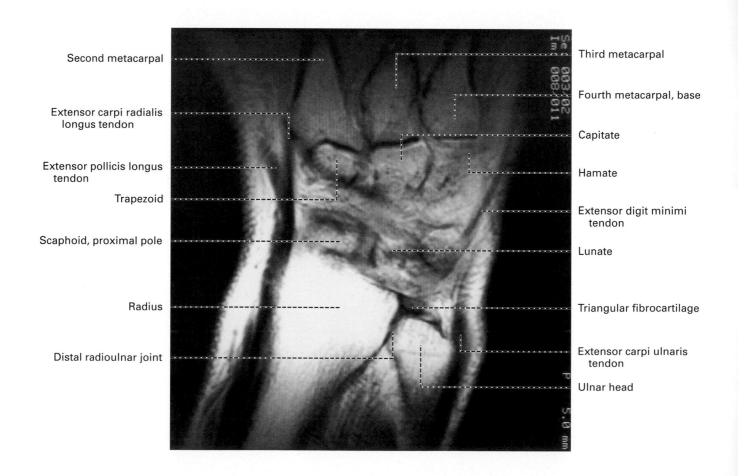

Second metacarpal

Extensor carpi radialis longus tendon

Extensor pollicis longus tendon

Trapezoid

Scaphoid, proximal pole

Radius

Distal radioulnar joint

Third metacarpal

Fourth metacarpal, base

Capitate

Hamate

Extensor digit minimi tendon

Lunate

Triangular fibrocartilage

Extensor carpi ulnaris tendon

Ulnar head

1. This section is through the posterior aspect of the carpal bones. There are no muscle or tendinous insertions on the dorsum of the carpus.

2. The extensor carpi ulnaris continues its course on the posteromedial aspect of the wrist toward its insertion on the base of the fifth metacarpal.

3. The extensor pollicis longus tendon can be seen coursing laterally toward the thumb.

4. The triangular fibrocartilage can be seen in this section. It extends between the medial aspect of the distal radius and styloid process of the ulna.

Figure 9.2.3

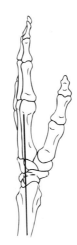

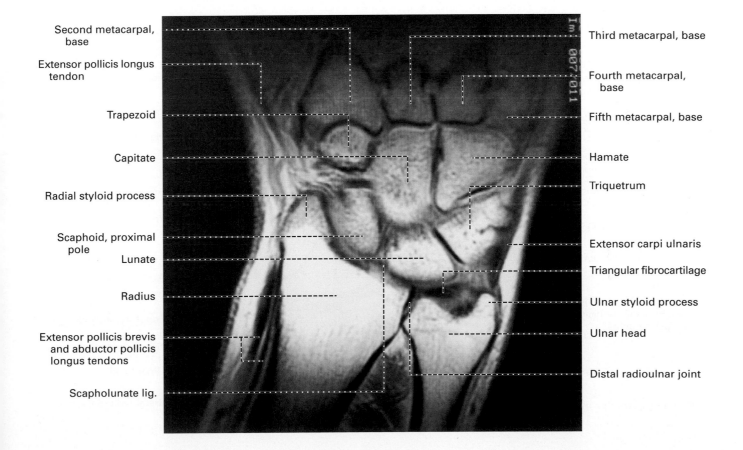

Second metacarpal, base

Extensor pollicis longus tendon

Trapezoid

Capitate

Radial styloid process

Scaphoid, proximal pole

Lunate

Radius

Extensor pollicis brevis and abductor pollicis longus tendons

Scapholunate lig.

Third metacarpal, base

Fourth metacarpal, base

Fifth metacarpal, base

Hamate

Triquetrum

Extensor carpi ulnaris

Triangular fibrocartilage

Ulnar styloid process

Ulnar head

Distal radioulnar joint

Figure 9.2.4

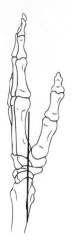

1. This section is through the distal radioulnar joint and triangular fibrocartilage.

2. Note the extensor carpi ulnaris tendon inserting at the base of the fifth metacarpal.

3. The extensor pollicis brevis and abductor pollicis longus tendons cross the lateral aspect of the wrist.

4. The pronator quadratus is seen in this section. It originates from the anterior surface of the distal one-fourth of the ulna and runs transversely to insert on the anterior surface of the radius.

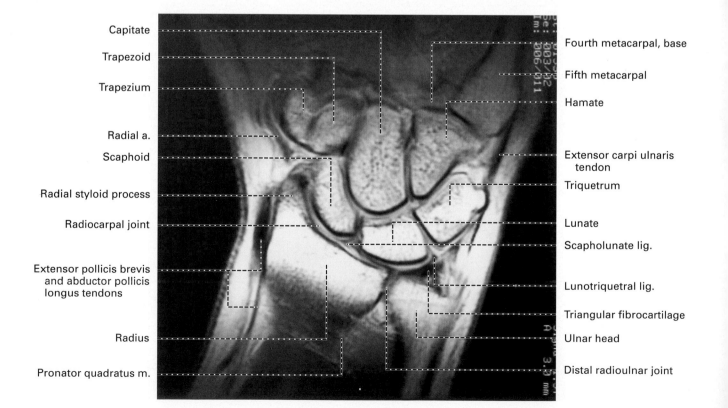

Capitate

Trapezoid

Trapezium

Radial a.

Scaphoid

Radial styloid process

Radiocarpal joint

Extensor pollicis brevis and abductor pollicis longus tendons

Radius

Pronator quadratus m.

Fourth metacarpal, base

Fifth metacarpal

Hamate

Extensor carpi ulnaris tendon

Triquetrum

Lunate

Scapholunate lig.

Lunotriquetral lig.

Triangular fibrocartilage

Ulnar head

Distal radioulnar joint

1. This section is through the floor of the carpal tunnel. It shows the triangular fibrocartilage.

2. The oblique head of the adductor pollicis muscle takes its origin mainly from the distal pole of the capitate.

3. The abductor digiti minimi muscle takes its origin from the pisiform.

4. The flexor pollicis brevis tendon is seen running adjacent to the first metacarpal toward its insertion on the proximal phalanx of the thumb.

5. Note the radial artery coursing through the snuff box between the navicular bone and the abductor pollicis longus tendon. The radial artery crosses from the volar aspect to the dorsal aspect of the wrist.

Figure 9.2.5

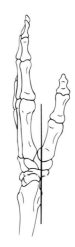

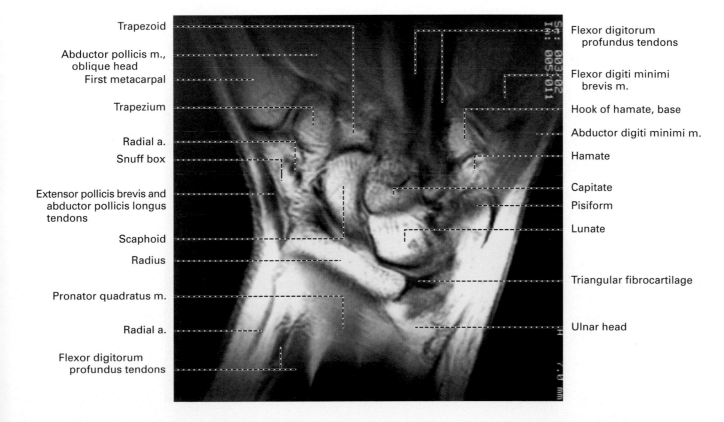

Trapezoid

Abductor pollicis m., oblique head
First metacarpal

Trapezium

Radial a.
Snuff box

Extensor pollicis brevis and abductor pollicis longus tendons

Scaphoid

Radius

Pronator quadratus m.

Radial a.

Flexor digitorum profundus tendons

Flexor digitorum profundus tendons

Flexor digiti minimi brevis m.

Hook of hamate, base

Abductor digiti minimi m.

Hamate

Capitate
Pisiform

Lunate

Triangular fibrocartilage

Ulnar head

Figure 9.2.6

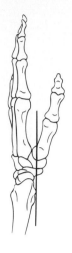

1. This section is through the carpal tunnel. It is bounded laterally by the scaphoid tuberosity and tubercle of the trapezium and medially by the pisiform bone and hook of the hamate.

2. Note the abductor pollicis longus as it inserts onto the base of the first metacarpal.

3. The flexor carpi ulnaris is seen in this section approaching its insertion on the pisiform bone.

4. Note the radial artery in the lateral aspect of the volar wrist before it enters the anatomic snuff box.

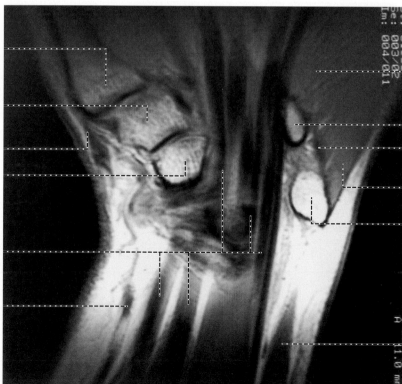

First metacarpal, base

Trapezium

Abductor pollicis longus tendon

Scaphoid tuberosity

Flexor digitorum profundus and superficialis tendons

Radial a.

Flexor carpi ulnaris tendon

Hook of hamate

Abductor digiti minimi m.

Pisohamate lig.

Pisiform

Flexor carpi ulnaris tendon

1. The carpal tunnel contains four flexor digitorum profundus tendons, four flexor digitorum superficialis tendons, the flexor pollicis longus tendon, and the median nerve.

2. The ulnar nerve and artery course along the lateral side of flexor carpi ulnaris. They enter the wrist region superficial to flexor retinaculum.

3. The flexor pollicis longus is seen taking a lateral course toward its insertion on the base of the distal phalanx of the thumb.

4. In this section, the flexor carpi ulnaris tendon is seen inserting on the pisiform.

Figure 9.2.7

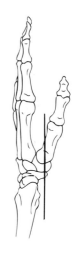

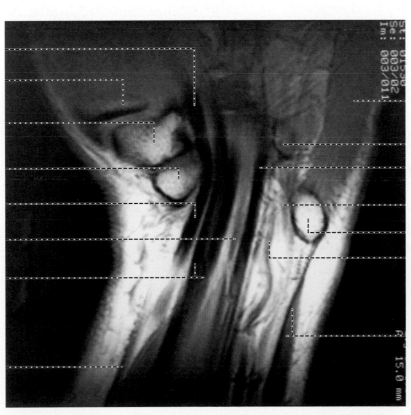

Flexor pollicis longus tendon

First metacarpal, base

Trapezium

Scaphoid tuberosity

Flexor pollicis longus tendon

Median n.

Flexor digitorum superficialis tendons

Flexor carpi radialis tendon

Abductor digiti minimus m.

Hook of hamate

Flexor digitorum superficialis tendon

Ulnar n.

Pisiform

Ulnar a.

Flexor carpi ulnaris tendon

Figure 9.2.8

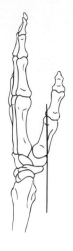

1. On the volar aspect of the wrist, the two most superficial tendons are those of palmaris longus and flexor carpi radialis.

2. The palmaris longus crosses the wrist superficial to the flexor retinaculum. Its tendon continues into the palm to become the palmar aponeurosis.

3. The flexor carpi radialis tendon crosses the wrist just volar to the scaphoid tuberosity and inserts onto the base of the second metacarpal.

4. The opponens pollicis is depicted in this section taking its origin from the flexor retinaculum and inserting on the shaft of the first metacarpal anteriorly.

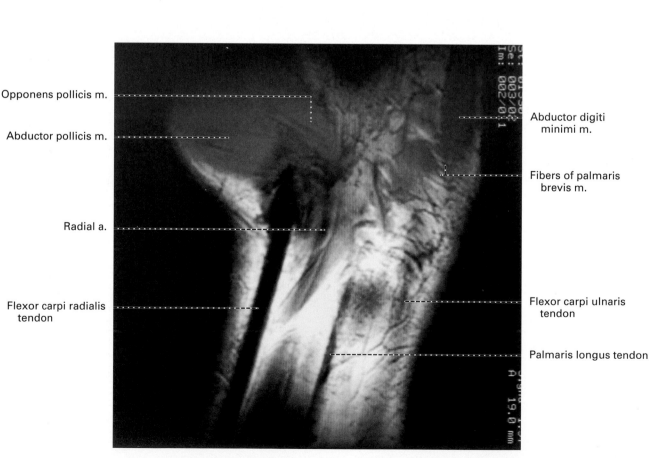

Figure 9.3.1

1. This section is through the medial aspect of the wrist. Included in this section is the pisiform bone, which is essentially a sesamoid bone.

2. Note the origin of the abductor digiti minimi from the pisiform. It courses distally to insert on the base of the proximal phalanx of the little finger.

3. The extensor carpi ulnaris tendon is seen in this section completing its insertion on the base of the fifth metacarpal.

4. The transversely arranged fibers of the palmaris brevis muscle are seen in this section. The muscle originates from the palmar aponeurosis and inserts into the skin on the ulnar border of the hand.

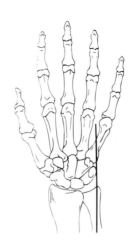

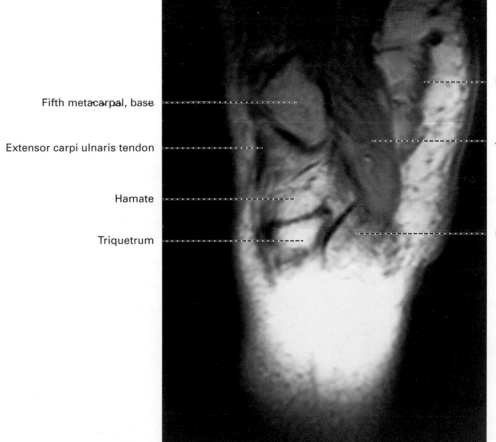

Fifth metacarpal, base

Extensor carpi ulnaris tendon

Hamate

Triquetrum

Palmaris brevis m.

Abductor digiti minimi m.

Pisiform

Figure 9.3.2

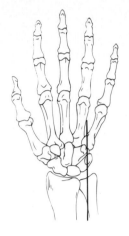

1. The medial boundary of the carpal tunnel is depicted in this section. It is formed by the pisiform bone and the hook of the hamate.

2. The tendon of extensor carpi ulnaris is seen traversing the ulnar groove on the posterior surface of the ulnar head.

3. Flexor carpi ulnaris tendon is noted inserting onto the pisiform.

4. The palmaris brevis muscle is seen as a thin muscle in the deep fascia of the palm superficial to the hypothenar muscles.

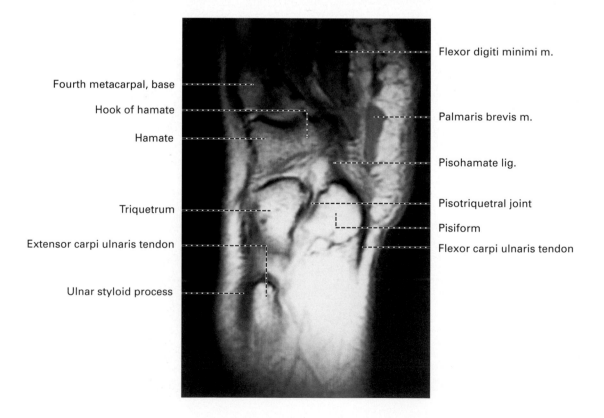

Fourth metacarpal, base

Hook of hamate

Hamate

Triquetrum

Extensor carpi ulnaris tendon

Ulnar styloid process

Flexor digiti minimi m.

Palmaris brevis m.

Pisohamate lig.

Pisotriquetral joint

Pisiform

Flexor carpi ulnaris tendon

1. This section is through the medial aspect of the carpal tunnel. The flexor digitorum profundus and superficialis tendons for the fifth digit are seen coursing distally.

2. The flexor carpi ulnaris tendon is seen prior to its insertion on the pisiform.

3. The triangular fibrocartilage, which extends between the medial aspect of the distal radius and the styloid process of the ulna, is depicted in this section.

4. Palmaris brevis is again depicted in this section. This muscle is innervated by the ulnar nerve.

Figure 9.3.3

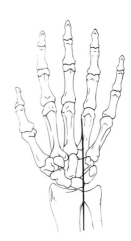

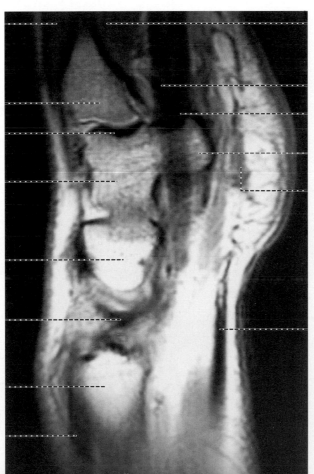

Third dorsal interosseus m.

Fourth metacarpal, base

Fourth carpometacarpal joint

Hamate

Triquetrum

Triangular fibrocartilage

Ulnar head

Extensor carpi ulnaris tendon

Third palmar interosseus m.

Flexor digitorum profundus tendon of the fifth digit

Flexor digitorum superficialis tendon of the fifth digit

Hook of hamate

Palmaris brevis m.

Flexor carpi ulnaris tendon

Figure 9.3.4

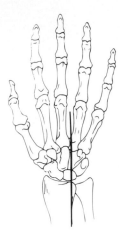

1. Note that the lunate articulates with both the radius and the triangular fibrocartilage proximally.

2. The triquetrum comes in contact with the triangular fibrocartilage when the wrist is in extreme adduction.

3. Note that the extensor tendon, depicted in this section posterior to the capitate and third metacarpal, is thinner than the flexor tendons.

4. The ulnar artery is seen superficial to the flexor tendon (and just beneath the palmaris brevis) where it enters the palm to form the superficial palmar arch.

5. Note the extensor digiti minimi tendon. In the wrist, it courses just lateral to the extensor carpi ulnaris tendon.

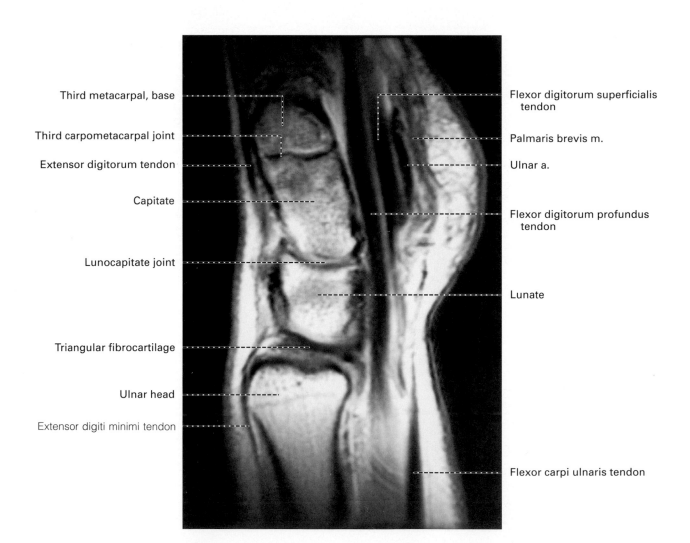

Third metacarpal, base	Flexor digitorum superficialis tendon
Third carpometacarpal joint	Palmaris brevis m.
Extensor digitorum tendon	Ulnar a.
Capitate	Flexor digitorum profundus tendon
Lunocapitate joint	Lunate
Triangular fibrocartilage	
Ulnar head	
Extensor digiti minimi tendon	Flexor carpi ulnaris tendon

1. This section is through the lateral portion of the triangular fibrocartilage before it attaches to the medial aspect of the distal radius.

2. The lunocapitate joint and capitate-third metacarpal joint are clearly depicted in this section. The capitate-third metacarpal joint is flat and barely allows any motion. The second carpometacarpal joint (shown in previous sections) also has very limited motion.

3. Note the well-developed flexor retinaculum bridging the carpal tunnel anterior to the flexor tendons.

4. Arterial branches of the deep palmar arch and dorsal carpal arch are depicted in this section.

Figure 9.3.5

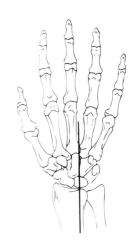

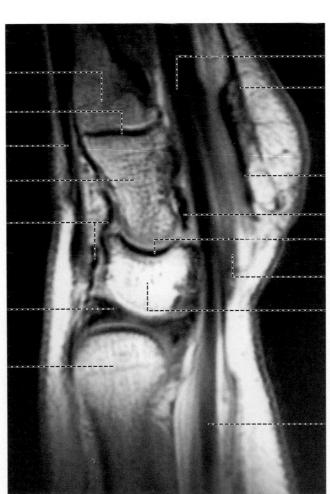

Third metacarpal, base

Third carpometacarpal joint

Extensor digitorum tendon

Capitate

Dorsal carpal arch, arterial branches

Triangular fibrocartilage

Lunate, head

Flexor digitorum profundus tendon

Palmar aponeurosis

Flexor retinaculum

Arterial palmar carpal branch

Lunocapitate joint

Flexor digitorum superficialis tendon

Lunate

Flexor digitorum profundus tendon

Musculature of the Hand

The intrinsic muscles of the hand are the subcutaneous muscle of the palm, muscles of the thumb, muscles of the little finger, lumbrical muscles, and interosseous muscles. Their origins and insertions are considered in the following table.

The median nerve supplies most of the muscles of the thenar region (thumb) and the lateral lumbrical muscles; the ulnar nerve supplies the muscles of the hypothenar region, interosseous muscles, medial lumbrical muscles, and two of the muscles of the thumb. No muscle bellies normally are found on the dorsum of the hand.

The movements of the hand are described in a different sense than is usual elsewhere. In regard to the four medial fingers (second to fifth), however, the terms *flexion* and *extension* are used in the usual sense. *Abduction* and *adduction* do not refer to the median plane of the body but rather to the axial line of the hand. The axial line runs through the middle digit, and abduction is movement away from this line. The first finger moves laterally or away from the middle finger, and the fourth and fifth fingers move medially or away from the middle finger. Adduction brings all the four fingers together or toward the middle finger. The thumb (or first digit) is placed at right angles to the palm and fingers. Flexion and extension of the thumb are movements in a plane parallel with the palm. Abduction is a forward movement, and adduction is a backward movement, at right angles to the palm. The thumb can rotate at the saddle-shaped carpometacarpal joint.

Table 10-1. Hand

Muscle	Origin	Insertion	Nerve Supply	Arterial Supply
Palmaris brevis	Ulnar border of palmar aponeurosis	Deep surface of the skin along the ulnar border of the palm	Ulnar n., superficial branch (C8, T1)	Ulnar, superficial branch
Abductor pollicis brevis	Palmar surface of flexor retinaculum, trapezium, and occasionally scaphoid	Radial side of base of proximal phalanx of the thumb	Recurrent branch of median n. (C8, T1)	Radial, superficial palmar branch
Opponens pollicis	Palmar surface of flexor retinaculum and tubercle of trapezium	Lateral part of palmar surface of the shaft of first metacarpal	Recurrent branch of median n. (C8, T1)	Radial, superficial palmar branch
Flexor pollicis brevis	Superficial head: trapezium, adjacent part of flexor retinaculum, and tendon sheath of flexor carpi radialis; deep head: trapezoid and capitate bones	Superficial head: lateral side of front of the base of the proximal phalanx; deep head: into a tendon of the superficial head	Recurrent branch of median n. and deep branch of the ulnar n. (C8, T1)	Radial, superficial palmar branch
Adductor pollicis brevis	Carpal head: flexor retinaculum, capitate, bases of second and third metacarpal; metacarpal head: palmar ridges of third metacarpal and capsules of the second, third, and fourth metacarpophalangeal articulations	Ulnar side of the front of the base of the proximal phalanx of the thumb	Recurrent branch of median n. (C8, T1)	Radial, superficial palmar branch
Abductor digiti minimi	Distal half of pisiform, pisihamate ligament, tendon of flexor carpi ulnaris, and frequently the flexor retinaculum	Two tendons: (1) ulnar side of base of the proximal phalanx of little finger and (2) aponeurosis of the extensor tendon of the little finger	Ulnar n., deep palmar division (C8, T1)	Ulnar, deep branch
Flexor digiti minimi brevis	Hook of the hamate and adjacent parts of flexor retinaculum	Ulnar side of the base of the proximal phalanx of the little finger	Ulnar n., superficial or deep palmar branch (C8, T1)	Ulnar, deep branch
Opponens digiti minimi	Distal border of hook of the hamate and adjacent flexor retinaculum	Medial surface of body and particularly onto the head of the fifth metacarpal	Ulnar n., deep palmar branch (C8, T1)	Ulnar, deep branch
Lumbrical	The two lateral lumbricals: radial and palmar sides of the first and second tendons of flexor digitorum profundus; the two medial lumbricals: adjacent side of the second and third tendons and the third and fourth tendons of flexor digitorum profundus	Into the radial border of the tendon of extensor digitorum on the back of the proximal phalanx	Median n., lateral two or three lumbricals; ulnar, deep palmar branch, medial one or two lumbricals (C8, T1)	Common digital arteries of superficial palmar arch
Interosseous	Palmar interosseous: anterior border of the shaft of the first, second, fourth, and fifth metacarpals. The first arises near the base and others arise from three-fourths of the shaft of the bone. Dorsal interosseous: adjacent sides of metacarpal bones in each metacarpal interspace	Into the expansion on the axial side of the corresponding digit. The first palmar interosseous is described frequently as a division of flexor brevis or adductor pollicis. The first dorsal interosseous usually inserts onto the proximal phalanx. The other three insert into the extensor expansion and proximal phalanx.	Ulnar n., deep palmar branch (C8, T1)	Radial, palmar metacarpal branches; dorsal metacarpal; and dorsal carpal rete

333

Figure 10.1.1

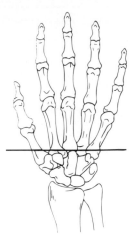

1. This section is through the bases of the metacarpal bones. The proximal ends of the interosseous muscles are depicted in this section.

2. On the volar aspect of the hypothenar muscles, the thin muscle fibers of the palmaris brevis muscle are seen within the superficial fascia.

3. The palmar aponeurosis is well developed in this section; it is a continuation of the palmaris longus muscle tendon.

4. Note that the transverse head of adductor pollicis takes its origin from the volar surface of the third metacarpal. The oblique head originates from the volar surface of the capitate and trapezoid.

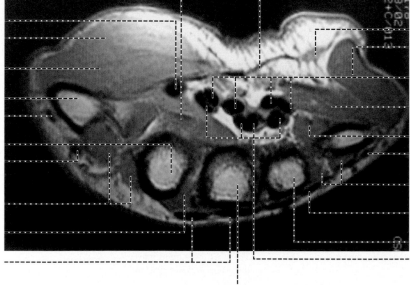

Adductor pollicis m.
Flexor pollicis longus tendon
Abductor and flexor pollicis brevis mm.
Opponens pollicis brevis m.
First metacarpal
Extensor pollicis brevis tendon
Second metacarpal
Extensor pollicis longus tendon
First dorsal interosseous m.
Second dorsal interosseous m.
Extensor digitorum and extensor indicis tendons

Palmar aponeurosis
Palmaris brevis m.
Abductor digiti minimi m.
Flexor digitorum superficialis tendons
Opponens digiti minimi m.
Volar interosseous m.
Tendon, extensor digiti minimi m.
Fourth dorsal interosseous m.
Tendon, extensor digitorum m.
Fourth metacarpal
Flexor digitorum profundus tendons
Third metacarpal

1. Between the palmar aponeurosis and the flexor digitorum superficialis tendons observe the neurovascular elements (not labeled). The arteries are the common palmar digital arteries, which are branches of the superficial palmar arch. The neural elements are common palmar digital nerves, which are branches of the ulnar and median nerves.

2. The superficial palmar arch is usually formed mainly by the ulnar artery and to a lesser extent by the superficial palmar branch of the radial artery. It gives three or four common digital branches, each of which divides into two proper palmar digital arteries. The proper palmar digital arteries supply the fingers.

3. The opponens pollicis muscle inserts on the lateral aspect of the shaft of the first metacarpal.

Figure 10.1.2

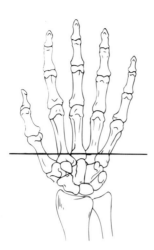

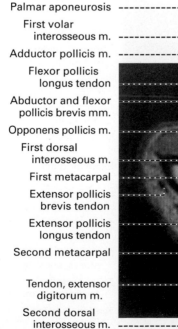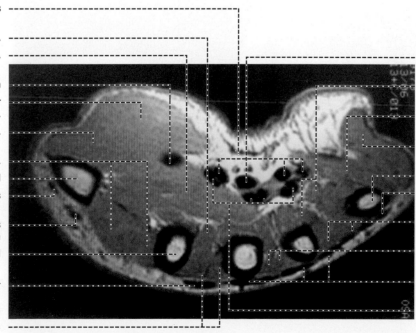

Palmar aponeurosis

First volar interosseous m.

Adductor pollicis m.

Flexor pollicis longus tendon

Abductor and flexor pollicis brevis mm.

Opponens pollicis m.

First dorsal interosseous m.

First metacarpal

Extensor pollicis brevis tendon

Extensor pollicis longus tendon

Second metacarpal

Tendon, extensor digitorum m.

Second dorsal interosseous m.

Flexor digitorum superficialis tendons

Second and third volar interosseous mm.

Opponens digiti minimi m.

Abductor digiti minimi m.

Fifth metacarpal

Tendon, extensor digiti minimi m.

Fourth dorsal interosseous m.

Third dorsal interosseous m.

Tendons, extensor digitorum m.

Flexor digitorum profundus tendons

Figure 10.1.3

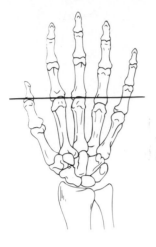

1. All the intrinsic muscles of the hand are depicted in this section.

2. All the thenar muscles (abductor pollicis brevis, flexor pollicis brevis, opponens pollicis) and the lateral two lumbricals are usually innervated by the median nerve.

3. The thenar muscles receive their nerve supply via the recurrent branch of the median nerve, which is quite superficial.

4. All the other intrinsic muscles of the hand are innervated by the ulnar nerve.

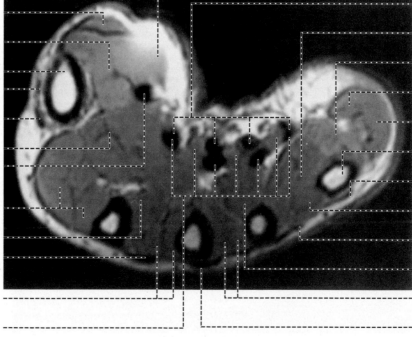

Flexor pollicis brevis m.
Abductor pollicis brevis m.
Opponens pollicis brevis m.
First metacarpal
Extensor pollicis brevis tendon
Extensor pollicis longus tendon
Adductor pollicis m.
Flexor pollicis longus tendon
First dorsal interosseous m.
First volar interosseous m.
Tendon, extensor digitorum m.
Second dorsal interosseous m.
Flexor digitorum profundus tendons and lumbrical mm.

Flexor digitorum superficialis tendons
Third volar interosseous m.
Opponens digiti minimi m.
Flexor digiti minimi brevis m.
Abductor digiti minimi m.
Fifth metacarpal
Extensor digiti minimi tendon
Fourth dorsal interosseous m.
Tendon, extensor digitorum m.
Second volar interosseous m.
Third dorsal interosseous m.
Tendon, extensor digitorum m.

1. Note that the flexor pollicis longus tendon takes an independent course from the other flexor tendons as it proceeds toward the thumb to insert on the base of the proximal phalanx.

2. The interosseous muscles are well developed in this section. There are three volar unipinnate interossei, which function as adductors, and four dorsal bipinnate interossei, which function as abductors. All the interossei are usually innervated by the ulnar nerve.

3. The extensor pollicis brevis and extensor pollicis longus muscles are coursing close together over the dorsum of the first metacarpal.

Figure 10.1.4

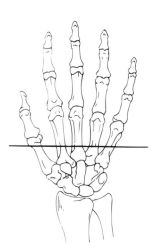

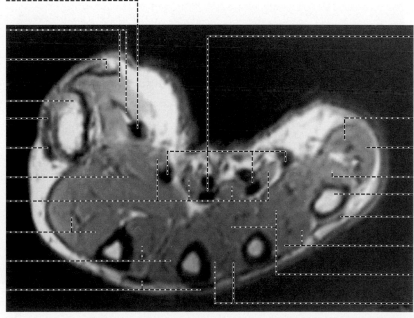

Flexor pollicis longus tendon
Opponens pollicis brevis m. and tendon
Abductor pollicis and flexor pollicis brevis m. and tendon
First metacarpal
Extensor pollicis brevis tendon
Extensor pollicis longus tendon
Adductor pollicis m.
Lumbrical mm.
First dorsal interosseous m.
Second dorsal interosseous m.
Tendons, extensor digitorum and extensor indicis mm.

Flexor digitorum superficialis and profundus tendons
Flexor digiti minimi brevis m.
Abductor digiti minimi brevis m.
Opponens pollicis m.
Fifth metacarpal
Tendon, extensor digiti minimi m.
Fourth dorsal interosseous m.
Third and second volar interosseous m.
Third dorsal interosseous m.

Figure 10.1.5

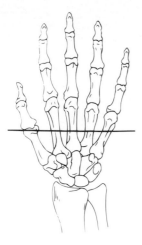

1. This section is through the head of the first metacarpal.

2. The lumbrical muscles are depicted in this section. There are four lumbricals in the hand, which originate from the lateral aspect of the flexor digitorum profundus tendons. They insert on the lateral side of the dorsal expansion of the corresponding digit.

3. The lateral two lumbricals are usually innervated by the median nerve and the medial two lumbricals by the ulnar nerve.

4. The abductor pollicis brevis and flexor pollicis brevis muscles have become tendinous as they approach their insertion on the base of the proximal phalanx of the thumb.

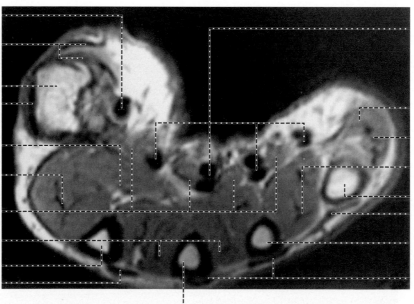

Flexor pollicis longus tendon

Abductor pollicis brevis and flexor pollicis brevis tendons

First metacarpal, head

Extensor pollicis longus and brevis tendon

Adductor pollicis m.

First dorsal interosseous m.

Lumbrical mm.

Second and third interosseous mm.

Second metacarpal

Extensor digitorum and extensor indicis tendons

Third metacarpal

Flexor digitorum superficialis and profundus tendons

Flexor digiti minimi brevis m.

Abductor digiti minimi m.

Fourth dorsal interosseous m.

Fifth metacarpal

Extensor digiti minimi m. tendon

Fourth metacarpal

Extensor digitorum tendons

1. This section is through the first carpometacarpal joint.

2. The flexor digit minimi brevis and abductor digiti minimi muscles have become mostly tendinous prior to their insertion at the base of the proximal phalanx of the little finger.

3. The flexor pollicis longus muscle now lies on the volar surface of the thumb; it will continue in this position until it inserts on the volar surface of the base of the distal phalanx.

4. Note the separate extensor tendons on the dorsum of the hand.

Figure 10.1.6

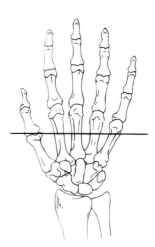

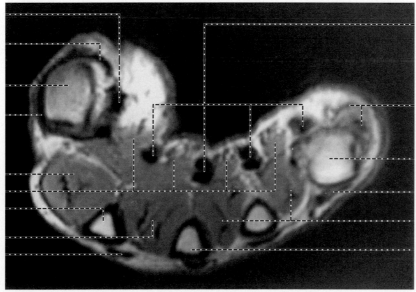

Flexor pollicis longus tendon

Tendon, abductor and opponens pollicis brevis mm.

First carpometacarpal joint

Extensor pollicis longus and brevis tendons

First dorsal interosseous m.

Lumbrical mm.

Second metacarpal

Second dorsal interosseous m.

Extensor digitorum and extensor indicis tendons

Flexor digitorum superficialis and profundus tendons

Tendons of flexor digiti minimi brevis and abductors digiti minimi mm.

Fifth metacarpal, head

Tendon of extensor digiti minimi m.

Third and fourth dorsal interosseous mm.

Third metacarpal

Figure 10.1.7

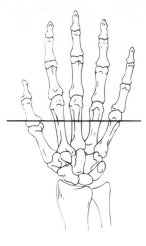

1. The extensor pollicis brevis tendon inserts onto the base of the proximal phalanx of the thumb.

2. The flexor digiti minimi brevis and abductor digit minimi muscles have become completely tendinous close to their insertion on the phalanx of the little finger.

3. The thumb is separating from the rest of the hand; it is functionally the most specialized digit in the hand.

4. The radial artery is the main blood supply to the dorsum of the hand.

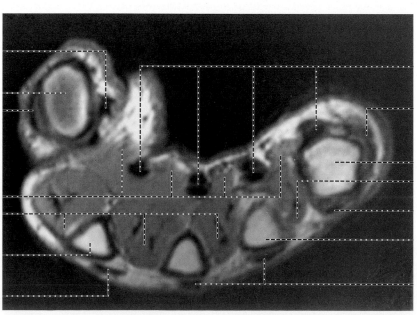

Flexor pollicis longus tendon

Thumb, base of proximal phalanx

Extensor pollicis longus and brevis tendon

Lumbrical mm.

First, second, and third dorsal interosseous mm.

Second metacarpal

Tendons of extensor digitorum and extensor indicis mm.

Flexor digitorum superficialis and profundus tendons

Tendons of flexor digiti minimi brevis and abductor digiti minimi mm.

Fifth metacarpal, head

Fourth dorsal interosseous m.

Tendon of extensor digiti minimi m.

Fourth metacarpal

Third and fourth extensor digitorum tendons

1. As the sections approach the fingers, the intrinsic muscles diminish in size and tendons become prominent.

2. The tendons of flexor digitorum superficialis and those of flexor digitorum profundus travel distally together and are difficult to separate in this section.

3. Note that the lumbrical muscles proceed distally on the radial side of the profundus tendons.

Figure 10.1.8

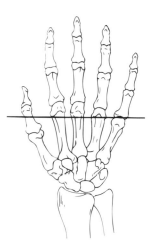

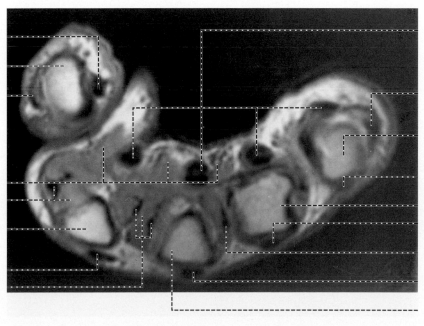

Flexor pollicis longus tendon

Thumb, proximal phalanx

Extensor pollicis longus tendon

Lumbrical mm.

First dorsal interosseous m. and tendon

Second metacarpal

Tendons of extensor digitorum and extensor indicis mm.

Second dorsal interosseous m. and tendon

Flexor digitorum superficialis and profundus tendons

Flexor and abductor digiti minimi brevis tendons

Fifth metacarpophalangeal joint space

Tendon of extensor digiti minimi m.

Fourth metacarpal head

Fourth finger, extensor digitorum tendon

Third dorsal interosseous m.

Third finger, extensor digitorum tendon

Third metacarpal

Figure 10.1.9

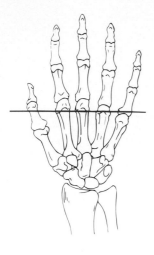

1. This section is through the distal palm.

2. The extensor tendons are flat and small compared with the flexor tendons.

3. At about this level, the hood and extensor expansions form.

4. The lumbricals, interossei, and extensor digitorum tendon of each digit merge to insert on the hood and dorsal expansion of each finger.

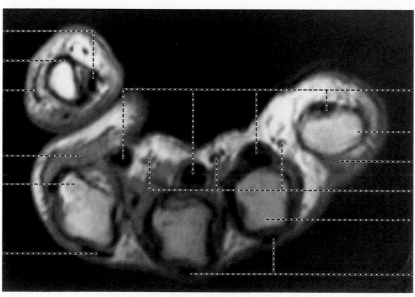

Flexor pollicis longus tendon

Thumb, proximal phalanx

Extensor pollicis longus tendon

First dorsal interosseous m.

Second metacarpal, head

Tendons of extensor digitorum and extensor indicis mm.

Flexor digitorum superficialis and profundus tendons

Fifth finger, base of proximal phalanx

Tendon of extensor digiti minimi m.

Common palmar digital aa., nn.

Fourth metacarpal

Extensor digitorum tendons

1. Note that beyond the metacarpophalangeal joint only tendons are present.

2. Note that the dorsal digital arteries are smaller than the palmar digital arteries.

Figure 10.1.10

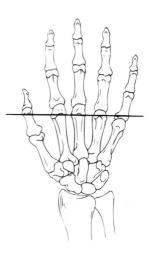

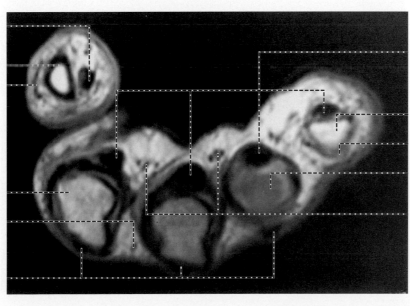

Flexor pollicis longus tendon

Thumb, proximal phalanx

Extensor pollicis longus tendon

Second metacarpal, head

Dorsal digital a.

Extensor digitorum tendons

Flexor digitorum superficialis and profundus tendons

Fifth finger, proximal phalanx

Tendon of extensor digiti minimi m.

Fourth metacarpophalangeal joint space

Common planar digital aa., nn.

Figure 10.1.11

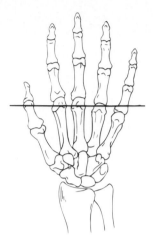

1. The dorsal expansion on the dorsum of the proximal phalanx of the fifth finger is identified.

2. Note the constant location of the common palmar digital arteries.

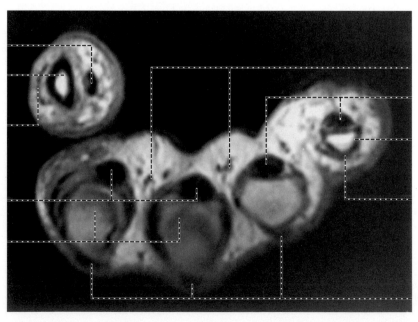

Flexor pollicis longus tendon

Thumb, proximal phalanx

Extensor pollicis longus tendon

Flexor digitorum superficialis and profundus tendons

Second and third fingers, carpometacarpal joints

Common palmar digital aa., nn.

Flexor digitorum superficialis and profundus tendons

Fifth finger, proximal phalanx

Dorsal expansion (hood)

Extensor digitorum tendons

1. This section is through the head of the proximal phalanx of the thumb.

2. The extensor pollicis longus and flexor pollicis longus tendons are flattened prior to their insertion on the base of the distal phalanx.

3. The little finger has separated from the rest of the palm.

Figure 10.1.12

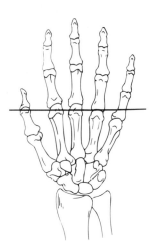

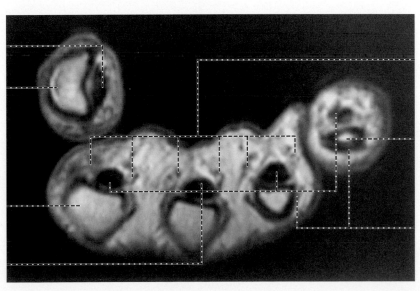

Flexor pollicis longus tendon

Head of proximal phalanx of thumb

Proximal phalanx, index finger

Flexor digitorum superficialis and profundus tendons

Palmar digital aa., nn.

Fifth finger, proximal phalanx

Dorsal expansions (hoods)

Figure 10.1.13

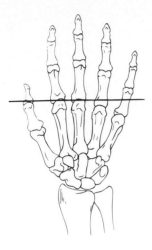

1. On the volar surface of the proximal phalanx of each finger the flexor digitorum superficialis splits into two bands, which proceed distally to insert on each side of the middle phalanx.

2. The flexor digitorum profundus tendon courses between the two bands of the flexor digitorum superficialis to insert on the base of the distal phalanx.

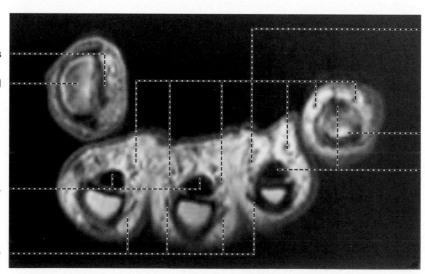

Flexor pollicis longus tendon

Thumb, interphalangeal

Index and third finger, flexor digitorum superficialis and profundus

Dorsal (extensor) expansions (hoods)

Second, third, fourth, and fifth fingers, palmar digital aa., nn.

Fifth finger, proximal phalanx

Fourth and fifth fingers, flexor digitorum superficialis and profundus

1. This section is through the fingers at the proximal phalanges.

2. The extensor pollicis longus has completed its insertion at the base of the distal phalanx of the thumb; the flexor pollicis longus is seen inserting at the base of the distal phalanx.

3. The dorsal expansions of the fingers are well developed on this section.

4. In the fingers, part of the extensor tendon inserts onto the base of the middle phalanx and the remainder inserts onto the base of the distal phalanx.

Figure 10.1.14

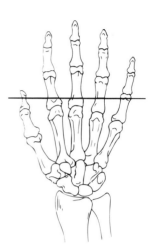

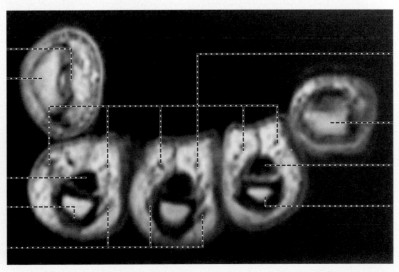

Flexor pollicis longus tendon, insertion

Thumb, base of distal phalanx

Second finger, flexor digitorum superficialis and profundus

Index finger, proximal phalanx

Dorsal (extensor) expansions (hoods)

Second, third, and fourth fingers, palmar digital aa., nn.

Fifth finger, head of proximal phalanx

Fourth finger, proximal phalanx

Fourth finger, flexor digitorum superficialis and profundus

CORONAL

Figure 10.2.1

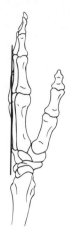

1. This coronal section is through the dorsal surface of the hand.

2. The extensor digitorum tendons for the long and ring fingers are depicted in this section.

3. Each of the extensor tendons merges into the hood and extensor expansion on the dorsum of the metacarpophalangeal joint and proximal phalanx.

4. The hood covers the head of the metacarpal, whereas the extensor expansion extends to the base of the middle phalanx.

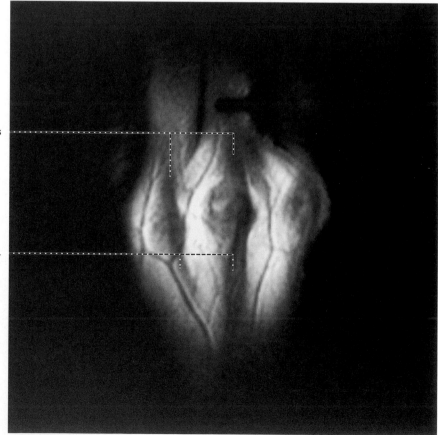

Dorsal expansions (hoods)

Long and ring fingers, extensor digitorum tendons

1. This section passes through the posterior aspects of the metacarpophalangeal joints of the second, third, and fourth fingers.

2. The second and third dorsal interosseous muscles are partially depicted in this section.

3. The second and third dorsal interossei, on either side of the third metacarpal, insert onto the base of the proximal phalanx of the long finger. The interosseous muscles also insert, in part, into the dorsal expansion.

Figure 10.2.2

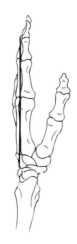

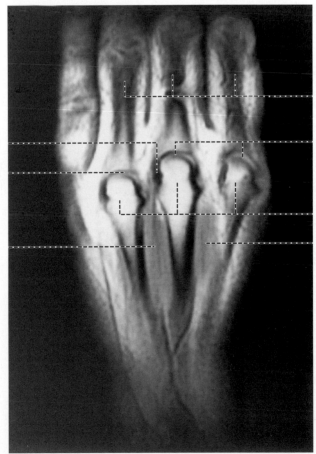

Tendon of third dorsal interosseous m.

Fourth metacarpophalangeal joint

Third dorsal interosseous m.

Long and ring fingers, dorsal expansions (hoods)

Second and third metacarpophalangeal joints

Second, third, and fourth metacarpal heads

Second dorsal interosseous m.

Figure 10.2.3

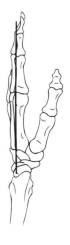

1. This section is through the proximal interphalangeal joints and some of the metacarpophalangeal joints of the fingers.

2. The dorsal interossei function as abductors; however, the part of the muscle inserting into the extensor functions in flexion of the metacarpophalangeal joints and extension of the proximal interphalangeal joints.

3. The second and third dorsal interosseous muscles insert on the base of the proximal phalanx of the long finger.

4. All the interosseous muscles originate from the shafts of the metacarpals.

5. The extensor carpi radialis tendon is seen inserting at the base of the third metacarpal.

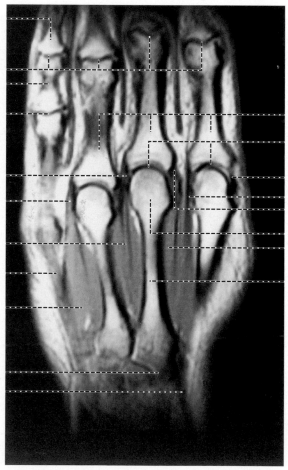

Left labels:
- Little finger, digital phalanx
- Proximal interphalangeal joints
- Middle phalanx
- Little finger, proximal interphalangeal joint
- Tendon of third dorsal interosseous m.
- Tendon of fourth dorsal interosseous m.
- Third dorsal interosseous m.
- Extensor digiti minimi tendon
- Fourth dorsal interosseous m.
- Third metacarpal, styloid process
- Extensor carpi radialis brevis tendon

Right labels:
- Proximal phalanges
- Metacarpophalangeal joints
- Tendon of first dorsal interosseous m.
- Tendon of first palmar interosseous m.
- Tendon of second dorsal interosseous m.
- Third metacarpal, head
- Second dorsal interosseous m.
- Third metacarpal

Figure 10.2.4

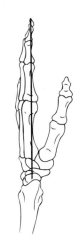

1. This section is through the volar aspect of the fingers.

2. The flexor tendons are seen on the volar surface of the proximal phalanges coursing toward their insertions. The flexor digitorum superficialis tendons insert onto the shafts of the middle phalanges, and the flexor digitorum profundus tendons insert at the bases of the distal phalanges.

3. The three volar interosseous muscles are clearly depicted in this section; they function as adductors of the fingers.

4. All the interossei are usually innervated by the ulnar nerve.

5. The extensor carpi ulnaris tendon is seen inserting onto the base of the fifth metacarpal.

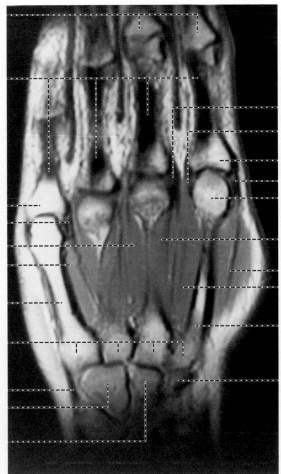

Index and long fingers, bases of proximal phalanges

Second through fifth fingers, flexor digitorum profundus tendons

Little finger, base of proximal phalanx

Tendon of the third palmar interosseous m.

Third dorsal interosseous m.

Third palmar interosseous m.

Fifth metacarpal

Second through fifth metacarpals,

Extensor carpi ulnaris tendon

Hamate

Capitate

Tendon of the second dorsal interosseous m.

Tendon of the first palmar interosseous m.

Index finger, base of proximal phalanx

Tendon of first dorsal interosseous m.

Second metacarpal, head

Second dorsal interosseous m.

First dorsal interosseous m.

First palmar interosseous m.

Second metacarpal

Trapezoid

Figure 10.2.5

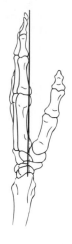

1. The flexor carpi radialis is demonstrated in this section as it inserts onto the base of the second metacarpal.

2. Note the origin of the transverse head of the adductor pollicis from the volar aspect of the third metacarpal shaft.

3. The deep palmar arch and some of its palmar metacarpal arterial branches are demonstrated in this section.

4. The abductor digiti minimi is demonstrated in this section inserting onto the base of the proximal phalanx of the little finger.

5. The opponens digiti minimi tendon is noted inserting on the medial aspect of the fifth metacarpal. It originates from the flexor retinaculum and hook of the hamate.

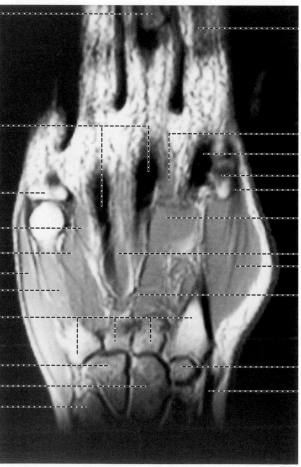

Long finger, middle phalanx

Index finger

Long and ring fingers, flexor digitorum profundus tendons

Lumbrical m.

Index finger, flexor digitorum profundus tendon

Second metacarpal, head

Little finger, base of proximal phalanx

Tendon of first dorsal interosseous m.

Fourth dorsal interosseous m.

Adductor pollicis m., transverse head

Third palmar interosseous m.

Lumbrical m.

First dorsal interosseous m.

Abductor digiti minimi m.

Opponens digiti minimi m.

Deep palmar arch

Second through fifth metacarpals, bases

Hamate

Trapezoid

Capitate

Flexor carpi radialis tendon

Triquetrum

1. This section passes through the long flexor tendons in the palm.

2. Note that the lumbrical muscles, which are seen originating from the radial side of flexor digitorum profundus tendons in the hand, insert into the lateral sides of the dorsal expansions.

3. The radial artery crosses from the volar to the dorsal aspect of the wrist.

Figure 10.2.6

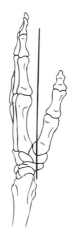

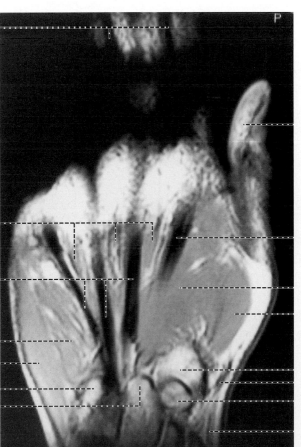

Index and long fingers, flexor digitorum tendons

Lumbrical mm.

Flexor digitorum profundus and superficialis tendons

Flexor digiti minimi m.

Abductor digiti minimi m.

Hook of hamate

Capitate

Thumb

Flexor digitorum tendons (profundus and superficialis)

Adductor pollicis m., oblique head

First dorsal interosseous m.

Second metacarpal, base
Extensor pollicis longus tendon

Trapezoid

Radial a.

Figure 10.2.7

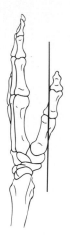

1. This section passes through the carpal tunnel; medially, the carpal tunnel is bounded by the pisiform and hook of the hamate. On the lateral side, the carpal tunnel is bounded by the scaphoid tuberosity and tubercle of trapezium.

2. The oblique and transverse heads of the adductor pollicis muscle converge to insert onto the base of the proximal phalanx medially.

3. Note that the medial sesamoid is situated within the tendon of the adductor pollicis.

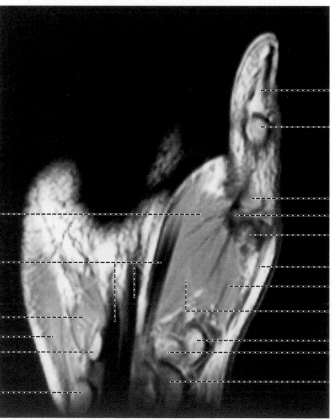

1. This section is through the thumb.

2. The fibers of palmaris brevis are quite superficial in the hypothenar aspect of the palm.

3. Note the insertion of the flexor pollicis longus tendon onto the base of the distal phalanx of the thumb.

4. Note the insertion of the flexor carpi ulnaris tendon onto the pisiform.

Figure 10.2.8

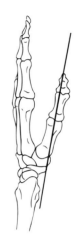

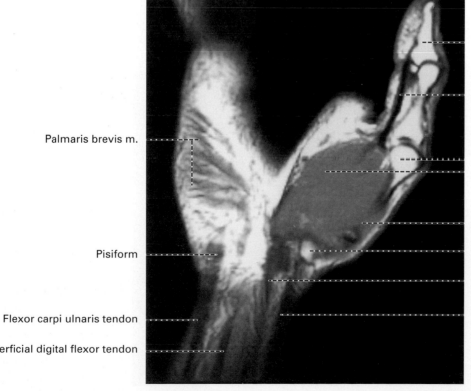

Thumb, distal phalanx

Flexor pollicis longus tendon

First metacarpal, head
Abductor pollicis brevis m.

Opponens pollicis m.

Trapezium

Palmaris longus tendon

Flexor carpi radialis tendon

Palmaris brevis m.

Pisiform

Flexor carpi ulnaris tendon

Superficial digital flexor tendon

Figure 10.2.9

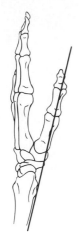

1. The flexor pollicis longus crosses the wrist through the carpal tunnel, where it is situated laterally.

2. Observe the articulation of the distal pole of the scaphoid tuberosity with the trapezium; trapezium articulates with the first metacarpal.

3. The abductor pollicis longus tendon is seen approaching its insertion at the base of the first metacarpal.

4. The lateral boundary of the carpal tunnel is depicted in this section. It consists of the scaphoid tuberosity and tubercle of trapezium.

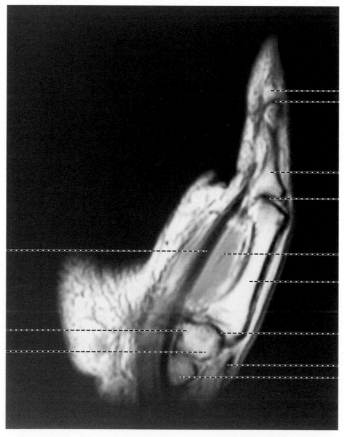

Thumb, distal phalanx
Interphalangeal joint

Thumb, proximal phalanx

Carpometacarpal joint

Flexor pollicis longus tendon

Flexor pollicis brevis m., deep head

First metacarpal

Tubercle of trapezium

First carpometacarpal joint

Trapezium

Abductor pollicis longus tendon
Scaphoid tuberosity

1. This section passes through the thenar eminence.

2. The flexor pollicis brevis and opponens pollicis muscles are clearly depicted in this section.

3. A sesamoid bone is seen in the tendon of the flexor pollicis brevis prior to its insertion onto the base of the proximal phalanx.

4. Note the insertion of the opponens pollicis muscle onto the shaft of the first metacarpal.

Figure 10.2.10

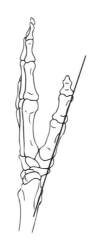

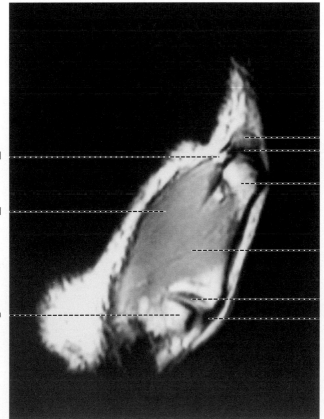

Lateral sesamoid

Flexor pollicis brevis m., superficial head

Trapezium

Thumb, base of proximal phalanx
Metacarpophalangeal joint

First metacarpal, head

Opponens pollicis m.

First carpometacarpal joint
Abductor pollicis longus tendon

Figure 10.2.11

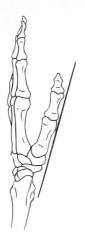

1. This is the most palmar section. It passes through the thenar eminence.

2. The flexor pollicis brevis and abductor pollicis brevis muscles, which constitute the thenar eminence, are depicted in this section.

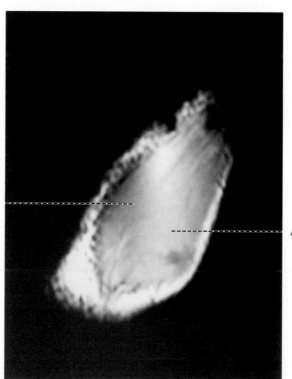

Flexor pollicis brevis m.

Abductor pollicis brevis m.

Figure 10.3.1

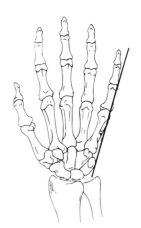

1. This section passes through the medial aspect of the hand. It depicts the fifth metacarpophalangeal joint and part of the hypothenar muscles.

2. The abductor and flexor digiti minimi muscles are depicted in this section. Both of these muscles insert on the base of the proximal phalanx medially.

3. The abductor digiti minimi originates from the pisiform bone and the flexor digiti minimi originates from the flexor retinaculum.

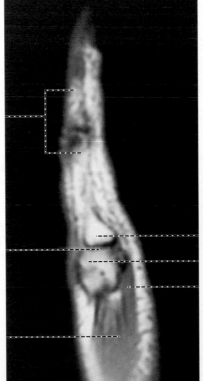

Little finger

Little finger, metacarpophalangeal joint

Abductor digiti minimi m.

Little finger, base of proximal phalanx

Fifth metacarpal, head

Flexor digiti minimi m.

Figure 10.3.4

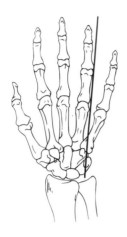

1. This section is through the base of the fifth metacarpal.

2. Note the thin fibers of the palmaris brevis muscle; this thin muscle is situated in the superficial fascia over the proximal portion of the hypothenar eminence.

3. Note the location of the superficial palmar arch in the palm. It is formed primarily by the ulnar artery.

4. The third palmar and fourth dorsal interosseous muscles are clearly depicted in this section.

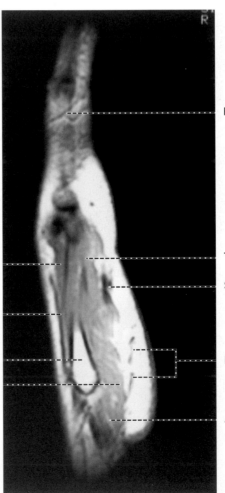

Ring finger

Fourth dorsal interosseous m.

Third palmar interosseous m.

Superficial palmar arch

Extensor digiti minimi tendon

Fifth metacarpal

Palmaris brevis m.

Opponens digiti minimi m.

Abductor digiti minimi m.

1. This section is through the ring finger. The base of the fifth metacarpal and its articulation with the hamate is also seen.

2. Note the insertion of the extensor carpi ulnaris onto the base of the fifth metacarpal.

3. The pisohamate ligament is partially outlined; it connects the pisiform to the hook of the hamate.

Figure 10.3.5

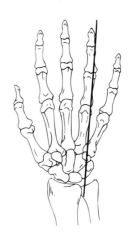

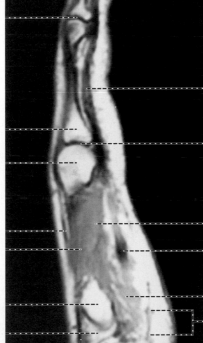

Middle phalanx

Proximal interphalangeal joint

Proximal phalanx

Fourth metacarpal, head

Extensor digitorum tendon

Fourth dorsal interosseous m.

Fifth metacarpal, base

Hamate

Extensor carpi ulnaris tendon

Triquetrum

Flexor digitorum profundus tendon

Flexor digitorum profundus and superficialis tendons

Metacarpophalangeal joint

Third palmar interosseous m.

Superficial palmar arch

Opponens digiti minimi m.

Palmaris brevis m.

Pisohamate lig.

Pisiform

Figure 10.3.6

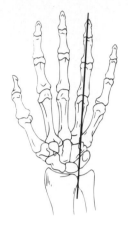

1. This section passes through the ring finger. The hook of the hamate is included in this section.

2. Note the ulnar artery crossing from the wrist to the palm just lateral to the pisiform. In this region, the ulnar artery travels with the ulnar nerve.

3. The flexor digitorum superficialis and profundus tendons are clearly depicted in this section.

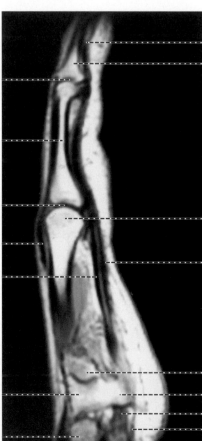

Proximal interphalangeal joint

Proximal phalanx

Metacarpophalangeal joint

Extensor digitorum tendon

Flexor digitorum profundus tendon

Hamate

Triquetrum

Flexor digitorum profundus tendon

Middle phalanx

Fourth metacarpal, head

Flexor digitorum superficialis tendon

Fourth metacarpal, base

Hook of hamate

Pisohamate lig.

Ulnar a.

1. This section passes between the third and fourth metacarpals.

2. The second palmar interosseous muscle is depicted in this section. It originates on the shaft of the fourth metacarpal laterally and inserts onto the base of the proximal phalanx of the ring finger.

3. The palmar aponeurosis is the continuation of the palmaris longus tendon.

Figure 10.3.7

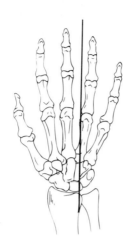

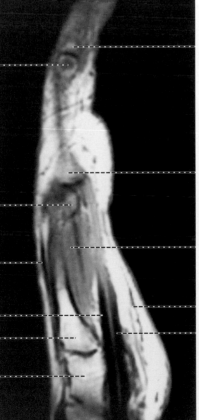

Ring finger, head of proximal phalanx

Ring finger, base of middle phalanx

Proximal phalanx, base

Fourth metacarpal, head

Second palmar interosseous m.

Extensor digitorum tendon

Palmar aponeurosis

Flexor digitorum profundus tendon

Flexor digitorum superficialis tendon

Fourth metacarpal, base

Hamate

Triquetrum

Figure 10.3.8

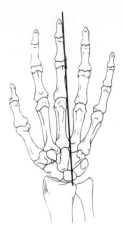

1. This section passes through the medial aspect of the long finger.

2. The flexor retinaculum is clearly depicted in this section. The flexor retinaculum forms the ventral or volar boundary of the carpal tunnel.

3. Medially, the carpal tunnel is bounded by the pisiform and hook of hamate. The carpal tunnel is bounded on the lateral side by the scaphoid tuberosity and tubercle of trapezium.

4. Note the palmar aponeurosis superficial to the flexor retinaculum and its distal extension into the palm.

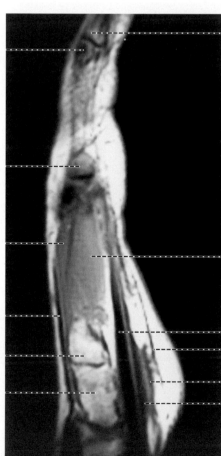

Long finger, head of proximal phalanx

Long finger, base of middle phalanx

Proximal phalanx, base

Third dorsal interosseous m.

Second palmar interosseous m.

Extensor digitorum tendon

Flexor digitorum profundus tendon

Fourth metacarpal, base

Palmar aponeurosis

Hamate

Flexor retinaculum

Flexor digitorum superficialis tendon

1. This section is through the long finger.

2. The relationship of the flexor digitorum superficialis tendon to the flexor digitorum profundus is clearly depicted in this section.

3. The third carpometacarpal joint is almost flat; therefore, little movement occurs at this joint.

4. The median nerve is seen immediately below the flexor retinaculum.

Figure 10.3.9

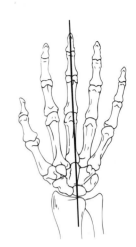

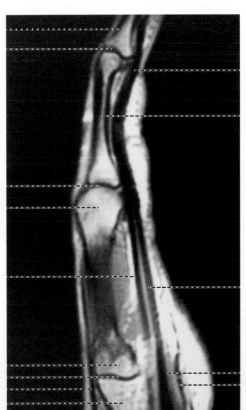

Middle phalanx

Proximal interphalangeal joint

Flexor digitorum profundus and superficialis tendons

Long finger, proximal phalanx

Long finger, metacarpophalangeal joint

Third metacarpal, head

Flexor digitorum profundus tendon

Flexor digitorum superficialis tendon

Third metacarpal, base
Third carpometacarpal joint
Extensor digitorum tendon
Capitate

Median n.
Flexor retinaculum

Lunate

Figure 10.3.10

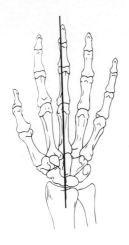

1. This section is through the lateral aspect of the long finger.

2. The transverse head of the adductor pollicis is seen originating from the palmar ridge (shaft) of the third metacarpal. The oblique head of the adductor pollicis (not seen in this section) arises from the volar aspect of the capitate and bases of the second and third metacarpals.

Long finger, middle phalanx

Proximal interphalangeal joint

Long finger, proximal phalanx

Long finger, metacarpophalangeal joint

Third metacarpal, head

Adductor pollicis m.

Third metacarpal

Flexor digitorum profundus and superficialis tendons

Extensor digitorum tendon

Flexor retinaculum

Capitate

Lunate

1. This section passes between the long and index fingers.

2. Abductor pollicis brevis is depicted in this section arising from the flexor retinaculum and the carpal bones below it.

3. The flexor pollicis longus is noted coursing distally toward the thumb.

4. The flexor carpi radialis crosses the wrist immediately volar to the scaphoid tuberosity.

5. Note the extensor carpi radialis brevis tendon inserting onto the base of the third metacarpal.

6. Note the lumbrical muscle arising from the flexor digitorum profundus tendon.

Figure 10.3.11

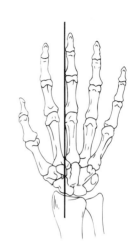

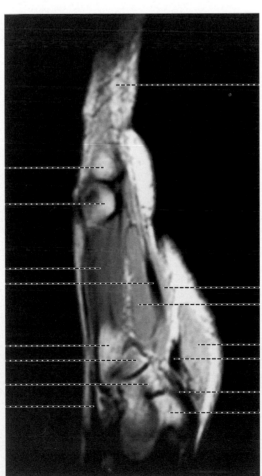

Long finger

Long finger, base of proximal phalanx

Third metacarpal, head

Second dorsal interosseous m.

Flexor digitorum profundus and superficialis tendons

Lumbrical m.

Adductor pollicis m.

Third metacarpal, base

Second metacarpal, base

Trapezoid

Extensor carpi radialis brevis

Abductor pollicis brevis m.

Flexor pollicis longus tendon

Flexor carpi radialis tendon

Scaphoid tuberosity

Figure 10.3.12

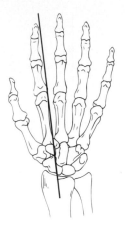

1. This section passes between the second and third metacarpals.

2. The flexor carpi radialis is seen approaching its insertion at the base of the second metacarpal.

3. The flexor pollicis longus is seen coursing along the thenar muscles toward the thumb. It lies between the deep and superficial heads of the flexor pollicis brevis muscle.

4. Note the extensor carpi radialis longus tendon as it inserts onto the base of the second metacarpal.

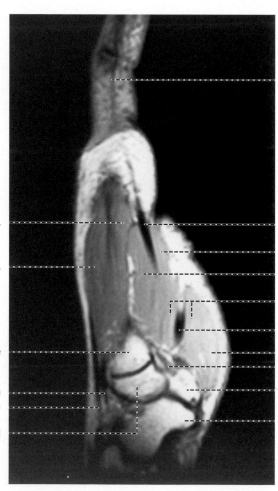

Index finger

First palmar interosseous m.

Flexor digitorum profundus and superficialis tendons

Lumbrical m.

Second dorsal interosseous m.

Adductor pollicis m.

Flexor pollicis brevis m., superficial and deep heads

Flexor pollicis longus tendon

Second metacarpal, base

Abductor pollicis brevis m.

Flexor carpi radialis tendon

Extensor carpi radialis longus tendon

Trapezium

Extensor indicis tendon

Scaphoid tuberosity

Trapezoid

1. This section is through the medial aspect of the index finger.

2. The extensor indicis tendon is seen on the dorsum of the hand coursing in the direction of the index finger.

3. The extensor pollicis longus tendon is depicted in this section as it veers laterally toward the thumb.

Figure 10.3.13

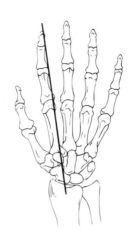

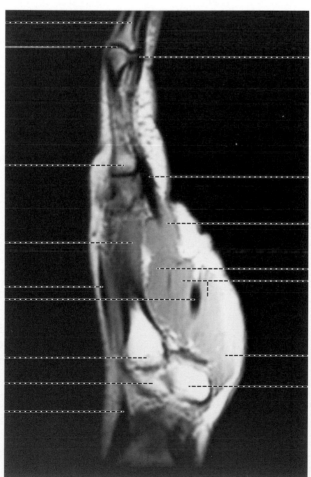

Index finger, middle phalanx
Index finger, proximal interphalangeal joint

Flexor digitorum profundus and superficialis tendons

Index finger, base of proximal phalanx

Flexor digitorum profundus and superficialis tendons

Lumbrical m.

First palmar interosseous m.

Adductor pollicis m.
Flexor pollicis brevis m., superficial and deep heads

Extensor indicis tendon
Flexor pollicis longus tendon

Second metacarpal, base

Abductor pollicis brevis m.

Trapezoid

Trapezium

Extensor pollicis longus tendon

Figure 10.3.14

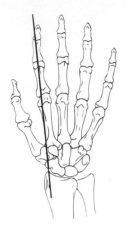

1. This section passes through the index finger.

2. The extensor indicis tendon is clearly depicted in this section.

3. Observe the radial artery as it crosses from the volar aspect to the dorsal aspect of the wrist.

4. The radial artery crosses dorsally through the anatomic snuff box, which is depicted in this section.

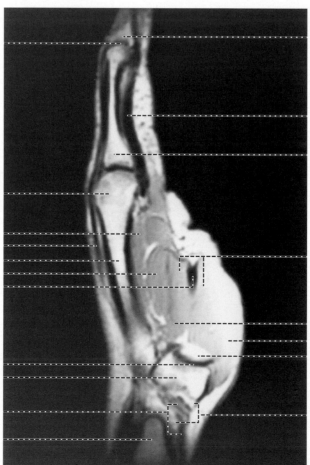

Proximal interphalangeal joint — Index finger, middle phalanx

Flexor digitorum profundus and superficialis tendons

Index finger, proximal phalanx

Second metacarpal, head

First palmar interosseous m.
Extensor indicis tendon
Second metacarpal
Adductor pollicis m.
Flexor pollicis longus tendon

Flexor pollicis brevis m., superficial and deep heads

Opponens pollicis m.
Abductor pollicis brevis m.
First metacarpal, base

First carpometacarpal joint
Trapezium

Radial a. — Snuff box

Radial styloid process

1. This section passes through the thenar eminence between the thumb and the index finger.

2. The abductor pollicis longus tendon is noted coursing toward its insertion on the base of the first metacarpal.

3. The extensor pollicis brevis tendon is seen just dorsal to the abductor pollicis longus tendon.

4. The extensor pollicis longus tendon is seen crossing the wrist in the direction of the thumb, where it inserts onto the base of the distal phalanx.

5. Observe the distal portion of the first dorsal interosseous muscle converging to insert on the bone of the proximal phalanx of the index finger.

Figure 10.3.15

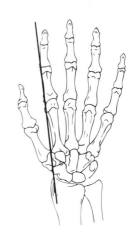

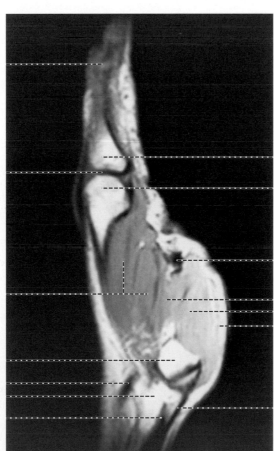

Index finger

Index finger, base of proximal phalanx

Index finger, metacarpophalangeal joint

Second metacarpal, head

Flexor pollicis longus tendon

First dorsal interosseus m.

Opponens pollicis m.
Flexor pollicis brevis m.
Abductor pollicis brevis m.

First metacarpal, base

Extensor pollicis longus tendon
Snuff box

Extensor pollicis brevis tendon

Abductor pollicis longus tendon

Figure 10.3.16

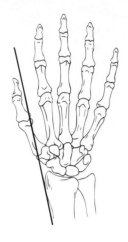

1. This section is through the base of the first metacarpal.

2. The abductor pollicis longus tendon is inserting at the base of the first metacarpal.

3. Note the tendon of the first dorsal interosseous muscle as it courses in the direction of the proximal phalanx, where it inserts on its base.

4. The extensor pollicis longus and brevis tendons are seen in this section; both are coursing in the direction of the thumb.

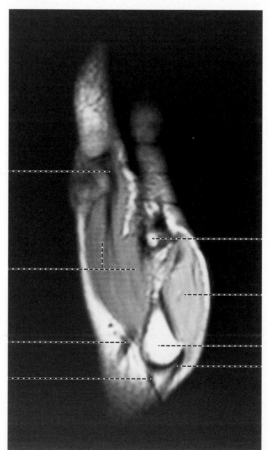

First dorsal interosseous tendon

First dorsal interosseous m.

Extensor pollicis longus tendon

Extensor pollicis brevis tendon

Medial sesamoid

Abductor pollicis brevis m.

First metacarpal, base

Abductor pollicis longus tendon

1. This section passes through the thumb.

Figure 10.3.17

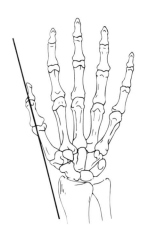

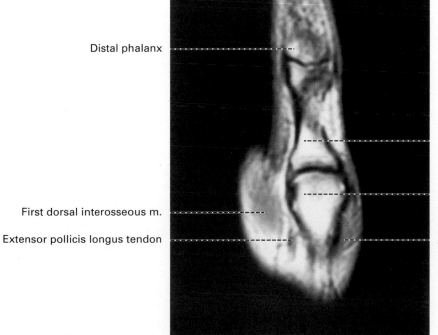

Distal phalanx

Proximal phalanx

First metacarpal, head

First dorsal interosseous m.

Extensor pollicis longus tendon

Abductor pollicis brevis m.

Chapter 11

THORAX AND HEART

Cardiac and Great Vessel MRI

MRI continues to increase in popularity in the evaluation of cardiac anatomy and in assessing those disease processes that affect the heart. The absence of a requirement for contrast media and radiation exposure make MRI attractive. The disadvantages are the time it takes to acquire the images, the narrow confines of the scanner gantry, and the degradation of the images by an irregular heart beat. Nevertheless, the advantages outweigh the disadvantages, and with newer refinements resulting in better resolution and with sequences that allow the acquisition of data in shorter time periods, MRI should grow in popularity and become an increasingly important imaging modality in the study of cardiac anatomy and function.

The most detailed anatomic images of the heart are obtained with T1 sequences. The ability of MRI to obtain images in axial, coronal, and sagittal planes has distinct advantages over CT, where the images can only be obtained in axial planes; if sagittal or coronal images are requested, it requires reformatting. The additional ability to acquire gradient refocused echo sequences has added another dimension to MRI by producing a bright signal in the blood pool. The latter will delineate vascular structures better than the black flow voids seen on T1 images. Another advantage to gradient refocused echo sequences is the ability to image the contracting heart and to observe wall motion abnormalities and valvular dysfunction.

Not only are cardiac relationships important but so too are the great vessel relationships; these structures are well seen on MRI. Aortic aneurysms and dissections can be distinctly seen. In addition, infants can be imaged and computer workstations can be used to assemble the MRI data into three-dimensional images. This allows radiologists, cardiologists, and surgeons to obtain excellent views of the sometimes complex relationships that occur in aortic aneurysms and in congenital heart disease.

The images in this chapter are representative of normal cardiac anatomy as seen in the axial, sagittal, and coronal planes. From these sequences it is hoped that a better appreciation of cardiac anatomy will be forthcoming.

1. This level is through the base of the neck.

2. The common carotid artery lies medial to the jugular vein.

3. A small portion of the subclavian arteries are identified but are partially obscured because of partial volume averaging.

Figure 11.1.1

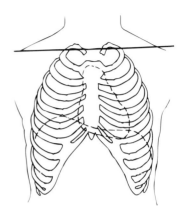

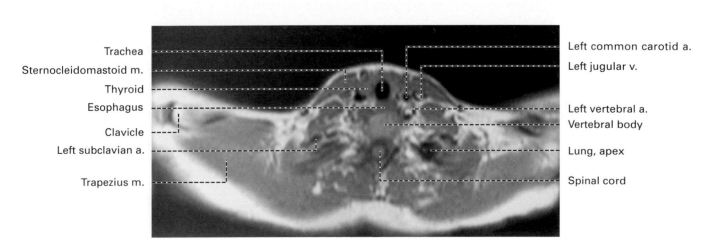

Trachea

Sternocleidomastoid m.

Thyroid

Esophagus

Clavicle

Left subclavian a.

Trapezius m.

Left common carotid a.

Left jugular v.

Left vertebral a.

Vertebral body

Lung, apex

Spinal cord

Figure 11.1.6

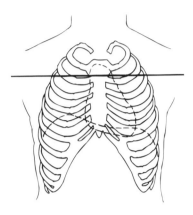

1. This level is at the aortic arch.

2. Medially, the tracheal bifurcation is becoming visible.

3. Anteriorly and to the right of the aorta is the superior vena cava.

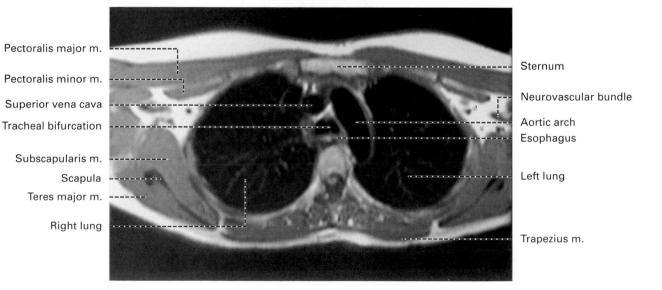

1 This slice is through the inferior aspect of the aortic arch.

2. The origins of the left and right mainstem bronchi are visible.

3. Some signal is seen in the superior vena cava due to slow flow.

Figure 11.1.7

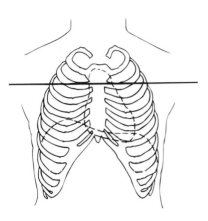

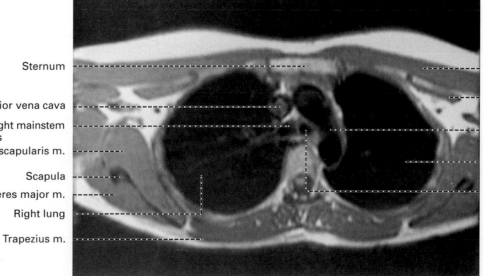

Sternum

Superior vena cava

Proximal right mainstem bronchus

Subscapularis m.

Scapula

Teres major m.

Right lung

Trapezius m.

Pectoralis major m.

Pectoralis minor m.

Aortic arch

Left lung

Proximal left mainstem bronchus

Figure 11.1.8

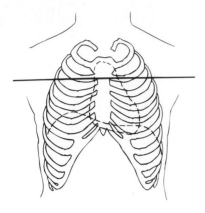

1. This slice is at the level of the aortic-pulmonary recess.

2. The aorta has divided into its ascending and descending divisions.

3. The bronchus to the right upper lobe is seen.

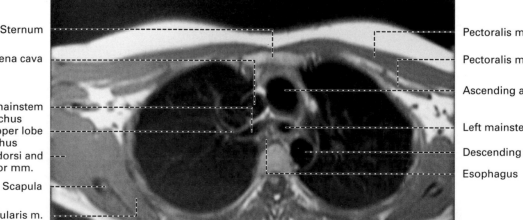

Sternum

Superior vena cava

Right mainstem bronchus
Right upper lobe bronchus
Latissimus dorsi and teres major mm.

Scapula

Subscapularis m.

Pectoralis major m.

Pectoralis minor m.

Ascending aorta

Left mainstem bronchus

Descending aorta

Esophagus

1, This section is at the level of the left pulmonary artery.

2. The left pulmonary artery is seen in profile as it loops up and over the left mainstem bronchus.

Figure 11.1.9

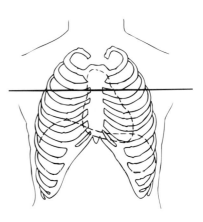

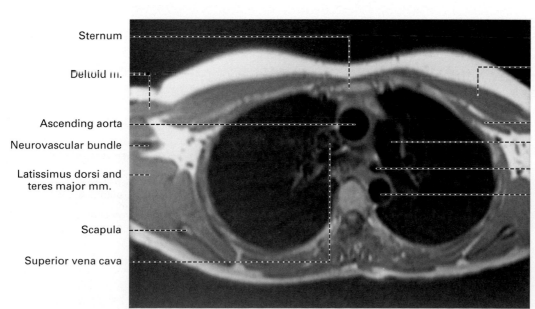

Sternum

Deltoid m.

Ascending aorta

Neurovascular bundle

Latissimus dorsi and teres major mm.

Scapula

Superior vena cava

Pectoralis major m.

Pectoralis minor m.

Left pulmonary a.

Left mainstem bronchus

Descending aorta

Figure 11.1.10

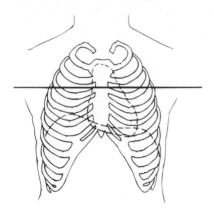

1. This section is through the right pulmonary artery.

2. Lateral to the descending aorta are the superior left pulmonary vein and left descending pulmonary artery.

3. The main pulmonary artery lies anteriorly.

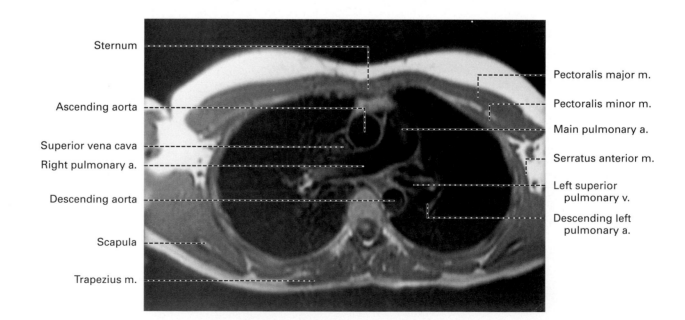

Sternum

Ascending aorta

Superior vena cava

Right pulmonary a.

Descending aorta

Scapula

Trapezius m.

Pectoralis major m.

Pectoralis minor m.

Main pulmonary a.

Serratus anterior m.

Left superior pulmonary v.

Descending left pulmonary a.

1. This slice is through the superior aspect of the left atrium.

2. The entrance of the right and left superior pulmonary veins can be seen.

3. The proximal main pulmonary artery can be seen in cross section.

4. The pulmonary valve is not readily identified on these images.

Figure 11.1.11

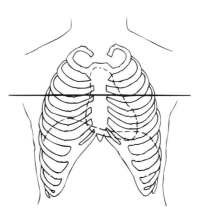

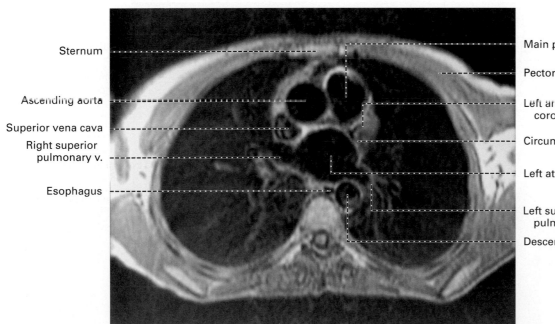

Sternum

Ascending aorta

Superior vena cava

Right superior
pulmonary v.

Esophagus

Main pulmonary a.

Pectoralis major m.

Left anterior descending
coronary a.

Circumflex coronary a.

Left atrium

Left superior
pulmonary v.

Descending aorta

Figure 11.1.12

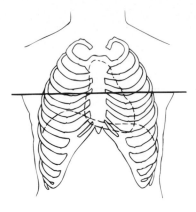

1. This section is through the lower aspect of the left atrium.

2. The right ventricular outflow tract can be identified anteriorly.

3. The right coronary artery can be identified in the epicardial fat.

4. The superior vena cava has been incorporated into the right atrium.

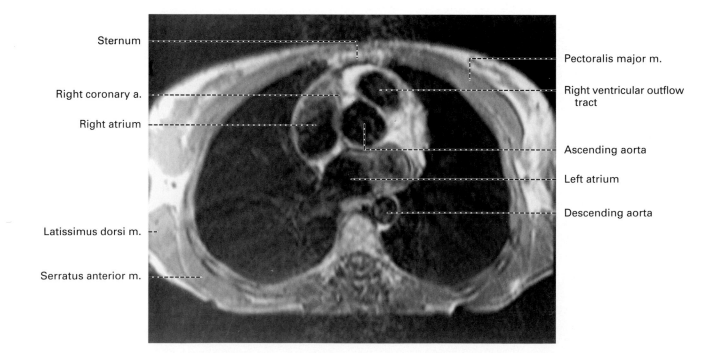

1. This section is at the level of the left ventricular outflow tract.

2. The sinuses of Valsalva are seen as slight dilatations of the aortic root.

3. The right coronary artery lies in the fat in the atrioventricular groove.

Figure 11.1.13

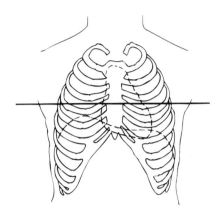

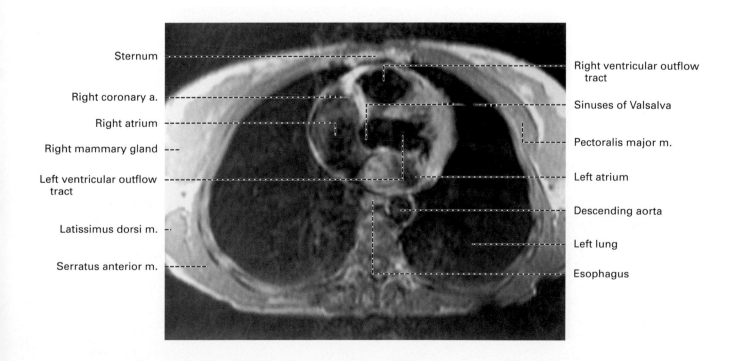

Figure 11.1.14

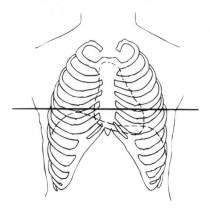

1. This section is through the superior aspect of the left ventricle.

2. The mitral valve annulus separates the lower part of the left atrium from the left ventricle.

3. The tricuspid valve is visible.

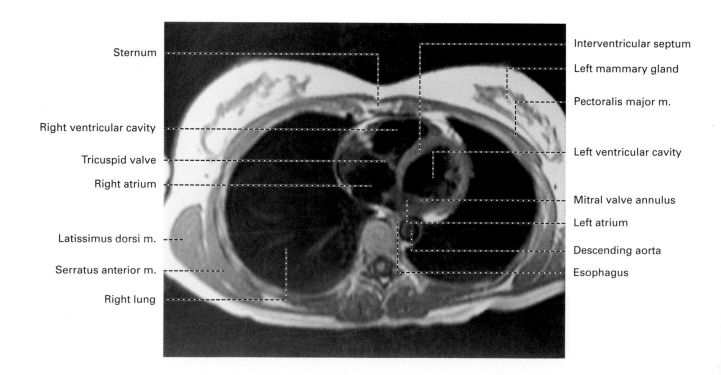

1. This section is through the mid body of the left ventricle.

2. The moderator band can be seen in the anterior aspect of the right ventricle.

Figure 11.1.15

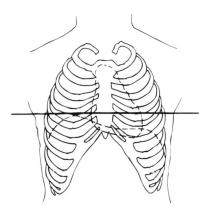

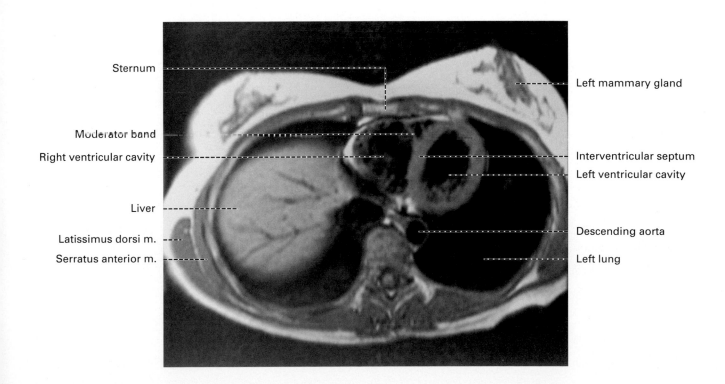

Sternum

Left mammary gland

Moderator band

Right ventricular cavity

Interventricular septum

Left ventricular cavity

Liver

Latissimus dorsi m.

Descending aorta

Serratus anterior m.

Left lung

Figure 11.1.16

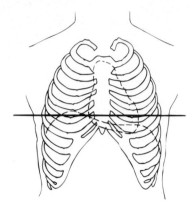

1. This section is through the inferior aspect of the left ventricle.

2. The right and left ventricular cavities are still identifiable.

3. The pericardium is seen as a dark stripe lateral to the left ventricle. Lateral to it is a linear structure with increased signal, which is fat lying on the surface of the pericardium. Fat is also seen anteriorly.

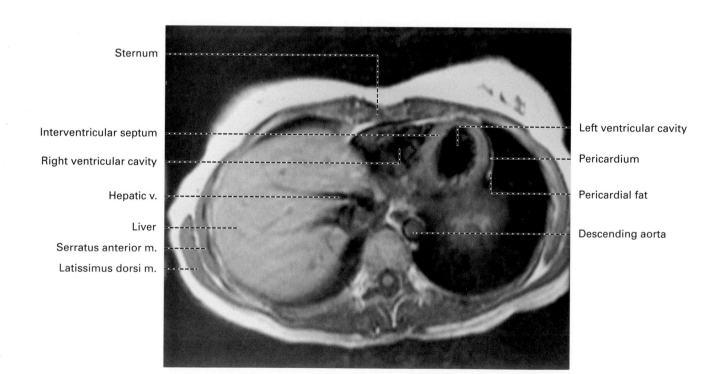

1. This section is through the apex of the left ventricle.

2. The right ventricle lies superiorly and is not seen.

3. The signal void to the right of the descending aorta is from the inferior vena cava.

Figure 11.1.17

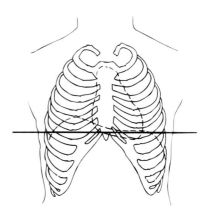

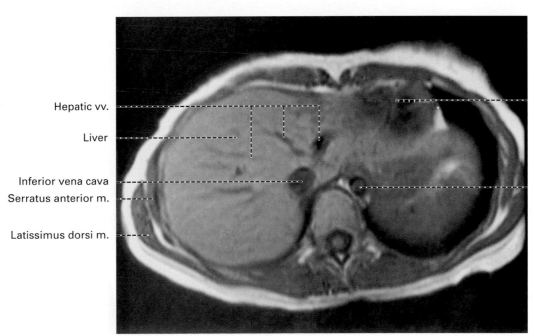

Hepatic vv.

Liver

Inferior vena cava

Serratus anterior m.

Latissimus dorsi m.

Left ventricular apex

Descending aorta

Figure 11.2.3

1. This section is at the level of the tracheal bifurcation and mid left atrium.

2. The superior pulmonary veins can be seen entering the left atrium.

3. Inferiorly, the hepatic veins are draining into the inferior vena cava.

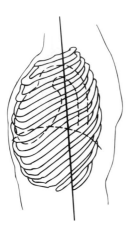

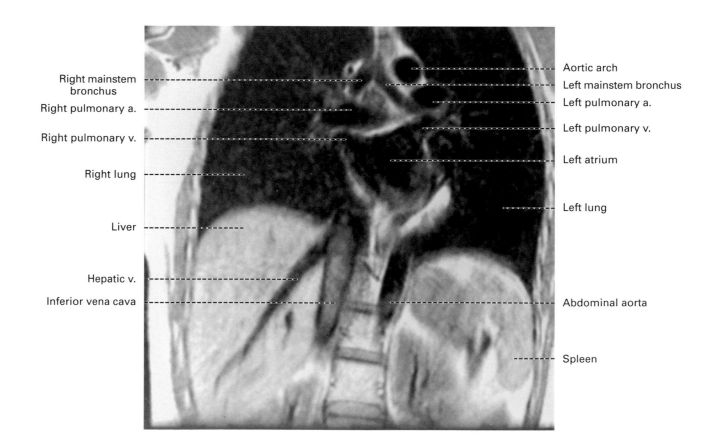

1. This section is at the level of the superior vena cava and pulmonary artery bifurcation.

2. The posterior aspect of the left and right atria are seen.

3. Inferiorly, the descending aorta and inferior vena cava are visualized.

Figure 11.2.4

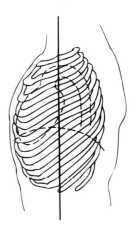

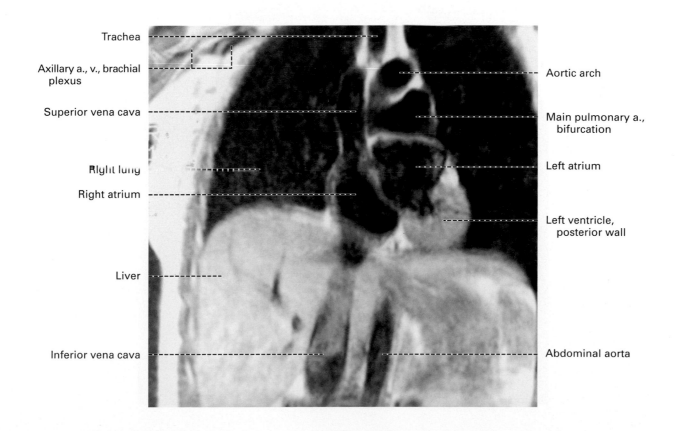

Trachea

Axillary a., v., brachial plexus

Superior vena cava

Right lung

Right atrium

Liver

Inferior vena cava

Aortic arch

Main pulmonary a., bifurcation

Left atrium

Left ventricle, posterior wall

Abdominal aorta

Figure 11.2.5

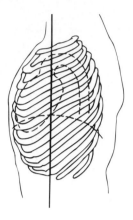

1. This section is at the level of the superior vena cava.

2. The left common carotid artery is seen coming off the aorta.

3. Inferiorly, both the inferior vena cava and descending aorta are visualized.

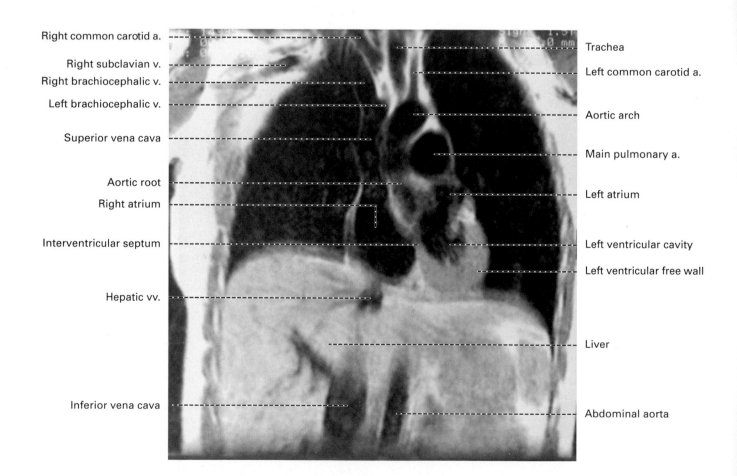

Right common carotid a.

Right subclavian v.

Right brachiocephalic v.

Left brachiocephalic v.

Superior vena cava

Aortic root

Right atrium

Interventricular septum

Hepatic vv.

Inferior vena cava

Trachea

Left common carotid a.

Aortic arch

Main pulmonary a.

Left atrium

Left ventricular cavity

Left ventricular free wall

Liver

Abdominal aorta

1. This section is through the aortic outflow tract.

2. The main pulmonary artery lies to the left of the aorta.

3. Part of the left atrial appendage can be seen.

4. The sinus of Valsalva can be identified.

Figure 11.2.6

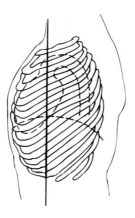

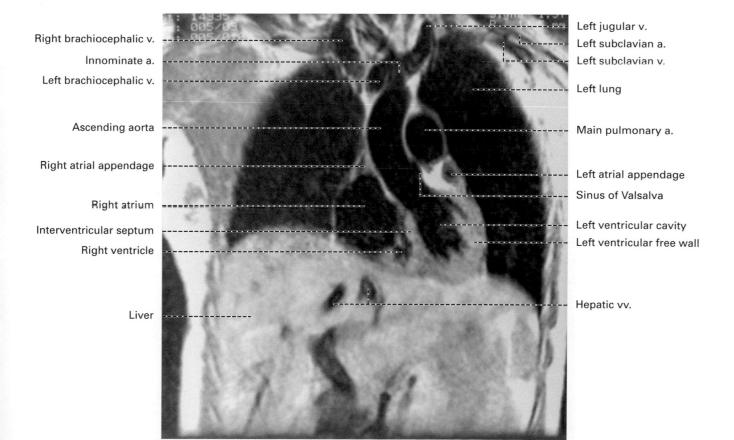

Right brachiocephalic v.

Innominate a.

Left brachiocephalic v.

Ascending aorta

Right atrial appendage

Right atrium

Interventricular septum

Right ventricle

Liver

Left jugular v.

Left subclavian a.

Left subclavian v.

Left lung

Main pulmonary a.

Left atrial appendage

Sinus of Valsalva

Left ventricular cavity

Left ventricular free wall

Hepatic vv.

Figure 11.2.7

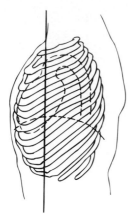

1. This section is through the main pulmonary artery and midportion of the left ventricle.

2. Part of the right atrium is seen lateral to the right ventricular outflow tract.

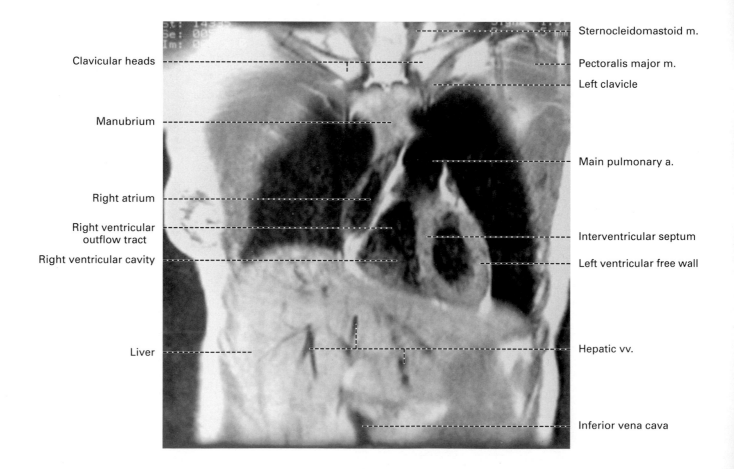

Label (left)	Label (right)
Clavicular heads	Sternocleidomastoid m.
Manubrium	Pectoralis major m.
Right atrium	Left clavicle
Right ventricular outflow tract	Main pulmonary a.
Right ventricular cavity	Interventricular septum
Liver	Left ventricular free wall
	Hepatic vv.
	Inferior vena cava

1. This section is through the right ventricular outflow tract ventral to the previous image.

2. The right ventricle, interventricular septum, and left ventricle are well visualized.

3. Hepatic veins are identifiable within the liver.

Figure 11.2.8

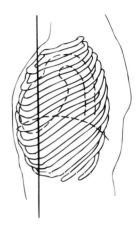

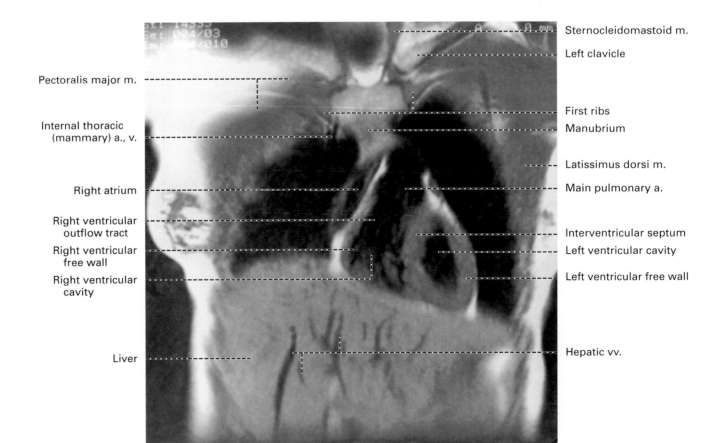

Pectoralis major m.	Sternocleidomastoid m.
Internal thoracic (mammary) a., v.	Left clavicle
Right atrium	First ribs
Right ventricular outflow tract	Manubrium
Right ventricular free wall	Latissimus dorsi m.
Right ventricular cavity	Main pulmonary a.
Liver	Interventricular septum
	Left ventricular cavity
	Left ventricular free wall
	Hepatic vv.

Chapter 12

ABDOMEN

Introduction

The abdomen is delimited superiorly by the hemidiaphragm and inferiorly by the false pelvis, the superior margin of which is defined by the iliac crests. The contents of the abdominal cavity are contained anteriorly and laterally by the lower thoracic ribs and abdominal wall musculature. The abdominal cavity is bordered posteriorly by the spine and paraspinous muscles.

The abdomen is divided anatomically into the intraperitoneal and extraperitoneal compartments. The intraperitoneal cavity contains the liver, spleen, gallbladder, and stomach, as well as loops of duodenum, small bowel, and colon. These are fixed to the abdominal walls by a number of peritoneal folds or reflections, by the small bowel mesentery, and by the transverse mesocolon. These define a number of spaces, primarily the subphrenic, subhepatic, paracolic, and subcolic, as well as the greater and lesser peritoneal cavities, which govern the initial spread of disease in the abdomen.

The retroperitoneum contains the pancreas, kidneys, ureters, and great vessels. It is subdivided by the perirenal fascia and lateroconal fascia into the anterior pararenal, posterior pararenal, and perirenal spaces, which limit or direct the initial spread of disease in the retroperitoneum.

In this section, important anatomic features of the abdominal viscera are identified. Although the individual intraperitoneal and extraperitoneal spaces of the abdomen cannot be visualized in the normal patient, these will be commented on where appropriate. The position of these spaces and compartments can usually be inferred. Knowledge of these anatomic structures is important in interpreting examinations in patients with disease.

Figure 12.1.1

1. This section extends through the confluence of the hepatic veins and the intrahepatic segment of the inferior vena cava.

2. The hepatic veins provide efferent drainage of the liver and are located within the intersegmental and interlobar fissures, outlining the segmental anatomy of the liver.

3. The right hepatic vein lies within the right intersegmental fissure, which separates the anterior and posterior segments of the right lobe of the liver.

4. The middle hepatic vein lies within the interlobar fissure, which separates the anterior segment of the right lobe and the medial segment of the left lobe of the liver.

5. The left hepatic vein lies within the left intersegmental fissure, which separates the medial and lateral segments of the left lobe of the liver.

6. Peritoneal reflections over the superior and posterior surfaces of the liver form the transversely oriented coronary ligaments and the sagittally oriented falciform ligament. These are not routinely visualized; however, they can limit or define the extent of subphrenic fluid collections.

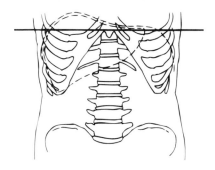

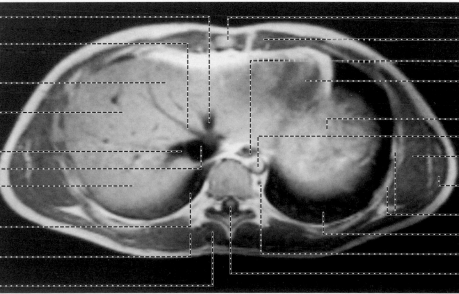

Left hepatic v.
Middle hepatic v.
Liver, left lobe medial segment
Liver, right lobe anterior segment
Right hepatic v.
Inferior vena cava
Liver, right lobe posterior segment
Right lung
Erector spinae mm.
Multifidus m.

Xiphoid process
Costal cartilage
Esophagus
Heart, diaphragmatic surface
Stomach, fundus
Aorta
Serratus anterior m.
Latissimus dorsi m.
Ribs
Left lung
Hemiazygos v.
Spinal cord

417

Figure 12.1.2

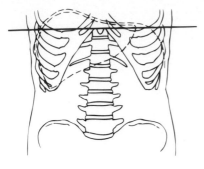

1. Note that the hepatic veins generally have a horizontal or horizontal oblique course on axial sections through the upper liver whereas the portal veins are oriented perpendicular to the plane of section.

2. The distal esophagus is visualized at this level. It often shows a peripheral ring of low- to intermediate-signal intensity arising from smooth muscle within the wall, and a central focus of either increased or decreased signal intensity corresponding to the mucosa and to the presence of either fluid or air within the lumen.

3. The diaphragm has three large openings: the vena cava foramen, the esophageal hiatus, and the aortic hiatus.

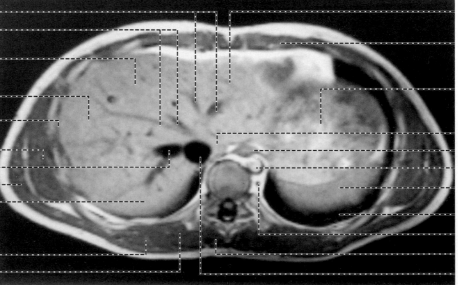

Left hepatic v.
Middle hepatic v.
Liver, left lobe medial segment
Liver, right lobe anterior segment
Intercostal mm.
Serratus anterior m.
Right hepatic v.
Latissimus dorsi m.
Liver, right lobe posterior segment
Iliocostalis lumborum m.
Longissimus thoracis m.

Liver, left lobe lateral segment
Costal cartilage
Stomach, fundus
Liver, caudate lobe
Esophagus
Aorta
Spleen
Left lung
Hemiazygos v.
Multifidus m.
Inferior vena cava

1. The superior portion of the caudate lobe is visualized at this level between the fissure for the ligamentum venosum and the inferior vena cava.

2. The spleen shows homogeneous low-signal intensity relative to the liver on heavily T1-weighted sequences.

3. The relative difference in signal intensity between the liver and spleen is a good indication of the degree of T1 weighting and thereby its expected sensitivity for liver metastases. The signal intensity of hepatic metastases often parallels that of the spleen.

4. The gastroesophageal junction is visualized at this level.

5. The wall of the gastric fundus will often appear abnormally thick in the collapsed stomach. Signal intensity within the normal gastric wall will parallel that of skeletal muscle on T1- and T2-weighted sequences.

6. Fat between the superior aspect of the fissure for the ligamentum venosum and the esophagus on this image, and on Figure 12.1.2, lies within the hepatoesophageal ligament, the superiormost extension of the lesser omentum.

Figure 12.1.3

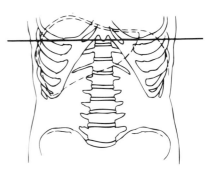

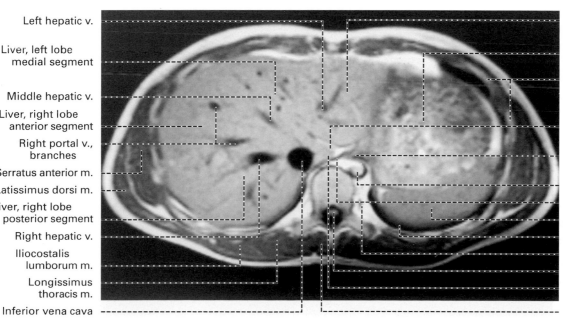

Left hepatic v.

Liver, left lobe medial segment

Middle hepatic v.

Liver, right lobe anterior segment

Right portal v., branches

Serratus anterior m.

Latissimus dorsi m.

Liver, right lobe posterior segment

Right hepatic v.

Iliocostalis lumborum m.

Longissimus thoracis m.

Inferior vena cava

Liver, left lobe lateral segment

Stomach, fundus

Ribs

Ligamentum venosum, fissure

Gastroesophageal junction

Aorta

Diaphragm, crus

Spleen

Left lung

Hemiazygos v.

Spinal cord

Liver, caudate lobe

Multifidus m.

Figure 12.1.14

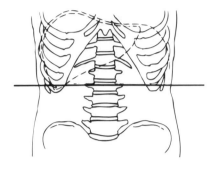

1. The right renal vein and both renal arteries are visualized at this level. The renal arteries originate from the aorta at about the level of the L1 or L2 vertebra.

2. The root of the small bowel mesentery extends from the distal transverse duodenum at its junction with the pancreas on the left at the level of L2 to the base of the cecum in the right iliac fossa. It crosses the duodenojejunal junction, third segment of the duodenum, aorta, inferior vena cava, right ureter, and right psoas muscle.

3. The small bowel mesentery supports the jejunum and ileum and contains the branches of the superior mesenteric vessels.

4. The small bowel mesentery provides anatomic continuity between the pancreas and loops of jejunum, ileum, and cecum.

Right renal a.

Superior mesenteric v.
Stomach, antrum
Pancreas, uncinate process

Inferior vena cava
Liver, right lobe
Colon, hepatic flexure
Duodenum, second portion
Right renal v.
Right kidney

Right renal pelvis

Right diaphragm, crus

Aorta

Stomach, air
Superior mesenteric a.
Stomach, body
Pancreas, body
Transverse colon
Left renal a.
Small intestine
Left renal pelvis
Descending colon
Left renal v.
Spleen
Latissimus dorsi m.
Left kidney, cortex
Left kidney, medulla
Left renal sinus
Quadratus lumborum m.
Psoas m.

1. The duodenojejunal junction and proximal loops of jejunum are visualized on this section.

2. The retroperitoneum is divided into three spaces: the anterior pararenal space, the perirenal space, and the posterior pararenal space. These are separated by the anterior and posterior renal fascia, which fuse laterally to form the lateroconal fascia.

3. The anterior pararenal space lies between the posterior parietal peritoneum and the anterior renal fascia. It contains the pancreas and segments of the duodenum and colon.

4. The perirenal space is defined anteriorly and posteriorly by the renal fascia. It contains the adrenal glands, kidneys, proximal renal collecting systems, and renal vessels.

5. The posterior pararenal space is limited by the posterior renal fascia and the transversalis fascia. It contains fat, which continues laterally to become the properitoneal fat.

6. The lateral margins of the psoas are outlined by perirenal fat at this level and by fat in the posterior pararenal space more inferiorly. Disease in these compartments can result in effacement of the psoas shadow on radiographs.

Figure 12.1.15

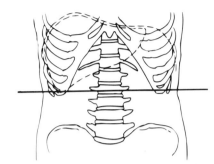

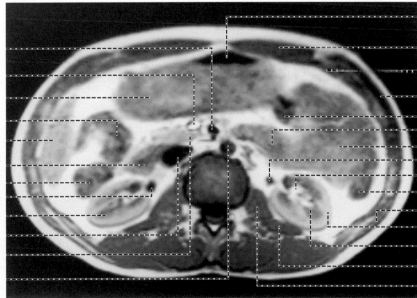

Superior mesenteric a.
Superior mesenteric v.
Stomach, antrum
Colon, hepatic flexure
Liver, right lobe
Duodenum, second portion
Ascending colon
Right renal pelvis
Right kidney
Inferior vena cava
Pancreas, uncinate process
Aorta

Stomach, air
Rectus abdominis m.
Transversus abdominis m.
External oblique m.
Transverse colon
Duodenojejunal junction
Jejunum
Left renal pelvis
Left renal sinus
Descending colon
Latissimus dorsi m.
Left kidney, cortex
Left kidney, medulla
Quadratus lumborum m.
Psoas m.

Figure 12.2.2

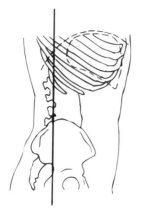

1. This section extends through the thoracic cord, kidneys, and sacroiliac joints.

2. The posterior superior surface of the liver is not covered by the peritoneum and is referred to as the "bare area." It is outlined superiorly and inferiorly by peritoneal reflections, the coronary ligaments.

3. This section extends obliquely through segments of the psoas muscles, the quadratus lumborum, and several of the intertransversarii muscles.

4. The psoas muscle originates from the transverse processes of all the lumbar vertebrae and from the superior and inferior margins of the lower thoracic vertebra and associated discs. The psoas muscle inserts with the tendon of the iliacus muscle onto the lesser trochanter of the proximal femur.

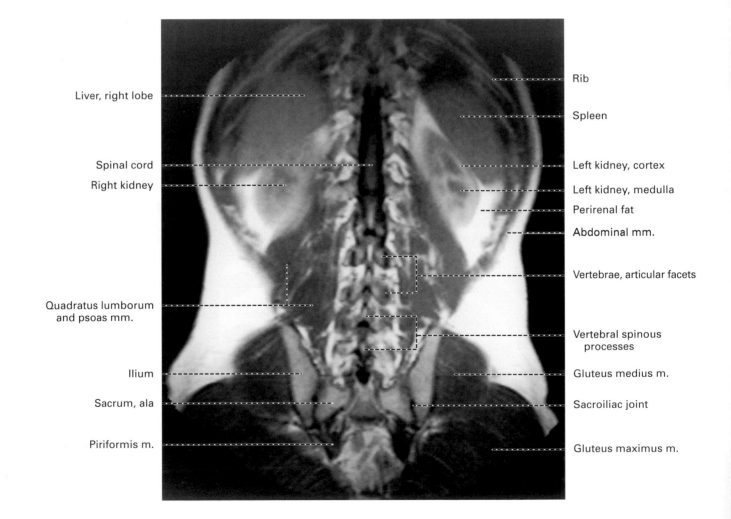

Liver, right lobe

Spinal cord

Right kidney

Quadratus lumborum and psoas mm.

Ilium

Sacrum, ala

Piriformis m.

Rib

Spleen

Left kidney, cortex

Left kidney, medulla

Perirenal fat

Abdominal mm.

Vertebrae, articular facets

Vertebral spinous processes

Gluteus medius m.

Sacroiliac joint

Gluteus maximus m.

1. The right subphrenic space is located between the diaphragm and the superior surface of the right lobe of the liver.

2. The posterior recess of the right subhepatic space (Morrison's pouch) is located between the right kidney and the inferior surface of the liver on this section.

3. The right subphrenic and right subhepatic spaces communicate around the lateral and anterior margins of the liver.

4. The diaphragmatic crura are visualized on this section and extend to the first three lumbar vertebrae on the right and the first two on the left.

5. The superior ligamentous portion of the sacroiliac joint is visualized on this section.

Figure 12.2.3

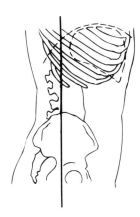

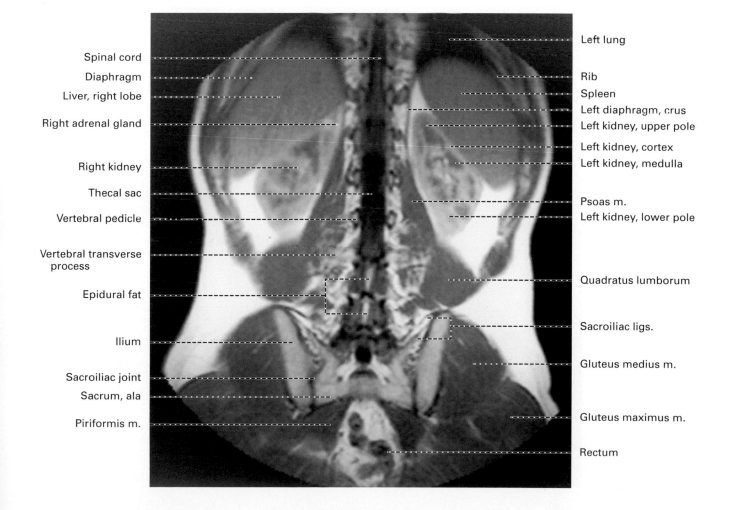

Figure 12.2.4

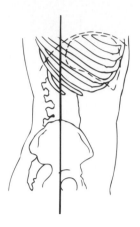

1 This section extends through both kidneys.

2. Corticomedullary differentiation is noted in the kidneys and should be seen in normal kidneys on heavily T1-weighted sequences. High-signal intensity within the renal sinus is secondary to fat.

3. Low-signal intensity is visualized within segments of the renal collecting systems bilaterally and is secondary to the long T1 relaxation associated with normal urine within the collecting systems.

4. The anterior portion of the sacroiliac articulation, the synovial (diarthrodial) portion of the joint, is visualized on this section.

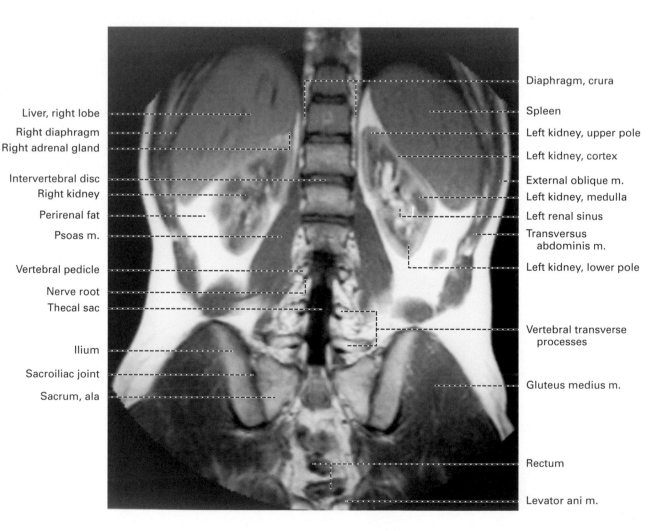

Liver, right lobe
Right diaphragm
Right adrenal gland
Intervertebral disc
Right kidney
Perirenal fat
Psoas m.
Vertebral pedicle
Nerve root
Thecal sac
Ilium
Sacroiliac joint
Sacrum, ala

Diaphragm, crura
Spleen
Left kidney, upper pole
Left kidney, cortex
External oblique m.
Left kidney, medulla
Left renal sinus
Transversus abdominis m.
Left kidney, lower pole
Vertebral transverse processes
Gluteus medius m.
Rectum
Levator ani m.

1. This section extends through the renal hila bilaterally.

2. The adrenal glands are visualized bilaterally within the suprarenal area of the perirenal spaces. The glands have an inverted Y contour.

3. The ascending and descending portions of the colon are visualized bilaterally and lie within the anterior pararenal space.

Figure 12.2.5

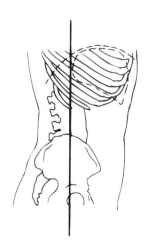

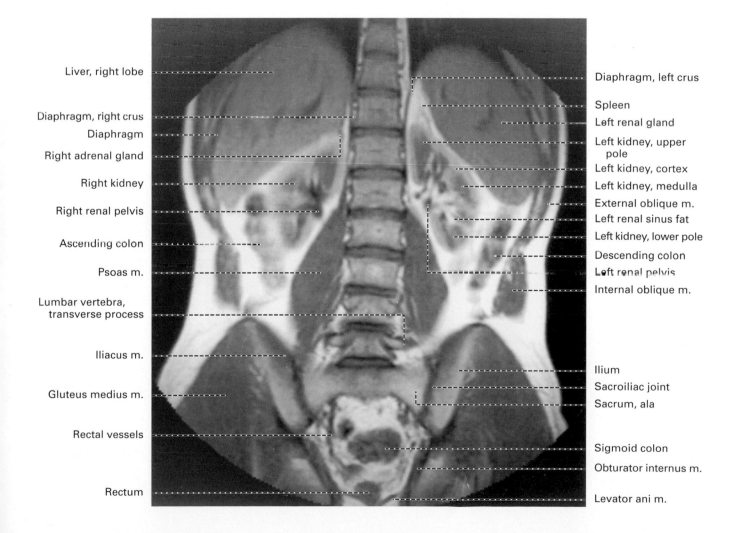

Liver, right lobe

Diaphragm, right crus
Diaphragm

Right adrenal gland

Right kidney

Right renal pelvis

Ascending colon

Psoas m.

Lumbar vertebra,
transverse process

Iliacus m.

Gluteus medius m.

Rectal vessels

Rectum

Diaphragm, left crus

Spleen
Left renal gland
Left kidney, upper
pole
Left kidney, cortex
Left kidney, medulla
External oblique m.
Left renal sinus fat
Left kidney, lower pole
Descending colon
Left renal pelvis
Internal oblique m.

Ilium
Sacroiliac joint
Sacrum, ala

Sigmoid colon
Obturator internus m.

Levator ani m.

Figure 12.2.6

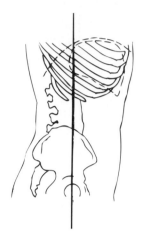

1. The anterior compartment of the right subhepatic space is related to the inferior surface of the liver and the gallbladder superiorly and is related to the hepatic flexure of the colon and the transverse mesocolon inferiorly.

2. The anterior compartment of the right subhepatic space communicates with the right subphrenic space laterally and superiorly and the right paracolic space inferiorly and laterally.

3. The right paracolic space communicates with the pelvis inferiorly, providing a conduit from the pelvis to the right subhepatic and right subphrenic spaces.

4. The left paracolic space is limited superiorly by the phrenicocolic ligament and communicates with the pelvis inferiorly.

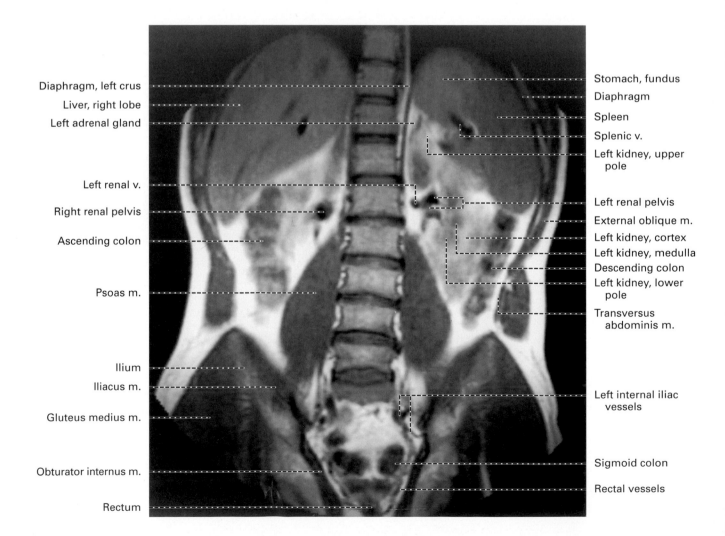

Figure 12.2.7

1. The right hepatic vein is visualized on this section and lies within the right intersegmental fissure, which separates the anterior and posterior segments of the liver.

2. The intrahepatic segment of the inferior vena cava is visualized well on this section; it is defined by the diaphragmatic and visceral surfaces of the liver. (Also see Fig. 12.2.8.)

3. The splenic vessels and the tail of the pancreas are visualized on this section; they lie within the lienorenal ligament.

4. The lateral margins of the distal psoas muscles on this section are outlined by fat in the postpararenal space. The lateral margins of the more cephalad psoas muscles are outlined by perirenal fat.

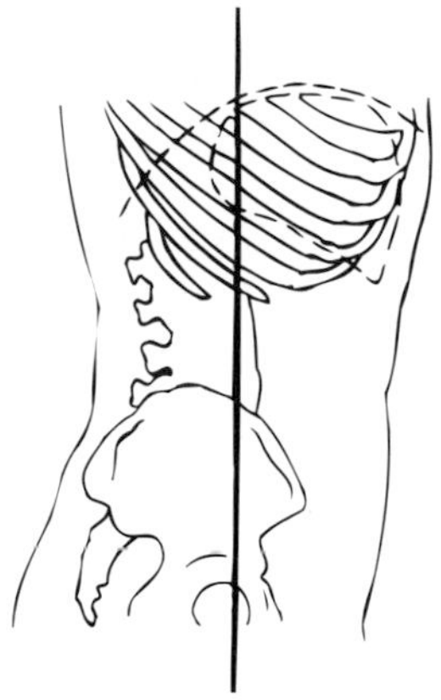

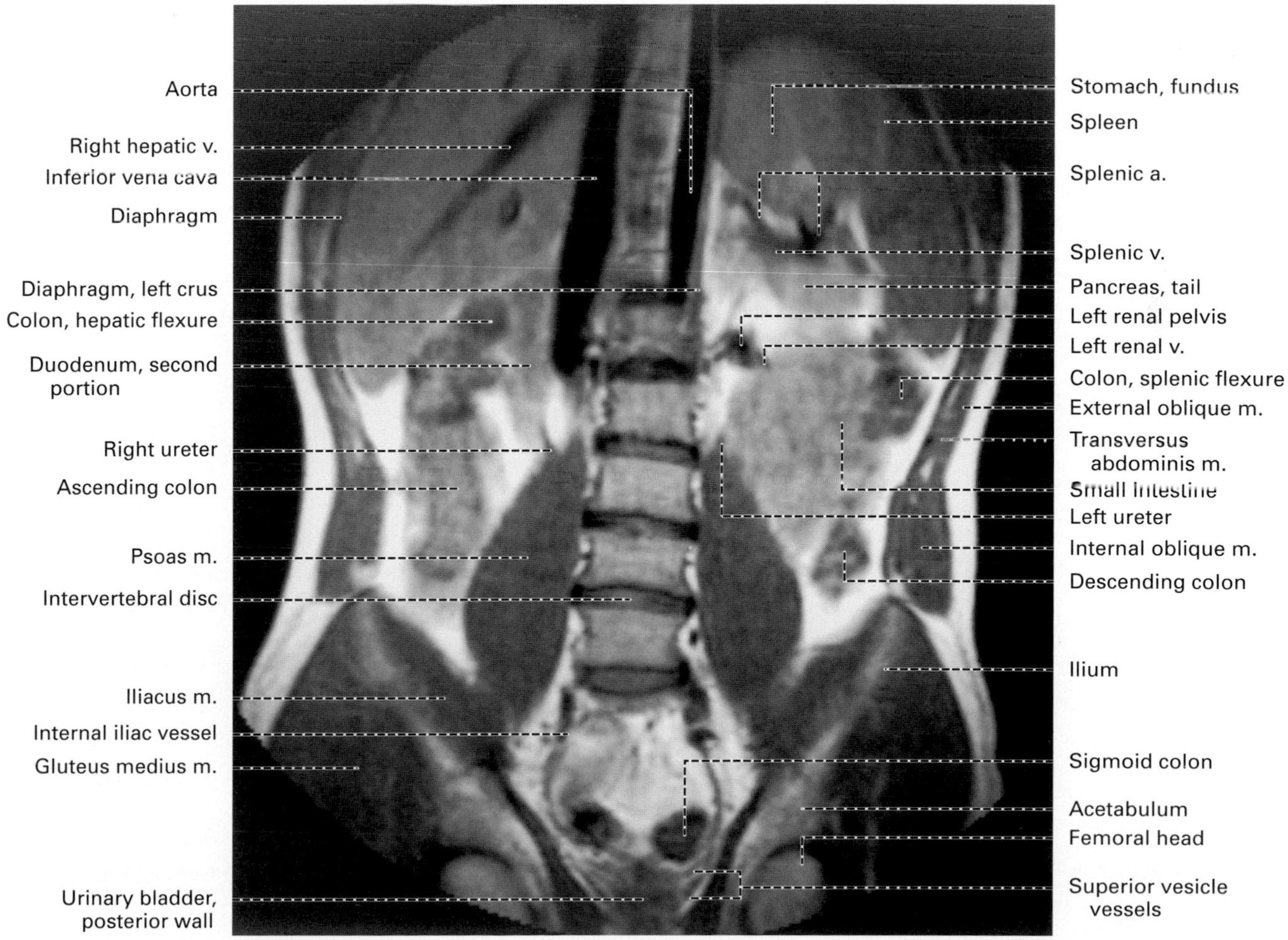
Aorta
Right hepatic v.
Inferior vena cava
Diaphragm
Diaphragm, left crus
Colon, hepatic flexure
Duodenum, second portion
Right ureter
Ascending colon
Psoas m.
Intervertebral disc
Iliacus m.
Internal iliac vessel
Gluteus medius m.
Urinary bladder, posterior wall
Stomach, fundus
Spleen
Splenic a.
Splenic v.
Pancreas, tail
Left renal pelvis
Left renal v.
Colon, splenic flexure
External oblique m.
Transversus abdominis m.
Small intestine
Left ureter
Internal oblique m.
Descending colon
Ilium
Sigmoid colon
Acetabulum
Femoral head
Superior vesicle vessels

Figure 12.2.8

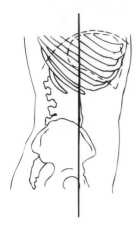

1. The caudate lobe of the liver is visualized medial to the inferior vena cava.

2. The caudate lobe projects into the lessor sac on the right. A superior recess of the sac extends posterior to the caudate lobe and often lies along the right lateral margin of the distal esophagus.

3. The transversus abdominis, the internal oblique, and the external oblique muscles can be identified on this section; they are members of the antero-lateral group of abdominal wall muscles.

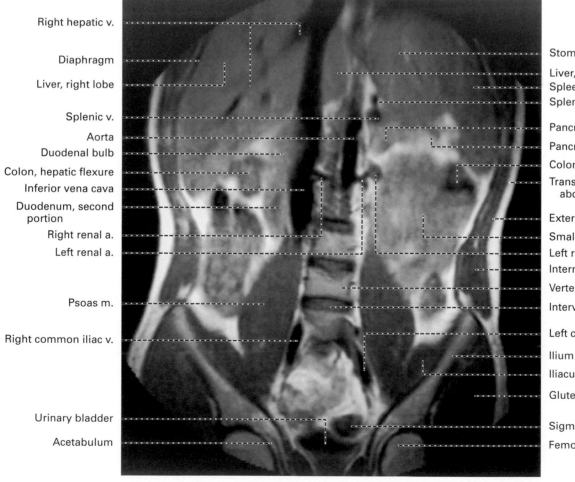

Right hepatic v.

Diaphragm

Liver, right lobe

Splenic v.

Aorta

Duodenal bulb

Colon, hepatic flexure

Inferior vena cava

Duodenum, second portion

Right renal a.

Left renal a.

Psoas m.

Right common iliac v.

Urinary bladder

Acetabulum

Stomach, fundus

Liver, caudate lobe

Spleen

Splenic a.

Pancreas, body

Pancreas, tail

Colon, splenic flexure

Transversus abdominis m.

External oblique m.

Small intestine

Left renal v.

Internal oblique m.

Vertebral body

Intervertebral disc

Left common iliac v.

Ilium

Iliacus m.

Gluteus medius m.

Sigmoid colon

Femoral head

1. The main portal vein is visualized on this section; its proximal segment lies within the porta hepatis and its distal segment descends within the hepatoduodenal ligament of the lesser omentum.

2. The three branches of the celiac axis—the hepatic, left gastric, and splenic arteries—can be identified on this section.

3. The left gastric artery, a branch of the celiac artery, extends superiorly along the lesser curve of the stomach, within the gastrohepatic segment of the lesser omentum.

4. The superior mesenteric artery is the second unpaired branch of the abdominal aorta. It can be seen originating from 0.5 to 2.0 cm below the celiac artery on this section.

5. Just caudal to the superior mesenteric artery, the renal arteries originate from the lateral borders of the aorta usually at the level of the L1 or L2 vertebra.

6. A groove is seen on the inferior surface of the caudate lobe and separates the papillary process medially from the caudate process of the caudate lobe laterally.

Figure 12.2.9

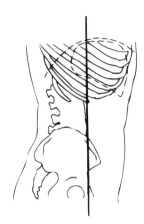

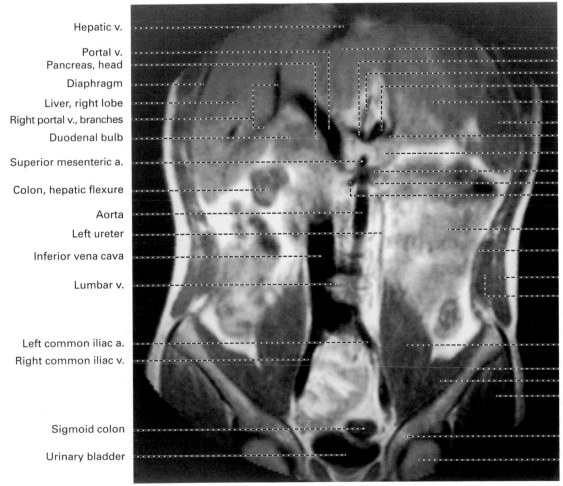

Hepatic v.

Portal v.
Pancreas, head
Diaphragm
Liver, right lobe
Right portal v., branches
Duodenal bulb

Superior mesenteric a.

Colon, hepatic flexure

Aorta
Left ureter
Inferior vena cava

Lumbar v.

Left common iliac a.
Right common iliac v.

Sigmoid colon
Urinary bladder

Liver, left lobe
Common hepatic a.
Left gastric a.
Celiac a.
Stomach, fundus

Spleen
Splenic a.
Pancreas

Left renal v.
Left renal a.
Right renal a.

Small intestine
Transversus abdominis m.
External oblique m.
Internal oblique m.

Psoas m.

Ilium
Iliacus m.
Gluteus medius m.

Acetabulum
Femoral head

Figure 12.2.16

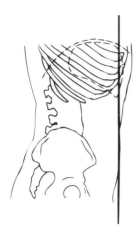

1. This section extends through the anterior thoracic and abdominal walls.

2. Low-signal intensity is noted within the lower thoracic costal cartilage.

3. A transverse tendinous insertion of the rectus abdominis is again noted.

4. The umbilicus is typically located at the level of the aortic bifurcation or at L3 to L4.

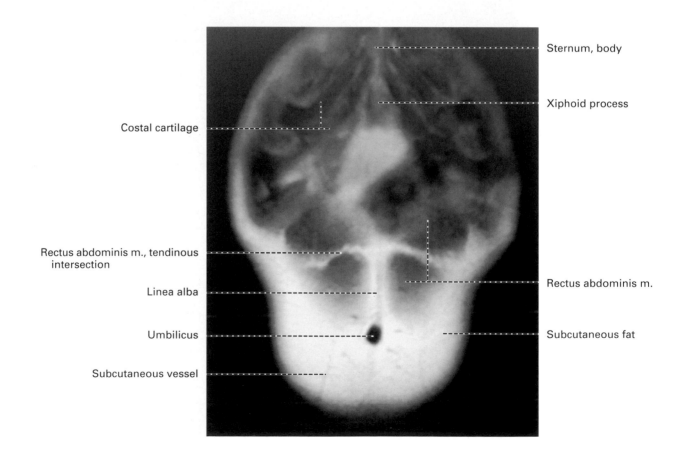

Figure 12.3.1

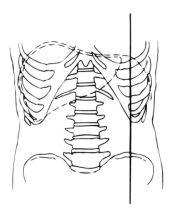

1. This section through the left abdomen extends through the spleen, gastric fundus, and left kidney.

2. The splenic artery and vein are visualized within the posterior substance of the tail of the pancreas.

3. The lesser sac is located anterior to the pancreas and posterior to the stomach. The lesser sac is limited on the left by the phrenicolienal ligament posteriorly and the gastrosplenic ligament anteriorly.

4. The lower part of the phrenicolienal ligament is called the lienorenal ligament; it extends from the splenic hilum to the anterior pararenal fat over the anterior aspect of the left kidney. The tail of the pancreas and the splenic vessels are visualized on this section; they are located between its leaves.

5. The gastrosplenic ligament extends from the greater curvature of the stomach to the splenic hilum on this section and contains the short gastric and left gastroepiploic vessels.

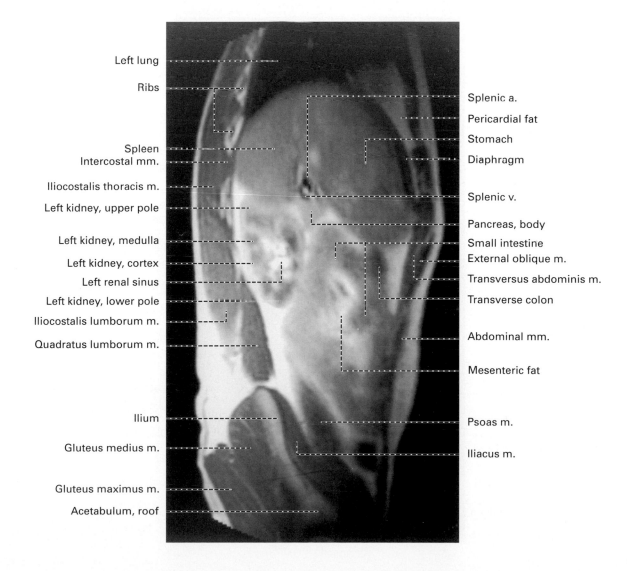

Left lung

Ribs

Spleen
Intercostal mm.

Iliocostalis thoracis m.

Left kidney, upper pole

Left kidney, medulla

Left kidney, cortex

Left renal sinus

Left kidney, lower pole

Iliocostalis lumborum m.

Quadratus lumborum m.

Ilium

Gluteus medius m.

Gluteus maximus m.

Acetabulum, roof

Splenic a.

Pericardial fat

Stomach

Diaphragm

Splenic v.

Pancreas, body

Small intestine
External oblique m.

Transversus abdominis m.

Transverse colon

Abdominal mm.

Mesenteric fat

Psoas m.

Iliacus m.

Figure 12.3.2

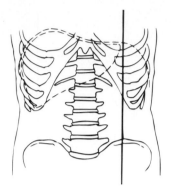

1. This section extends through the erector spinae, quadratus lumborum, iliacus, and psoas muscles posteriorly.

2. The iliocostalis lumborum muscle, the lateralmost component of the erector spinae complex, is seen on this section; it arises from a common origin, the sacrum and iliac bones, and inserts onto the lower six thoracic ribs.

3. The quadratus lumborum muscle attaches to the iliolumbar ligament and adjacent iliac crest inferiorly and to the transverse processes of the upper four lumbar vertebrae and twelfth thoracic rib superiorly.

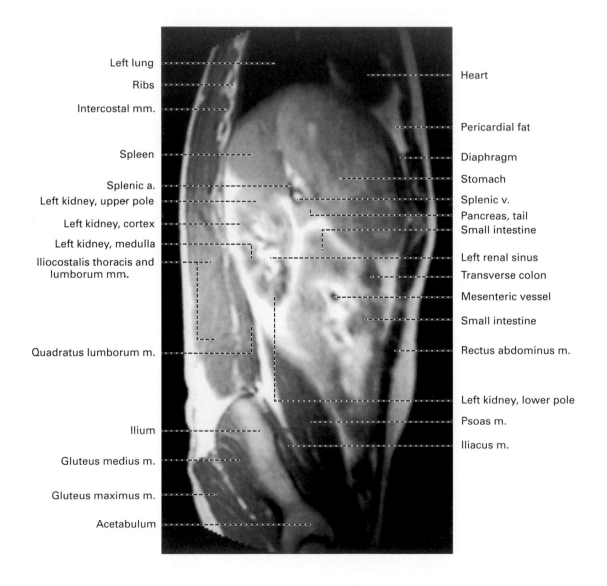

1. This le[...]
creas, [...]

2. The lef[...]
in the [...]

3. The lef[...]
within [...]

4. This se[...]
tor spi[...]
sacrum[...]
sacrosp[...]
ribs an[...]

5. The tra[...]
from th[...]

1. This section passes through the stomach, body of the pancreas, and renal hilum.

2. The body of the pancreas and splenic vessels are retroperitoneal on this section, lying within the anterior pararenal space.

3. The lesser sac is located anterior to the pancreas and posterior to the stomach.

4. The left kidney is noted in the perirenal space of the retroperitoneum. There is normal corticomedullary differentiation and high-signal intensity associated with fat in the renal hilum.

5. The upper pole of the kidney usually lies more posterior and medial than the lower pole as in this case.

Figure 12.3.3

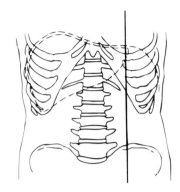

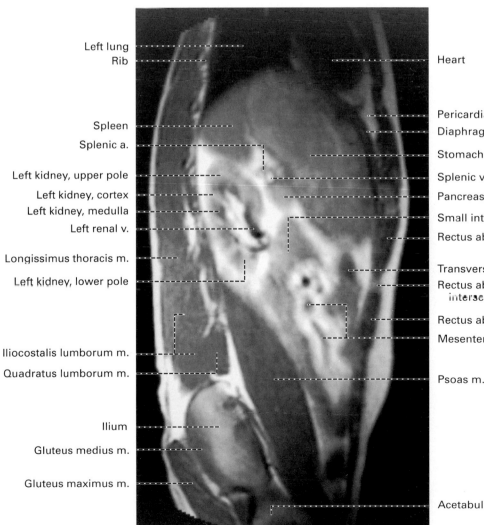

Figure 12.3.16

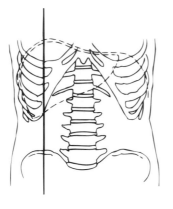

1. This section extends through the liver, right kidney, and hepatic flexure of the colon.

2. Fat is visualized within the proximal gallbladder fossa.

3. The quadrate lobe is defined by the gallbladder fossa and fissure for the ligamentum teres and is contiguous with the medial segment of the liver superiorly.

4. The anterior and posterior branches of the right portal vein are visualized on this section.

5. The ascending and posterior curves of the hepatic flexure of the colon are retroperitoneal and are located within the anterior pararenal space.

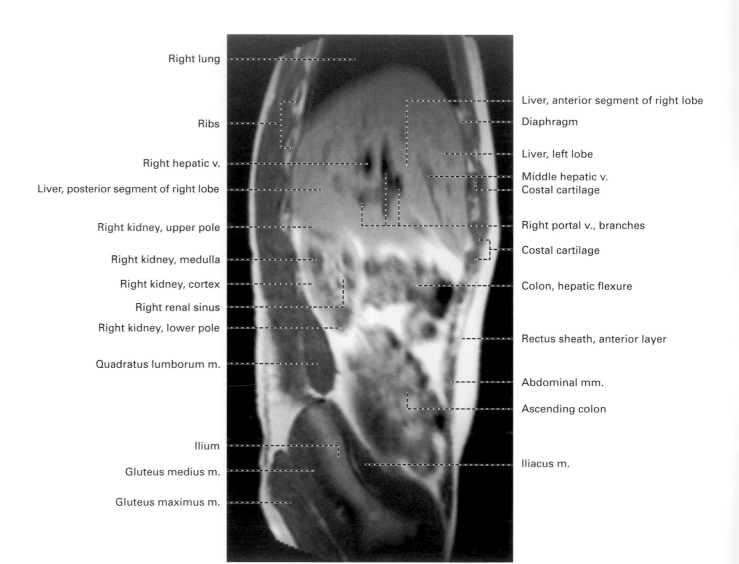

Right lung

Ribs

Right hepatic v.

Liver, posterior segment of right lobe

Right kidney, upper pole

Right kidney, medulla

Right kidney, cortex

Right renal sinus

Right kidney, lower pole

Quadratus lumborum m.

Ilium

Gluteus medius m.

Gluteus maximus m.

Liver, anterior segment of right lobe

Diaphragm

Liver, left lobe

Middle hepatic v.
Costal cartilage

Right portal v., branches

Costal cartilage

Colon, hepatic flexure

Rectus sheath, anterior layer

Abdominal mm.

Ascending colon

Iliacus m.

Chapter 13

FEMALE PELVIS

Introduction

In this section on the female pelvis, the illustrations and discussions are directed exclusively to the pelvic viscera, the peritoneal reflections, and extraperitoneal fascia that are specific to the female pelvis. The abdominal wall muscles, posterior pelvic wall muscles, paraspinous muscles, muscles of the hip, and femoral muscle groups are discussed in the section on the male pelvis.

Loops of small bowel are normally seen in the anterior aspect of the pelvic cavity and are related to the dome of the urinary bladder. The sigmoid colon and rectum including the anal canal are seen within the posterior pelvis. The distal ureters, urinary bladder, and urethra reside in the pelvis. The female reproductive organs including the uterus, ovaries, and vagina are also illustrated.

Peritoneal reflections over the dome of the urinary bladder, uterus, and rectum form the paravesical recesses, the vesicouterine recess, and rectouterine fossa. The cul-de-sac of the rectouterine fossa is limited laterally by peritoneal reflections over the uterosacral ligaments. The peritoneal reflection over the uterus forms the broad ligament, which contains the parametrium, uterine arteries, uterine tubes, uterine and round ligaments, epoophoron, and paroophoron. It is also related to the ureters and ovaries.

The pelvic cavity is limited by the pelvic diaphragm, urogenital diaphragm, and peritoneal structures as in the male. The perineum contains the distal urethra, the vulva, and the anus in the female.

1. This section extends through the uterine fundus and both ovaries. The uterus is retroverted in this subject.

2. The uterus is divided into the body, or corpus, a narrow isthmus, and the cervix. The segment of the corpus that lies above the uterine tubes is called the fundus. The uterus shows homogeneous intermediate-signal intensity on T1-weighted sections.

3. The fallopian tubes (not seen) extend from the superior angle of the uterus to the side of the pelvis. Each is suspended by a mesenteric peritoneal fold, the mesosalpinx.

4. The round ligament of the uterus arises ventral and caudal to the uterine tubes; it passes along the lateral wall of the pelvis, through the inguinal canal, and contributes to the substance of the labia majora.

5. The ovaries are visualized within the ovarian fossae, which are shallow depressions in the pelvic sidewall just below the bifurcation of the iliac vessels. The ovaries will often be displaced or ectopic in parous patients.

6. The ovaries are attached to the broad ligament of the uterus by the meso-varium, to the uterine tube by the ovarian fimbriae, to the pelvic sidewall by the suspensory ligament, and to the uterus by the ligament of the ovary. The ligament of the ovary arises dorsal and caudal to the uterine tube.

Figure 13.1.1

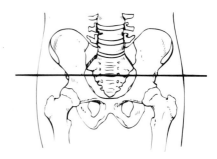

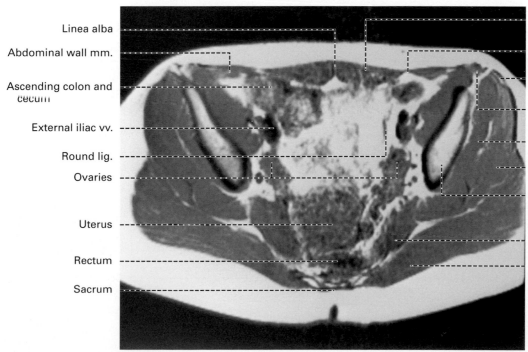

Linea alba

Abdominal wall mm.

Ascending colon and cecum

External iliac vv.

Round lig.

Ovaries

Uterus

Rectum

Sacrum

Rectus abdominis m.

Linea semilunaris

Tensor fasciae latae m.

Sartorius m.

Gluteus minimus m.

Gluteus medius m.

Innominate bone

Piriformis m.

Gluteus maximus m.

Figure 13.1.2

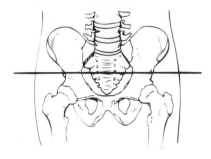

1. This section extends through the uterine corpus and both ovaries.

2. The uterus, ovaries, and adjacent loops of bowel show intermediate-signal intensity on T1-weighted sections and can be difficult to separate from each other.

3. The body of the uterus, or uterine corpus, is seen on this section.

4. The broad ligaments of the uterus are fibrous sheets covered by peritoneum that extend from the sides of the uterus to the floor and sidewall of the pelvis. Together with the uterus they separate the intraperitoneal cavity of the pelvis into the vesicouterine and rectouterine fossae.

5. The broad ligaments of the uterus contain the parametrium, uterine arteries, uterine tubes, proximal round ligaments, epoophoron, and paroophoron. They are also related to the ureters and ovaries.

6. The more distal segment of the round ligament can be visualized coursing along the pelvic sidewall, medial to the external iliac arteries, to exit the pelvis through the inguinal canal on more caudal sections.

7. The proximal rectum is visualized dorsal to the uterus.

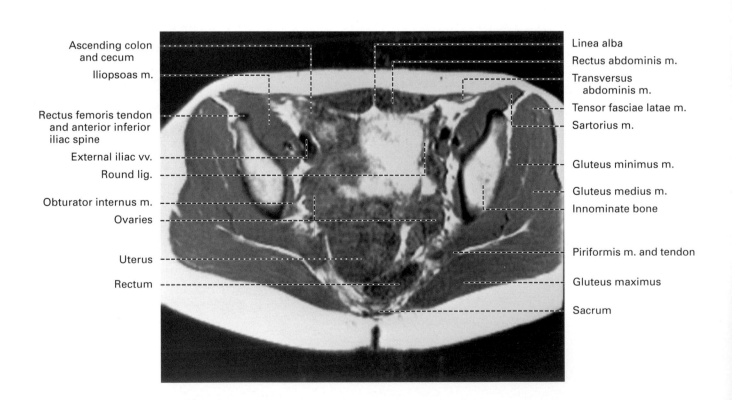

Ascending colon and cecum
Iliopsoas m.
Rectus femoris tendon and anterior inferior iliac spine
External iliac vv.
Round lig.
Obturator internus m.
Ovaries
Uterus
Rectum

Linea alba
Rectus abdominis m.
Transversus abdominis m.
Tensor fasciae latae m.
Sartorius m.
Gluteus minimus m.
Gluteus medius m.
Innominate bone
Piriformis m. and tendon
Gluteus maximus
Sacrum

1. This section extends through the uterine cervix, vaginal fornices, urinary bladder, and rectum.

2. The uterine cervix is divided into a supravaginal segment and the portio cervix, which protrudes into the vaginal vault.

3. The vagina is a muscular tube that extends from the level of the cervix to the perineum. The vagina can be divided anatomically into thirds. The upper third includes the vaginal fornices.

4. Fibrous tissue surrounding the anterior and lateral aspects of the supravaginal cervix is termed the parametrium.

5. The uterine arteries are visualized within the parametrium, lateral to the vaginal fornices and uterine cervix. The uterine arteries enter the uterus at the level of the uterine isthmus. The isthmus represents the junction of the uterine corpus and cervix and is located at the level of the internal cervical os, which can be identified on T2-weighted sections.

6. The peritoneum reflects over the dome of the urinary bladder, then onto the corpus uteri forming the vesicouterine recess.

7. Peritoneum covers the dorsal surface of the uterus and upper vagina. It reflects onto the rectum to form the rectouterine fossa. Peritoneal reflections over the uterosacral ligaments limit the rectouterine fossa bilaterally delineating the true cul-de-sac.

8. The cardinal ligaments (not seen) are fibrous sheets of subserosal fascia that extend from the lateral margins of the lower cervix and vagina to the lateral wall of the pelvis. They represent a deep continuation of the broad ligaments.

Figure 13.1.3

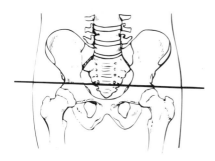

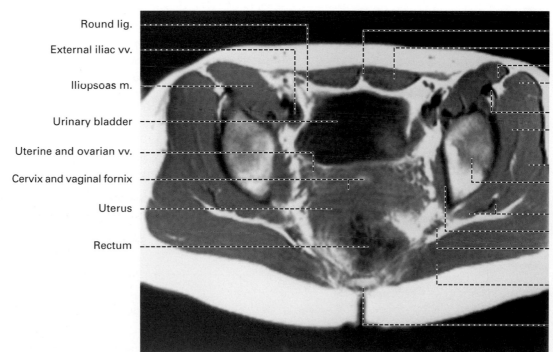

Round lig.
External iliac vv.
Iliopsoas m.
Urinary bladder
Uterine and ovarian vv.
Cervix and vaginal fornix
Uterus
Rectum

Linea alba
Rectus abdominis m.
Sartorius m.
Tensor fasciae latae m.
Rectus femoris tendon
Gluteus minimus m.
Gluteus medius m.
Innominate bone
Piriformis m. and tendon
Obturator internus m.
Superior gluteal vessels and sciatic n.
Gluteus maximus m.
Sacrum

Figure 13.1.4

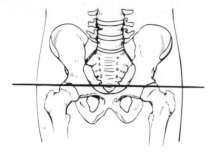

1. This section extends through the urinary bladder, vagina, and distal rectum.

2. The vagina is a muscular tube that extends from the vestibule to the uterine cervix. Reflections of the vagina onto the cervix form the anterior and posterior fornices. The perineal opening of the vagina is called the vestibule.

3. The anterior and posterior walls of the vagina are typically in contact with one another, resulting in a C- or H-shaped contour.

4. The levator ani and coccygeus muscles can be identified posterior and lateral to the vagina and rectum. These muscles form the pelvic diaphragm as well as the principal support for the pelvic organs.

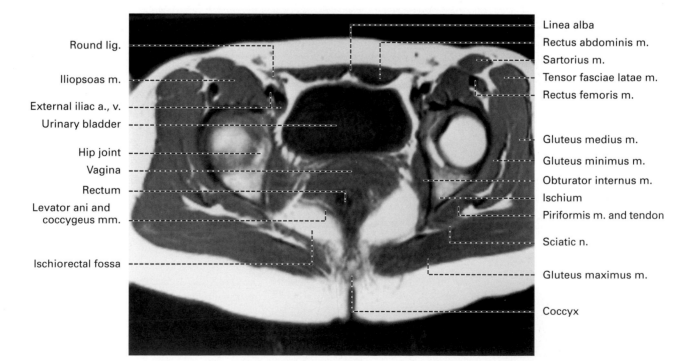

1. This section includes the vagina, urinary bladder, and anus.

2. This section extends through the middle one-third of the vagina, which is usually located at the level of the base of the urinary bladder.

3. The margins of the vagina, anus, and levator ani muscles are not delineated well as each shows intermediate-signal intensity on T1-weighted images, isointense with muscle. The urinary bladder is seen better due to low-signal intensity associated with urine in the bladder lumen.

4. The anal canal begins where the ampulla of the rectum narrows; it is normally 2.5 to 4.0 cm long.

5. The levator ani muscles are bordered bilaterally by fat within the ischiorectal fossae.

Figure 13.1.5

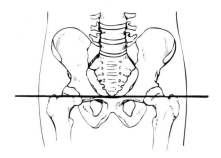

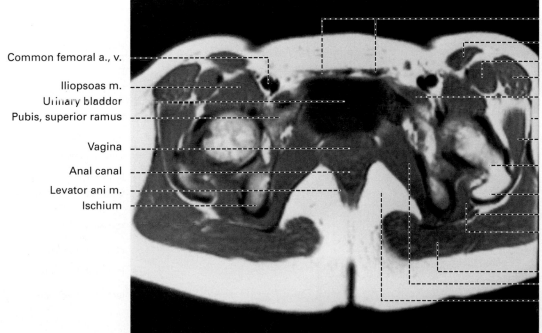

Common femoral a., v.

Iliopsoas m.
Urinary bladder
Pubis, superior ramus

Vagina

Anal canal

Levator ani m.
Ischium

Rectus abdominis m.

Sartorius m.

Rectus femoris m.

Tensor fasciae latae m.

Pectineus m.

Fascia lata

Gluteus medius m. and tendon

Femoral neck

Greater trochanter

Sciatic n.

Inferior gemellus and obturator internus mm., tendon

Gluteus maximus m.
Obturator internus m.

Ischiorectal fossa

Figure 13.1.6

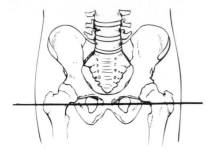

1. This section extends through the vagina, urethra, and anal canal.

2. The female urethra is about 4 cm long. It penetrates the urogenital diaphragm at this level through the genital hiatus.

3. This section extends through the lower one-third of the vagina, which is usually located at the level of the urethra, below the base of the urinary bladder. The lower third of the vagina is distinctive in that disease in this area will often spread along the pudendal chain or into the inguinal area.

4. Anatomic detail of the urethra, vagina, and anal canal is not visible as each of these structures shows homogeneous intermediate-signal intensity on T1-weighted sections.

5. Fat within the ischiorectal fossa outlines the posterior margin of the levator ani muscles.

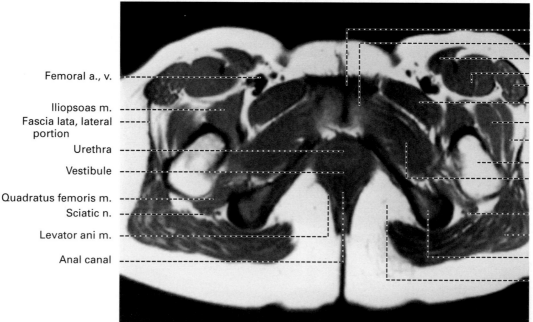

1. This section extends through the perineum, distal urethra, vestibule of the vagina, and distal anal canal.

2. The perineum is an anatomic space superficial to the pelvic and urogenital diaphragm, defined by the pubic arch, tip of the coccyx, inferior rami of the pubis and ischium, and the sacrotuberous ligament.

3. The clitoris is composed of the corpora cavernosa, each of which is attached to the pubic ramus and ischia, and each of which is invested with an ischiocavernosus muscle.

4. The lower end of the vagina is surrounded by the erectile tissue of the bulb of the vestibule.

5. The puborectalis muscular sling is seen around the distal anal canal at this level.

Figure 13.1.7

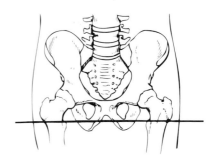

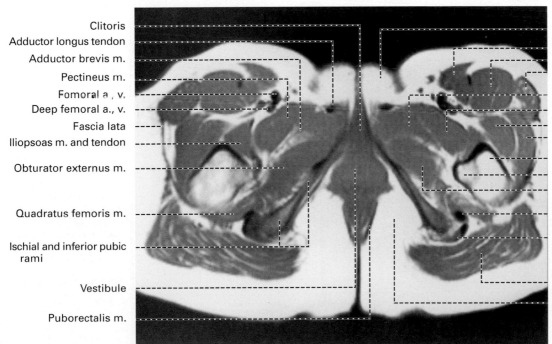

Clitoris	Mons pubis
Adductor longus tendon	Sartorius m.
Adductor brevis m.	Rectus femoris m.
Pectineus m.	Tensor fasciae latae m.
Fomoral a , v.	Adductor brevis m.
Deep femoral a., v.	Pectineus m.
Fascia lata	Vastus intermedius m.
Iliopsoas m. and tendon	Vastus lateralis m.
Obturator externus m.	Femur
	Lesser trochanter
	Obturator externus m.
Quadratus femoris m.	Semimembranosus tendon
Ischial and inferior pubic rami	Semitendinosus and long head of biceps femoris tendons
Vestibule	Gluteus maximus m.
Puborectalis m.	Ischiorectal fossa

Figure 13.1.8

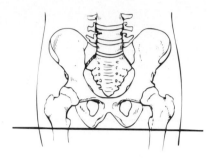

1. This section extends through the perineum.

2. Low-signal intensity is seen with the labia minora.

3. High-signal intensity is seen with fat in the labia majora.

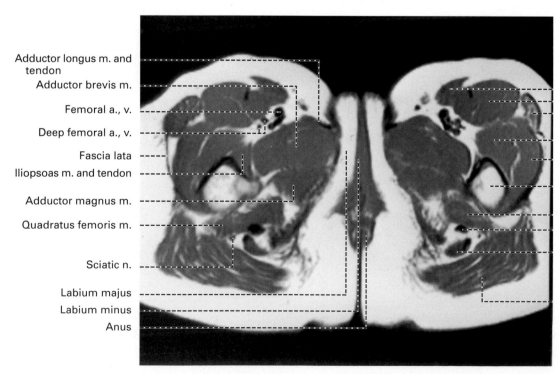

1. This is a T2-weighted section through the pelvis of a suject with an anteverted uterus.

2. This section extends through the posterior aspect of the uterine corpus, the posterior aspect of the uterine cervix, and the ovaries.

3. Intermediate-signal intensity is seen within the peripheral myometrium of the uterine corpus.

4. Low-signal intensity is seen within the posterior cervical stroma.

5. The posterior vaginal fornix inserts into the posterior cervix. It shows low-signal intensity on these images and is difficult to separate from low signal associated with the adjacent cervix and rectum.

6. The ovaries show heterogeneous signal intensity. Foci of high-signal intensity are associated with the presence of prefollicular cysts. The ovarian stroma shows heterogeneous intermediate- to low-signal intensity.

7. The right ovary is seen well on this section. Except for a single prefollicular cyst, the left is difficult to separate from the adjacent sigmoid colon.

8. Low-signal intensity can generally be seen within the bowel wall and is associated with smooth muscle. Signal intensity within the lumen will vary with the contents.

Figure 13.1.9

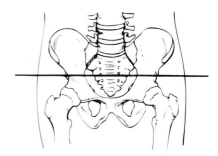

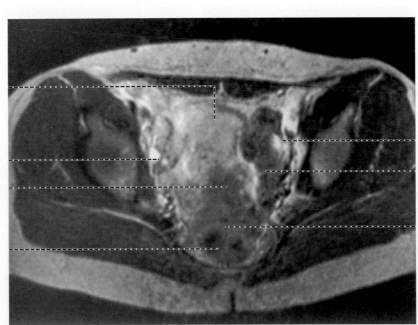

Peripheral myometrium with uterine corpus

Right ovary with follicular and prefollicular cysts

Cervical stroma

Rectum

Prefollicular cysts in left ovary

Sigmoid colon

Vagina, posterior fornix

Figure 13.1.10

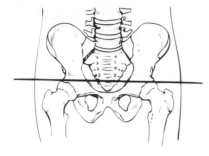

1. This section extends through the anteverted uterus, ovaries, and rectum.

2. The zonal anatomy of the uterus is demonstrated on T2-weighted images. High-signal intensity is seen within the endometrial canal, low-signal intensity within the transitional zone or basal layer of the myometrium, and intermediate-signal intensity within the peripheral myometrium. The appearance of the uterus on these images will vary throughout the menstrual cycle and can be less distinct in postmenopausal patients.

3. Serpiginous foci of increased and decreased signal intensity are seen within the parametrium and are associated with the uterine and ovarian vessels. The uterine vessels enter at the level of the isthmus.

4. The supravaginal segment of the cervix and the portio cervix, which extends into the vaginal vault, can be seen on this section. Either two or three zones of signal intensity can be seen within the cervix on T2-weighted sections.

5. The posterior vagina and lateral insertions of the vagina into the cervix can be seen. Low-signal intensity is seen within the vaginal wall and is associated with the muscular layer of the vaginal wall. With progression of the menstrual cycle through the proliferative phase to the early secretory phase, there are progressive changes in the vagina. There is an increase in the thickness of a central layer of high-signal intensity associated with the mucosal portion of the vaginal wall, and there is an increase in the signal intensity of the muscular portion of the wall.

5. High-signal intensity is seen within two small prefollicular cysts in the right ovary. The intermediate-signal intensity stroma is difficult to discern from intermediate-signal intensity within the parametrium on this section.

6. High-signal intensity is seen within a larger follicular cyst and two small prefollicular cysts in the left ovary. Follicular cysts can normally measure up to 2 cm in diameter. The intermediate-signal intensity stroma can be seen in the left ovary on this section.

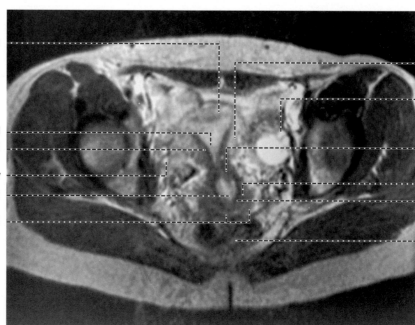

Uterine fundus — Myometrium, peripheral zone — Left ovary — Endometrial canal — Myometrium, junctional zone — Right ovary — Uterine isthmus and internal os — Endocervical canal — Cervical stroma — External os — Vagina, posterior wall — Rectum

1. This section extends through the dome of the urinary bladder, uterus, upper one-third of the vagina, and rectum.

2. Intermediate-signal intensity is seen within the peripheral myometrium of the uterine corpus.

3. Low-signal intensity is seen within the cervical stroma.

4. A focus of high signal within the vaginal vault is most likely related to a nabothian cyst on the portio cervix.

5. Low-signal intensity is seen within the anterior fornix, anterior wall, and posterior wall of the vagina.

Figure 13.1.11

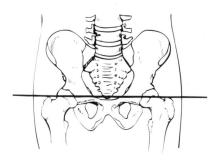

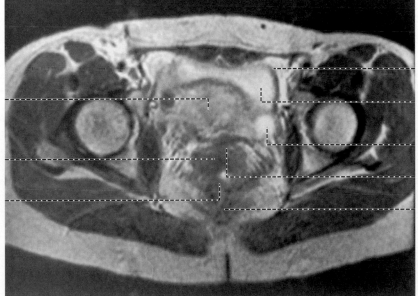

Uterine corpus

Uterine cervix

Vagina, posterior wall

Urinary bladder, muscular wall

Urinary bladder, lumen

Left ovary

Vagina, anterior wall and fornix

Rectum

Figure 13.1.12

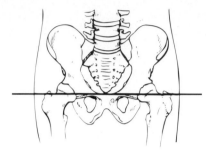

1. This section extends through the urinary bladder, vagina, and rectum.

2. High signal is seen with urine in the bladder lumen on T2-weighted sections. Low-signal intensity is seen within the muscular layer of the bladder wall.

3. Low-signal intensity is seen within the walls of the vagina. Increased signal associated with the mucosal portion of the vaginal wall is minimal on these sections.

4. High signal is seen within the vascular paracolpos.

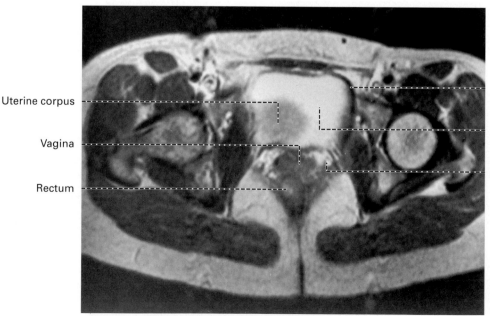

Uterine corpus

Vagina

Rectum

Urinary bladder, muscular wall

Urinary bladder, lumen

Paracolpos vv.

1. This section extends through the base of the urinary bladder, middle one-third of the vagina, and distal rectum.

2. High-signal intensity is again seen with urine in the bladder lumen.

3. Intermediate- to high-signal intensity is seen within the central aspect of the vagina and is associated with the mucosal layer of the vagina and the vaginal contents. Low-signal intensity is again seen with the muscular portion of the vaginal wall.

4. A target pattern of signal intensity is seen within the rectum. There is a central focus of high-signal intensity associated with the rectal mucosa and rectal contents. There is a central ring of low-signal intensity associated with the lamina propria and muscularis mucosa. A peripheral ring of high signal is associated with the submucosal tissue deep to the muscularis mucosa. A more peripheral ring of low signal is associated with the muscularis propria.

5. The low-signal intensity levator ani is outlined by high-signal intensity within the paracolpos and by fat in the ischiorectal fossae.

Figure 13.1.13

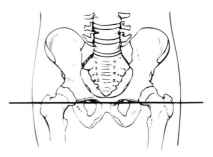

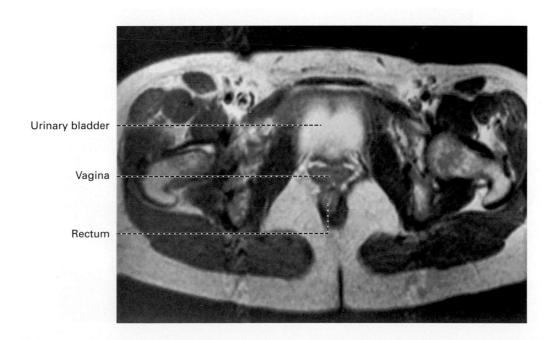

Urinary bladder

Vagina

Rectum

Figure 13.1.14

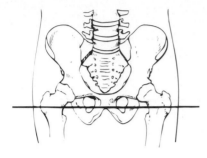

1. This section extends through the urethra, one-third of the vagina, and anus.

2. The urethra shows a targetlike pattern of signal intensity. There is a central focus of low-signal intensity that corresponds to the epithelium, an inner ring of intermediate-signal intensity corresponding to spongy erectile tissue in the submucosal layer, and a peripheral ring of low-signal intensity corresponding to the outer ring of urethral muscle.

3. The lower one-third of the vagina is located at the level of the urethra. The lymphatics arising from the lower vagina will often drain into the pudendal and inguinal areas.

4. A target pattern of signal intensity is seen within the anal canal.

5. Low-signal intensity is seen with the levator ani muscle.

6. Anatomic details at the level of the urethra are delineated on T2-weighted sequences in contrast to those on T1-weighted sections.

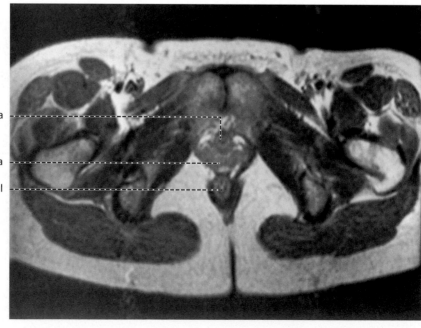

Urethra

Vagina

Anal canal

1. This section extends through the clitoris, distal urethra, introitus, and distal rectum.

2. Both crura of the clitoris are visualized on this section. These show a central area of intermediate- to high-signal intensity associated with the central vascular erectile tissue and a peripheral rim of low-signal intensity associated with the tunica albuginea.

3. A low-signal intensity ring is seen with the distalmost aspect of the urethra.

4. Intermediate-signal intensity is seen within the central aspect of the introitus and is presumably associated with the mucosa and mucosal secretions. Peripheral low-signal intensity is seen with the distal muscularis.

5. Fat is seen within the ischiorectal fossa.

Figure 13.1.15

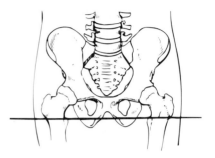

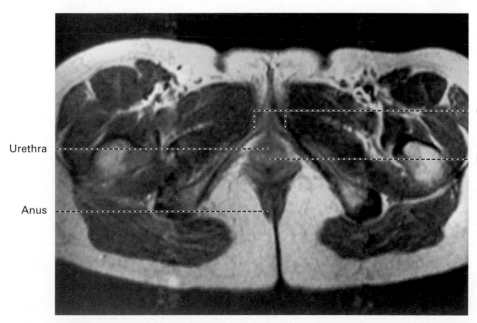

Urethra

Anus

Clitoris, crura

Introitus

Figure 13.2.1

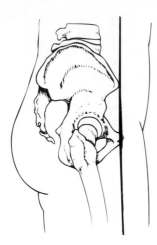

1. This section extends through the most anterior portion of the pelvis.

2. High-signal intensity is seen with fat in the mons pubis.

3. Note the umbilicus, the tendinous insertions of the rectus abdominis muscles, the tendinous origins of the sartorius and tensor fasciae latae muscles, and the superficial epigastric vessels.

4. The inguinal ligament can be seen on this section.

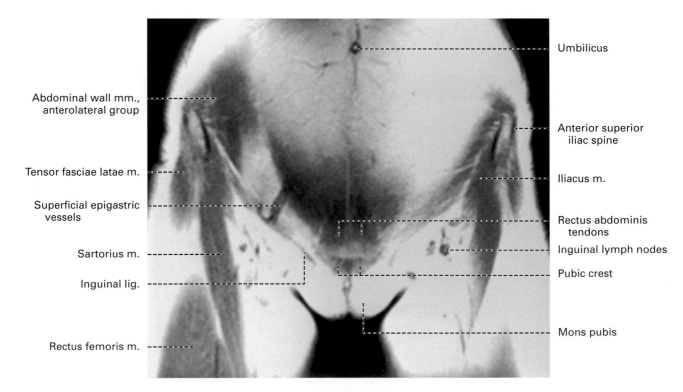

Abdominal wall mm., anterolateral group

Tensor fasciae latae m.

Superficial epigastric vessels

Sartorius m.

Inguinal lig.

Rectus femoris m.

Umbilicus

Anterior superior iliac spine

Iliacus m.

Rectus abdominis tendons

Inguinal lymph nodes

Pubic crest

Mons pubis

1. This section extends through the anterior pelvic cavity and perineum.

2. Intermediate-signal intensity is seen within the clitoris.

3. High signal is seen with fat within the labia majora.

4. Low-signal intensity is seen with urine in the urinary bladder. The dome of the urinary bladder is covered with peritoneum. Laterally, this peritoneum reflects onto the pelvic sidewall, forming the shallow paravesical fossae.

5. Note the cecum, loops of small bowel within the pelvis, the distal iliac and proximal femoral vessels, the iliopsoas muscles, muscles of the gluteal region, and muscles of the anterior and medial femoral compartments.

Figure 13.2.2

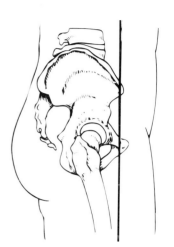

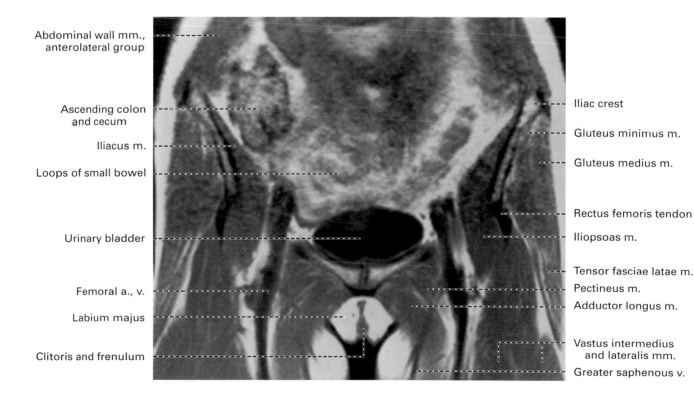

Abdominal wall mm., anterolateral group

Ascending colon and cecum

Iliacus m.

Loops of small bowel

Urinary bladder

Femoral a., v.

Labium majus

Clitoris and frenulum

Iliac crest

Gluteus minimus m.

Gluteus medius m.

Rectus femoris tendon

Iliopsoas m.

Tensor fasciae latae m.

Pectineus m.

Adductor longus m.

Vastus intermedius and lateralis mm.

Greater saphenous v.

Figure 14.1.8B

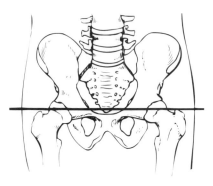

1. This is a T2-weighted section at the same level as the image in Figure 14.1.8A.

2. High-signal intensity is again noted with urine within the urinary bladder.

3. High-signal intensity is also noted with urine within the bladder neck. Low-signal intensity on the margins of the bladder neck is associated with muscle within the bladder floor and internal urethral sphincter.

4. The prostate gland consists primarily of the central and transitional zones at the level of the base. Low-signal intensity is seen within the central aspect of the prostate gland on T2-weighted images, although high-signal intensity nodules can be seen with adenomatous hyperplasia of the transitional zone.

5. The high-signal intensity rim on the periphery of the prostate gland at this level is due in part to visualization of a small portion of the peripheral zone and to partial voluming of the proximal seminal vesicles.

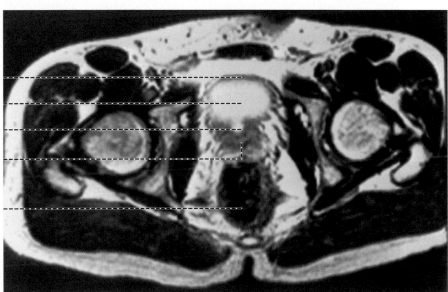

Urinary bladder, muscular wall

Urinary bladder lumen

Urinary bladder neck

Prostate gland, base

Rectum

1. This section extends through the pelvis at the level of the pubic bones, body of the prostate, and coccyx.

2. Posteriorly, the prostate gland is separated from the rectum by the rectovesical fascia of Denonvilliers.

3. The insertions of the gluteus medius and the greater tuberosities are again noted.

4. The extent of the obturator internus muscle is appreciated best on this section. It arises from the inner surface of the anterolateral wall of the pelvis, passes through the lesser sciatic foramen, and inserts onto the anterior part of the medial aspect of the greater tuberosity.

5. The lesser sciatic foramen is defined anteriorly by the tuberosity and body of the ischium, superiorly by the spine of the ischium and the sacrospinous ligament, and posteriorly by the sacrotuberous ligament.

6. The inferior gemellus muscle blends with the obturator internus tendon lateral to the lesser sciatic foramen. The inferior gemellus muscle originates from the tuberosity of the ischium and blends with the tendon of the obturator internus muscle to insert onto the greater tuberosity.

7. The pelvic origins of the medial femoral muscles are visualized on sections through the lower pelvis. These include the pectineus, gracilis, and adductor muscles.

8. The proximal pectineus muscle is seen on this section. It arises from the pectineal line of the pubis and inserts onto the medial aspect of the proximal femur from the lesser trochanter to the linea aspera.

Figure 14.1.9

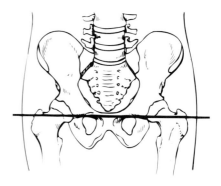

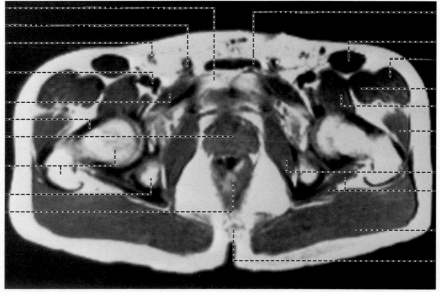

Pubic bone
Spermatic cord
Superficial epigastric a., v.
Common femoral vessels
Pectineus m.
Iliofemoral lig.
Prostate gland
Femoral head and greater tuberosity
Innominate bone
Rectum

Rectus abdominis mm. and tendon
Sartorius m.
Tensor fasciae latae m.
Rectus femoris m.
Iliopsoas m.
Gluteus minimus and medius mm. and tendons
Obturator internus m.
Gemellus mm. and obturator internus tendon
Gluteus maximus
Coccyx

Figure 14.1.10

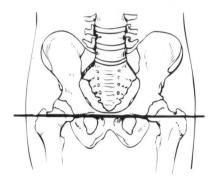

1. This is a T2-weighted image through the pelvis at the level of the body of the prostate.

2. Anatomically, the gland is separated into an anterior fibromuscular zone, a central zone, a transitional zone, and a peripheral zone.

3. Focal high-signal intensity is visualized within the prostatic segment of the urethra in the central aspect of the gland.

4. Low-signal intensity anterior to the urethra corresponds to the fibromuscular zone of the prostate.

5. Intermediate-signal intensity is seen within the central aspect of the prostate gland and corresponds to the transitional and central zones of the prostate. The central and transitional zones of the prostate each show intermediate-signal intensity on T2-weighted images and cannot be distinguished from one another. The central zone does not extend, however, below the level of the verumontanum.

6. High-signal intensity is seen within the normal peripheral zone. This is outlined by a thin low-signal intensity capsule.

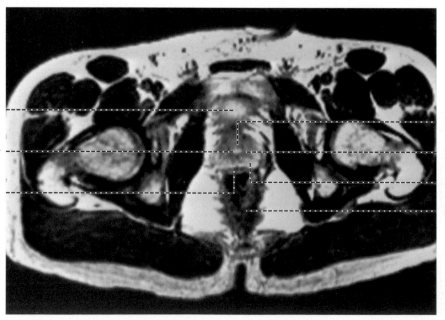

Urinary bladder

Urethra, prostatic segment

Prostatic capsule

Prostate, fibromuscular zone

Prostate, transitional/ central zone

Prostate, peripheral zone

Rectum

1. This section extends through the pelvis at the level of the apex of the prostate gland, pubic symphysis, and ischial tuberosities.

2. Anteriorly, the prostate gland is separated from the pubis by the space of Retzius, which contains fat and the prostatic venous plexus of Santorini.

3. This anal canal is seen within the posterior pelvis. It is normally 2.5 to 4.0 cm long beginning where the ampulla of the rectum narrows, at about the level of the apex of the prostate in males.

4. The suspensory ligament of the penis is visualized on this section.

5. The obturator externus muscle is seen at this level. It originates from the anterior pelvis and obturator membrane, passes behind the neck of the femur, and inserts onto the trochanteric fossa of the femur.

6. The pelvic diaphragm is a muscular sling that encloses the abdominopelvic cavity inferiorly; together with the urogenital diaphragm and perineal structures, it supports the pelvic viscera.

7. The levator ani muscles form the principal part of the pelvic diaphragm. They arise from the pubis, the obturator fascia, and the ischial spines, and insert posteriorly onto the lower two segments of the coccyx, the anococcygeal raphe, the external anal sphincter, and the perineal body. The medial aspects of the levator ani muscles outline a midline opening, the genital hiatus, through which the urethra and anal canal exit.

Figure 14.1.11

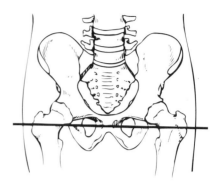

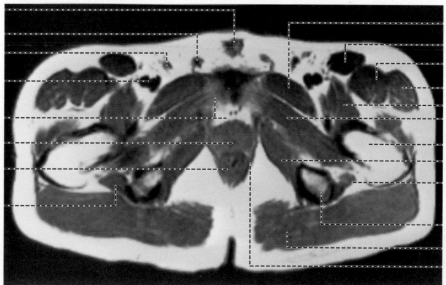

Suspensory lig.
Spermatic cord
Superficial epigastric a., v.
Common femoral a., v.
Pubic bone and retropubic space of Retzius
Prostate gland
Anal canal
Inferior gemellus m.

Pectineus m.
Sartorius m.
Rectus femoris m.
Tensor fasciae latae m.
Iliopsoas m.
Obturator externus m.
Femur
Obturator internus m.
Inferior gemellus and quadratus femoris mm.
Ischial tuberosity
Gluteus maximus m.
Levator ani m.

Figure 14.1.12

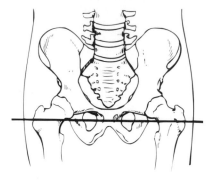

1. This is a T1-weighted image through the apex of the prostate gland.

2. The urethra is visualized within the central aspect of the gland and is surrounded anteriorly by the low-signal intensity fibromuscular zone, and both laterally and posteriorly by the high-signal intensity peripheral zone.

3. Low-signal intensity is seen within the muscular walls of the anal canal.

4. The levator ani muscles are outlined posteriorly by high signal associated with fat within the ischiorectal fossae.

5. The ischiorectal fossa is an anatomic space delimited anteriorly by the posterior borders of the transverse perinei superficialis and profundus muscles, posteriorly by the gluteus maximus muscle and sacrotuberous ligament, laterally by the obturator internus muscle and ischial tuberosity, and medially by the pelvic diaphragm and external anal sphincter muscles.

6. The ischiorectal fossa contains fat, the inferior rectal vessels and nerves, and the internal pudendal vessels.

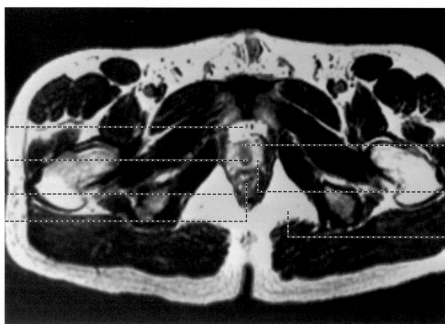

Retropubic space of Retzius

Urethra, prostatic segment

Levator ani m.

Anal canal

Prostate gland, fibromuscular zone

Prostate gland, peripheral zone

Ischiorectal fossa

1. This section extends through the lower margin of the pubis, the membranous urethra, and the ischial tuberosities.

2. The insertions of the iliopsoas muscles onto the lesser trochanter are seen on this and subsequent sections.

3. The origins of the adductor muscles (longus, brevis, and magnus) are seen on this section.

4. The adductor muscles originate from the pubis and inferior pubic ramus and insert onto the medial aspect of the femur.

5. The levator ani muscles and ischiorectal fossae are noted again.

6. The proximal origin of the vastus lateralis can be seen on this section. This muscle belongs to the anterior femoral group, which also includes the sartorius, rectus femoris, vastus intermedius, and vastus medialis muscles.

Figure 14.1.13

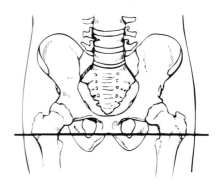

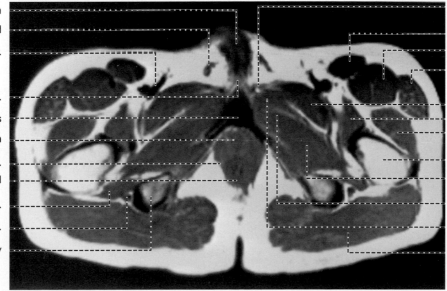

Penis, dorsum
Spermatic cord
Common femoral a., v.

Penis, suspensory lig.
Pubic symphysis
Membranous urethra

Levator ani m.
Anal canal

Quadratus femoris m.

Sciatic n.

Ischial tuberosity

Adductor longus tendon
Sartorius m.
Rectus femoris m.
Tensor fasciae latae m.
Pectineus m.
Iliopsoas m.
Vastus lateralis m.
Femur
Obturator externus m.
Adductor magnus m.
Adductor brevis m.
Gluteus maximus m.

Figure 4.1.14

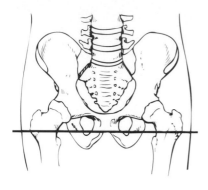

1. This is a T2-weighted section through the membranous urethra.

2. The membranous urethra shows a zonal pattern of signal intensity: a central low-signal intensity dot corresponds to the epithelium, an intermediate ring of higher signal intensity to submucosa, and a peripheral ring of low-signal intensity to the outer striated muscle.

3. The anal canal shows a more complex targetlike pattern of signal intensity: a central focus of low-signal intensity corresponding to the contents of the lumen, a central intermediate-signal intensity ring to the mucosa and secretions, a central ring of low-signal intensity to the muscularis mucosa, an outer ring of intermediate-signal intensity to the submucosa, and a peripheral low-signal intensity ring to the muscularis propria.

4. High-signal intensity is seen within the corpora cavernosa of the penis.

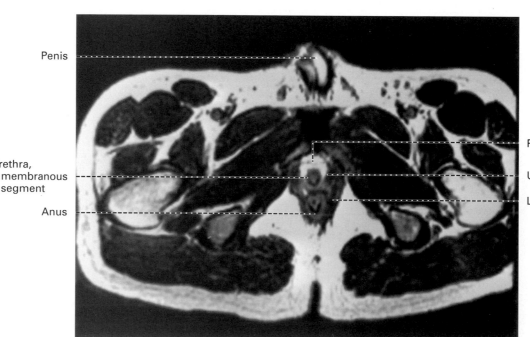

1. This section extends through the urogenital diaphragm and ischial rami.

2. The medial femoral muscles can be identified on this section. From front to back these are the adductor longus, adductor brevis, and adductor magnus muscles medially and the pectineus muscle laterally.

3. The common tendinous origin of the hamstring muscles from the ischial tuberosity is seen. These muscles and tendons can be separated on more caudal sections.

4. The transverse perinei superficialis muscles can be identified on this section; they mark the posterior margin of the urogenital diaphragm.

5. The urogenital diaphragm, or deep perineal compartment, is defined by the superior and inferior fascia of the urogenital diaphragm and contains the transverse perinei profundus muscle. It also contains the sphincter urethrae, the membranous portion of the urethrae, the bulbourethral glands, internal pudendal vessels, and the deep dorsal vein and dorsal nerve of the penis.

6. The perineal body is the central tendinous point of the perineum. It is a fibromuscular mass located between the bulb of the penis, anus, and transverse perinei muscles.

7. The corpora cavernosa penis and ischiocavernosus muscles are seen on this section and are discussed with Figure 14.1.16.

8. The origin of the superficial epigastric vessels from the femoral vessels can be seen on this section.

Figure 14.1.15

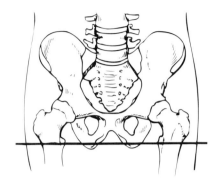

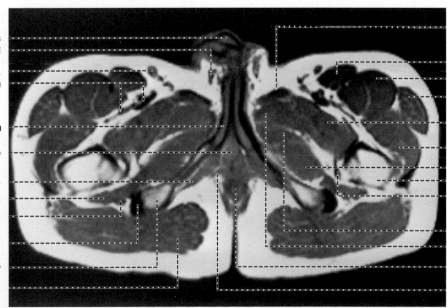

Penis
Spermatic cord

Great saphenous v.
Femoral a., v., with
proximal deep
femoral a.

Corpora cavernosum
penis
Penis, bulb

Ischial cavernosus m.
Quadratus femoris m.
Sciatic n.
Posterior femoral
mm., tendinous
origin
Ischial tuberosity

Gluteus maximus m.

Adductor longus m.

Sartorius m.
Rectus femoris m.
Tensor fasciae latae
m.
Pectineus m.

Vastus lateralis m.

Obturator externus m.
Femur
Medial femoral
circumflex vessel

Adductor magnus m.
Adductor brevis m.

Anal canal

Transverse perinei
superficialis m.

Figure 14.1.16

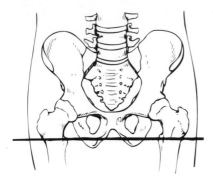

1. This T2-weighted image extends through the urogenital diaphragm and penis.

2. The penis is composed of two lateral masses, the corpora cavernosa penis, and a median mass, the corpus spongiosum penis.

3. The corpora cavernosa penis are visualized well on these sections. They show intermediate- to high-signal intensity on T2-weighted sections in the normal subject. They are enclosed by a low-signal intensity capsule, the tunica albuginea, and by Buck's fascia; these structures cannot be separated on MRI.

4. Proximally, the corpora cavernosa penis are enclosed by the ischiocavernosus muscles.

5. The spongiose segment of the male urethra can be seen as a central ring of intermediate-signal intensity within the superior aspect of the bulb of the penis.

6. The male urethra is usually 17.5 to 120 cm long and is divided into the prostatic, membranous, and spongiose segments.

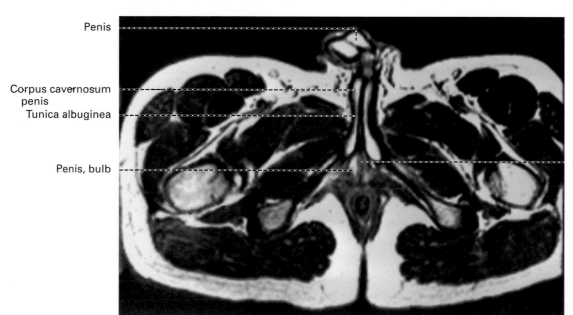

Penis

Corpus cavernosum penis

Tunica albuginea

Penis, bulb

Urethra, spongiose segment

1. This section is at the level of the perineum or superficial perineal compartment and includes the bulb of the penis, the ischial rami, and the lesser trochanter of the femur.

2. The superficial perineal compartment contains the bulbospongiosus body and muscle, the ischiocavernosus bodies and muscles, the transverse perinei superficialis muscle, and the perineal vessels and nerves.

3. The biceps femoris, semitendinosus, and semimembranosus are seen just caudal to the ischial tuberosities. They all originate on the tuberosity of the ischium and contribute to extension of the hip and knee.

4. The spermatic cords are visualized on Figures 14.1.9 through 14.1.18; they are composed of the cremasteric muscles, the ductus deferens, the arteries of the ductus and testes, and the pampiniform venous plexus.

5. The quadratus femoris muscles are seen on this section. They originate from the upper external border of the ischial tuberosity and insert onto a small tubercle on the posterior aspect of the femur.

6. The most proximal origin of the vastus intermedius is seen on this section.

Figure 14.1.17

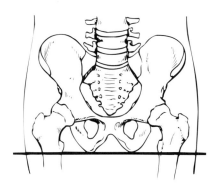

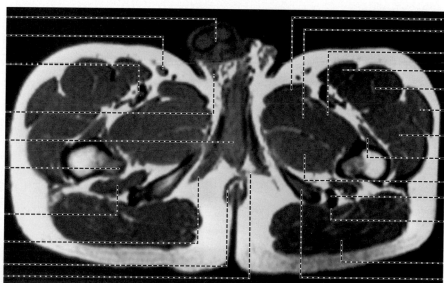

Penis
Greater saphenous v.
Superficial femoral a., v.
Spermatic cord
Penis, corpus spongiosum
Proximal femur, lesser trochanter
Quadratus femoris m.
Ischial cavernosus m.
Anal canal
Perineum, superficial transverse m.

Adductor longus m.
Adductor brevis m.
Pectineus m.
Sartorius m.
Rectus femoris m.
Tensor fasciae latae m.
Vastus lateralis m.
Vastus intermedius m.
Adductor magnus m.
Semimembranosus tendon
Semitendinosus and biceps femoris tendons
Gluteus maximus m.
Ischial ramus

Figure 14.2.3

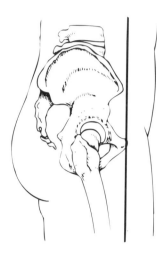

1. This section extends through the anterior pelvis at the level of the common femoral vessels and pubis.

2. Several loops of bowel are visualized within the pelvic cavity. Loops of small bowel, the cecum, and sigmoid colon are normally found within the pelvis.

3. The tendinous origin of the tensor fasciae latae muscle from the anterior iliac crest is seen on this section. It inserts distally into the iliotibial tract of the fascia lata.

4. The pubic crest and the most anterior aspect of the origin of the pectineus muscle from the pectin pubis can be seen.

5. The origins of the inferior epigastric and deep circumflex iliac vessels from the external iliac vessels can be seen, as can the femoral vessels distal to the inguinal ligament.

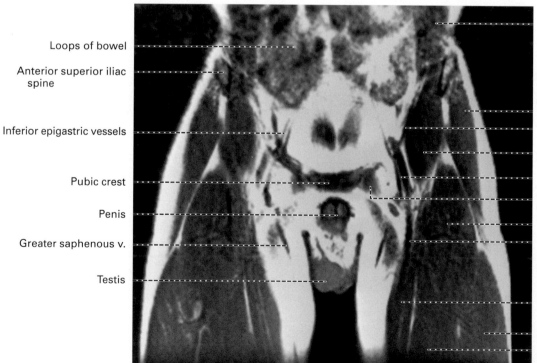

Loops of bowel

Anterior superior iliac spine

Inferior epigastric vessels

Pubic crest

Penis

Greater saphenous v.

Testis

Abdominal wall mm.

Tensor fasciae latae m.

Deep circumflex iliac vessels
Iliopsoas m.

Common femoral vessels

Pectineus m.

Rectus femoris m.

Femoral a.

Sartorius m.

Vastus lateralis m.

Vastus intermedius m.

1. This section extends through the anterior pelvic cavity, pubis, and urinary bladder.

2. Loops of small bowel and the cecum are visualized within the pelvic cavity. The cecum usually lies within the right iliac fossa or the true pelvis. It is enveloped entirely by peritoneum, although in 5 percent it is attached posteriorly to the iliac fascia by connective tissue.

3. This section extends through the iliacus muscle and the iliopsoas muscle as it exits the pelvic cavity.

4. The pectineus and adductor longus muscles of the medial thigh can be seen.

5. The pectineus muscle arises from the pectineal line of the pubis and inserts onto the medial aspect of the proximal femur from the lesser trochanter to the linea aspera.

6. The adductor longus muscle is the most anterior of the three adductor muscles. It arises by a flat narrow tendon (see axial sections) from the anterior pubis and courses inferiorly, posteriorly, and laterally within the medial thigh to insert onto the linea aspera of the middle one-third of the femur.

7. The distal aspect of the external iliac vessels and the proximal femoral vessels are again noted.

Figure 14.2.4

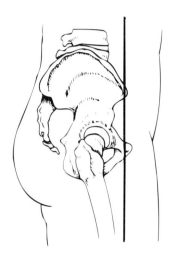

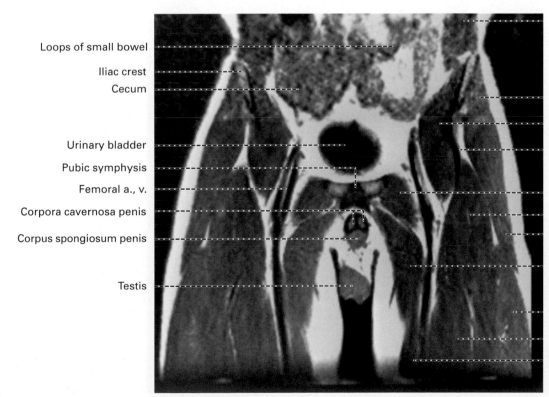

Figure 14.2.5

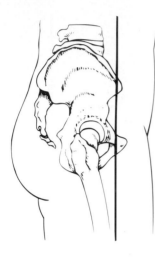

1. This section extends through the anterior pelvic cavity at the level of the anterior inferior iliac spine, with visualization of the urinary bladder and pubic symphysis.

2. Loops of small bowel, the cecum, and ascending colon are noted in the pelvic cavity.

3. The tendinous origin of the rectus femoris muscle from the anterior inferior iliac spine can be seen. The rectus femoris muscle courses along the anterior aspect of the thigh and contributes to the quadriceps tendon.

4. The most anterior origins of the gluteus medius and gluteus minimus muscles from the iliac crest and iliac fossa can be seen.

5. The proximal origins of the pectineus and adductor longus muscles are seen again.

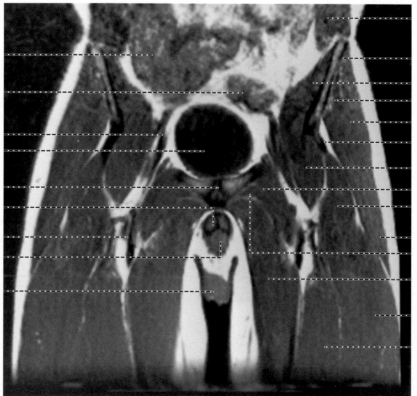

Cecum and ascending colon

Sigmoid colon

External iliac a., v.
Urinary bladder

Pubic symphysis

Corpus cavernosum penis

Deep femoral a., v.

Corpus spongiosum

Testis

Anterolateral abdominal wall mm.

Iliac bone

Iliacus m.
Gluteus minimus m.

Gluteus medius m.
Rectus femoris tendon

Iliopsoas m.

Pectineus m.
Rectus femoris m.

Tensor fasciae latae m.
Obturator externus m.

Adductor longus m.

Vastus lateralis m.

Vastus intermedius m.

1. This section extends through the anterior pelvic cavity, the urinary bladder, and the base of the penis.

2. The psoas muscle, iliacus muscle, and combined iliopsoas muscle course over the anterior hip joint.

3. The proximal portions of the medial femoral muscles are noted. The anteriormost origin of the adductor brevis muscle from the ischial ramus is seen. The pectineus, adductor longus, and adductor magnus muscles are identified in the more distal thigh.

4. The most anterior aspect of the origin of the obturator externus muscle from the ischial ramus, ischial tuberosity, and obturator membrane is seen. The obturator externus muscle courses laterally to insert onto the trochanteric fossa of the femur.

5. Several anterior femoral muscles are noted. The reflected tendon of the proximal rectus femoris is seen above the lateral acetabulum. The vastus intermedius and vastus lateralis muscles are seen in the more distal thigh.

6. The external iliac vessels are seen medial to the psoas muscles. The femoral vessels are located between the anterior medial groups of thigh muscles.

Figure 14.2.6

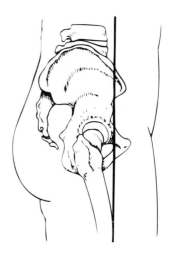

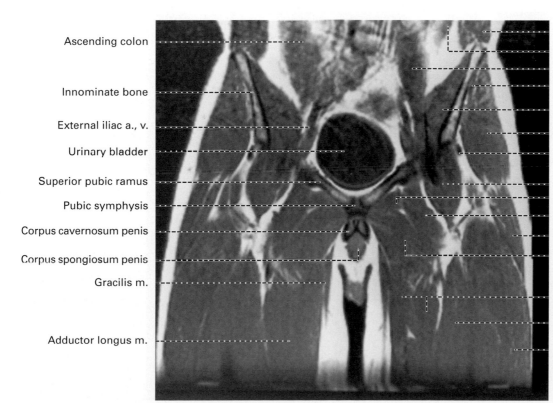

Ascending colon

Innominate bone

External iliac a., v.

Urinary bladder

Superior pubic ramus

Pubic symphysis

Corpus cavernosum penis

Corpus spongiosum penis

Gracilis m.

Adductor longus m.

Abdominal wall mm.

Descending colon

Psoas m.

Gluteus minimus m.

Iliacus m.

Gluteus medius m.

Rectus femoris m., reflected tendon

Iliopsoas m.

Obturator externus m.

Pectineus m.

Tensor fasciae latae m.

Adductor brevis m.

Adductor longus m.

Vastus intermedius m.

Vastus lateralis m.

Figure 14.2.7

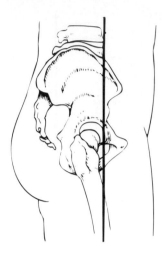

1. This section extends through the pelvic cavity in the coronal plane at the level of the anterior acetabulum.

2. Anterolateral abdominal wall muscles can be seen at the superior margin of the figure.

3. The psoas major and iliacus muscles form the posterior muscular wall of the pelvis.

4. Several of the medial femoral muscles are seen, including the pectineus, adductor brevis, adductor longus, and gracilis muscles. The gracilis muscle arises from the lower part of the body of the pubis and inserts onto the medial aspect of the proximal tibia as part of the pes anserinus.

5. Several of the anterior femoral muscles are seen, including the vastus intermedius and lateralis muscles.

6. The obturator externus, gluteus medius, and gluteus minimus muscles of the gluteal region are noted.

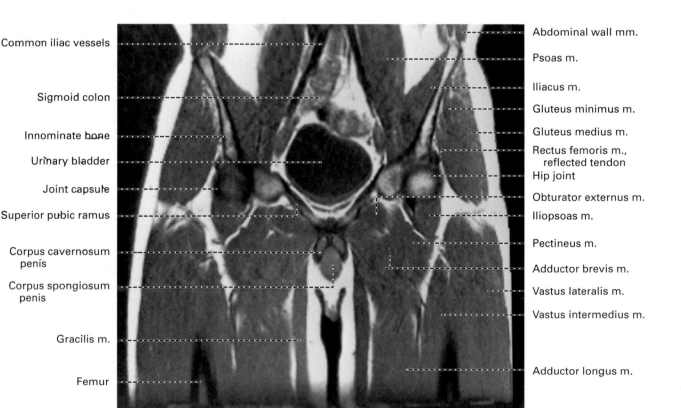

Common iliac vessels

Sigmoid colon

Innominate bone

Urinary bladder

Joint capsule

Superior pubic ramus

Corpus cavernosum penis

Corpus spongiosum penis

Gracilis m.

Femur

Abdominal wall mm.

Psoas m.

Iliacus m.

Gluteus minimus m.

Gluteus medius m.

Rectus femoris m., reflected tendon

Hip joint

Obturator externus m.

Iliopsoas m.

Pectineus m.

Adductor brevis m.

Vastus lateralis m.

Vastus intermedius m.

Adductor longus m.

1. This section extends through the urinary bladder, the obturator foramen, and the hip joints.

2. Except for a small groove at the top, the obturator foramen is covered by the fibrous obturator membrane. This membrane is outlined medially by the lateral border of the obturator internus muscle and laterally by the medial border of the obturator externus.

3. The most anterior portion of the levator ani muscle is seen. The levator ani muscles form the principal component of the pelvic diaphragm or pelvic floor. They arise from the posterior aspect of the pubis, the inner surface of the ischial spines, and tendinous arches connecting the two. The pelvic diaphragm is perforated by the urethra and anus through the genital hiatus.

4. The anterior aspect of the urogenital diaphragm can be seen on this section. It spans the space between the ischial rami and contains the transverse perinei profundus muscle.

5. The urinary bladder rests on the pelvic diaphragm. It is supported by the pelvic diaphragm, by the urogenital diaphragm, and by structures in the perineum.

6. Low-signal intensity on the inferior margins of the corpora cavernosa penis and corpus spongiosum penis is seen.

7. The intermediate-signal intensity band within the superior joint space of the hip corresponds primarily to hyaline cartilage over the superior acetabulum.

Figure 14.2.8

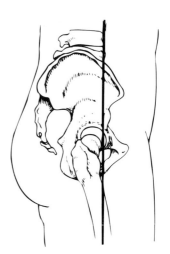

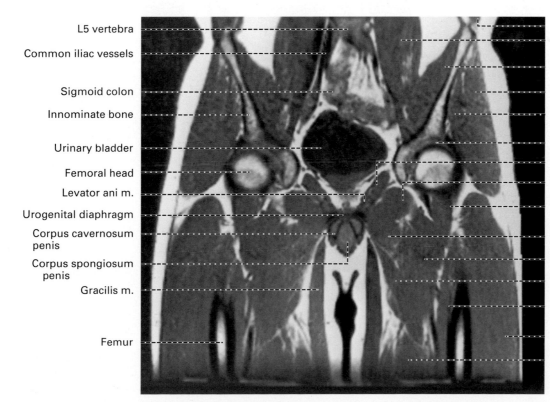

L5 vertebra	Abdominal wall mm.
Common iliac vessels	Psoas m.
	Iliacus m.
Sigmoid colon	Gluteus medius m.
Innominate bone	Gluteus minimus m.
Urinary bladder	Hip joint
Femoral head	Obturator internus m.
Levator ani m.	Obturator externus m.
Urogenital diaphragm	Iliopsoas m.
Corpus cavernosum penis	Adductor magnus m.
Corpus spongiosum penis	Adductor brevis m.
Gracilis m.	Adductor magnus m.
	Vastus intermedius m.
	Vastus lateralis m.
Femur	Adductor longus m.

Figure 14.2.9

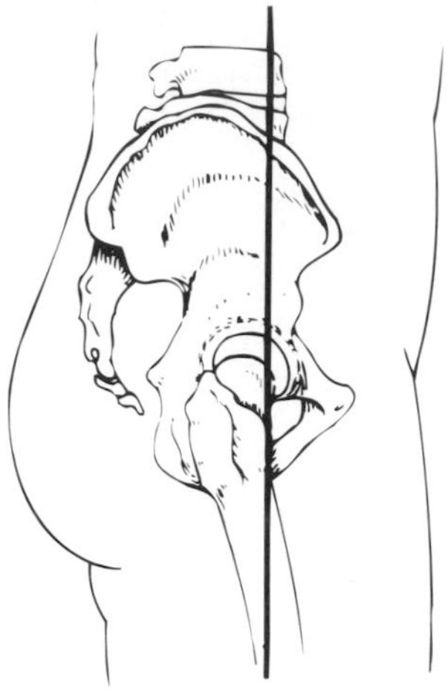

1. This section extends through the urinary bladder, anterior aspect of the prostate, urogenital diaphragm, bulb of the penis, and medial femoral muscles.

2. The structure of the urogenital diaphragm can be discerned on this section. A central band of intermediate-signal intensity corresponds to the transverse perinei profundus muscle. Low-signal intensity outlining the superior and inferior margins of the muscle represent the superior and inferior fascia of the urogenital diaphragm and define the deep perineal compartment.

3. The deep perineal compartment contains the transverse perinei profundus muscle, the sphincter urethrae, the membranous portion of the urethrae, the bulbourethral glands, internal pudendal vessels, and the deep dorsal vein and dorsal nerve of the penis.

4. The medial femoral muscles are delineated on this section. The origins of the adductor brevis and adductor magnus muscles can be separated on this section below the origin of the obturator externus muscle. The gracilis and pectineus muscles are also seen.

5. Low-signal intensity on the lateral margin of the superior acetabulum corresponds to the acetabular labrum and the joint capsule.

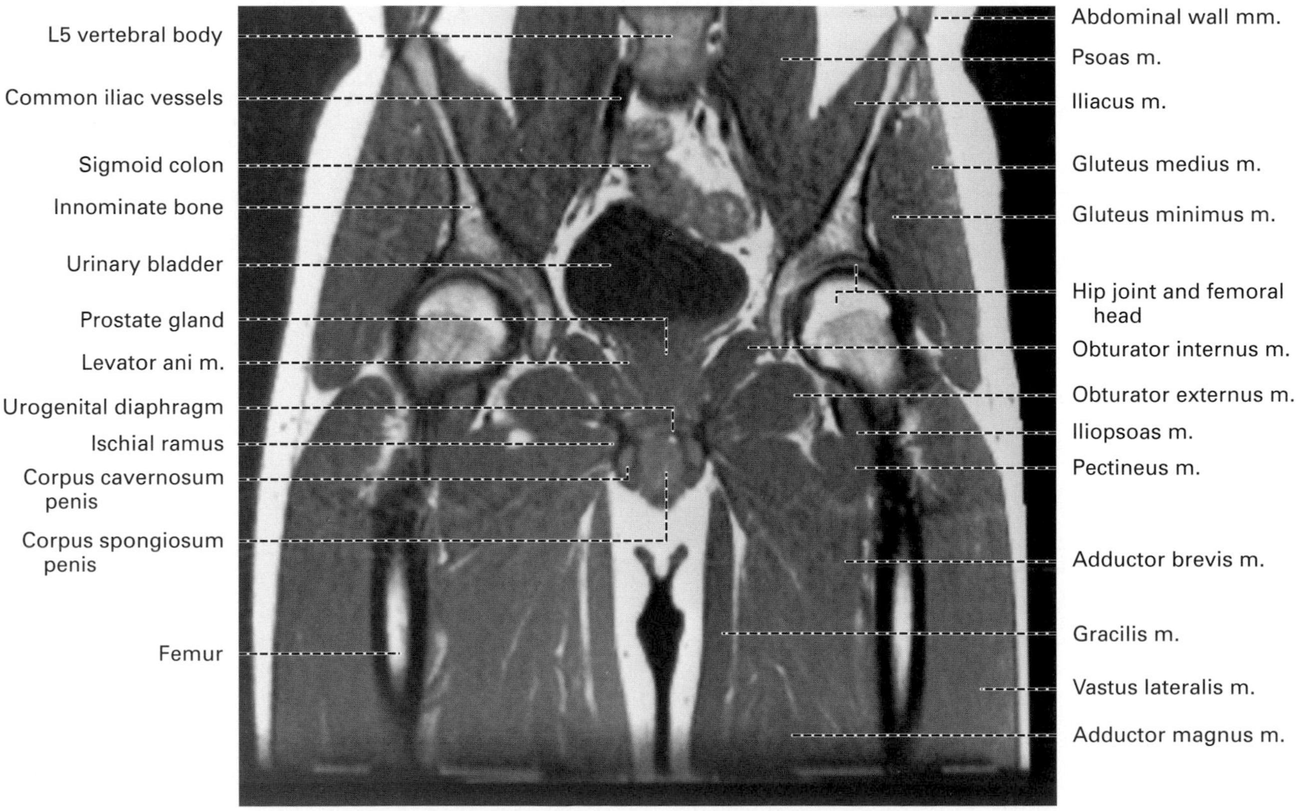
L5 vertebral body
Common iliac vessels
Sigmoid colon
Innominate bone
Urinary bladder
Prostate gland
Levator ani m.
Urogenital diaphragm
Ischial ramus
Corpus cavernosum penis
Corpus spongiosum penis
Femur
Abdominal wall mm.
Psoas m.
Iliacus m.
Gluteus medius m.
Gluteus minimus m.
Hip joint and femoral head
Obturator internus m.
Obturator externus m.
Iliopsoas m.
Pectineus m.
Adductor brevis m.
Gracilis m.
Vastus lateralis m.
Adductor magnus m.

1. This section extends through the pelvic cavity at the level of the sacral promontory. It extends through the urinary bladder, urogenital diaphragm, membranous urethra, and bulb of the penis.

2. Superiorly, the bladder is covered by peritoneum. Laterally, this peritoneum reflects onto the pelvic sidewall forming the shallow paravesical fossae.

3. The inferior aspect of the prostate is defined as the apex, the midportion as the body, and the superior aspect as the base. The prostate can also be divided into a middle and two lateral lobes.

4. The urethra penetrates the levator ani and urogenital diaphragm through the genital hiatus. Fibrous tissue within the hiatus is derived from the inferior and superior fascia of the urogenital diaphragm.

5. The levator ani muscles are difficult to separate from the lateral margin of the prostate on this section. The urogenital diaphragm can be visualized inferior to the prostate and lateral to the membranous urethra. Intermediate-signal intensity within the compartment is again noted; it corresponds to the transverse perinei profundus muscle. Low-signal borders correspond to the superior and inferior fascia of the urogenital diaphragm.

6. The bulb of the penis is seen below the urogenital diaphragm; it contains the most proximal portion of the spongiose component of the urethra.

Figure 14.2.10

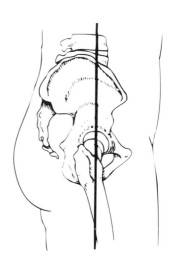

L5 vertebral body

L5–S1 intervertebral disc

Internal iliac vessels

Sigmoid colon

Urinary bladder

Prostate gland

Urethra, membranous segment

Transverse perinei profundus m. and fasciae

Corpus cavernosum penis

Corpus spongiosum penis

Levator ani m.

Abdominal wall mm.

Psoas m.

Iliacus m.

Gluteus medius m.

Gluteus minimus m.

Innominate bone

Femoral head and hip joint

Obturator internus m.

Obturator externus m.

Iliopsoas m.

Ischial ramus

Pectineus m.

Femur

Adductor magnus m.

Gracilis m.

Vastus lateralis m.

Figure 14.2.11

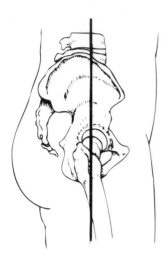

1. This section extends through the pelvic cavity at the level of the hips, posterior urinary bladder, and lesser trochanter of the femur.

2. The pelvic cavity contains a loop of sigmoid colon. The sigmoid normally lies within the pelvis. It is completely surrounded by peritoneum and is attached by an extensive mesentery, the sigmoid mesocolon.

3. The joint spaces of the hips are visualized well. Intermediate-signal intensity within the superior aspect of the hip joint is secondary to hyaline cartilage. High-signal intensity within the medial joint space is associated with the fatty pulvinar.

4. The insertions of the obturator externus into the trochanteric fossa of the femur, of the iliopsoas tendon onto the lesser trochanter, and of the gluteus minimus tendon onto the greater trochanter are seen on this section.

5. The ischiocavernosus and bulbospongiosus muscles are difficult to separate at this level. Both structures show intermediate-signal intensity on T1-weighted images.

6. This section is at the level of the posterior margin of the urogenital diaphragm. The transverse perinei superficialis muscle is difficult to separate from other structures on this image.

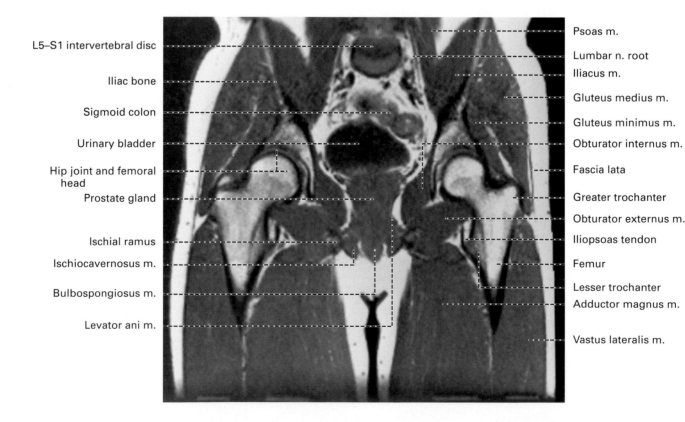

L5–S1 intervertebral disc
Iliac bone
Sigmoid colon
Urinary bladder
Hip joint and femoral head
Prostate gland
Ischial ramus
Ischiocavernosus m.
Bulbospongiosus m.
Levator ani m.

Psoas m.
Lumbar n. root
Iliacus m.
Gluteus medius m.
Gluteus minimus m.
Obturator internus m.
Fascia lata
Greater trochanter
Obturator externus m.
Iliopsoas tendon
Femur
Lesser trochanter
Adductor magnus m.
Vastus lateralis m.

1. This section extends through the pelvic cavity, the rectosigmoid colon, the posterior wall of the urinary bladder, and the anal canal.

2. The pelvic cavity contains a loop of distal sigmoid colon.

3. Foci of low-signal intensity around the proximal seminal vesicles are related to the perivesicle venous plexus.

4. The anterior recesses of the ischiorectal fossae are seen at this level. The anterior recesses are bordered medially by the levator ani muscle, laterally by the obturator internus, and anteriorly by the transverse perinei profundus and superficialis muscles.

5. The gluteus medius, gluteus minimus, piriformis, obturator internus, gemelli, and obturator externus muscles of the gluteal area are identified on this section.

6. The insertions of the gluteus medius, piriformis, obturator internus, gemelli, and obturator externus muscles onto the greater tuberosity are seen.

7. The low-signal intensity fascia lata (not labeled) is visualized superficial to the gluteus medius muscle and greater tuberosity.

Figure 14.2.12

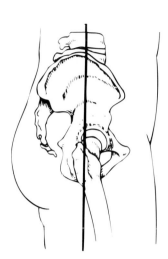

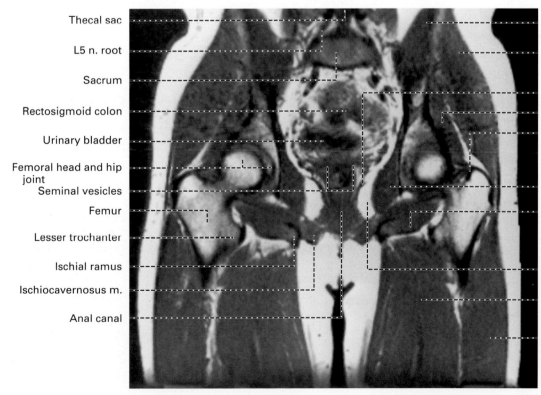

Thecal sac
L5 n. root
Sacrum
Rectosigmoid colon
Urinary bladder
Femoral head and hip joint
Seminal vesicles
Femur
Lesser trochanter
Ischial ramus
Ischiocavernosus m.
Anal canal

Iliacus m.
Gluteus medius m.
Levator ani m.
Gluteus minimus m.
Tendinous insertions of piriformis, obturator internus, and gemelli mm.
Obturator internus m.
Obturator externus and quadratus femoris mm.
Anterior recess, ischiorectal fossa
Adductor magnus m.
Vastus lateralis m.

Figure 14.2.13

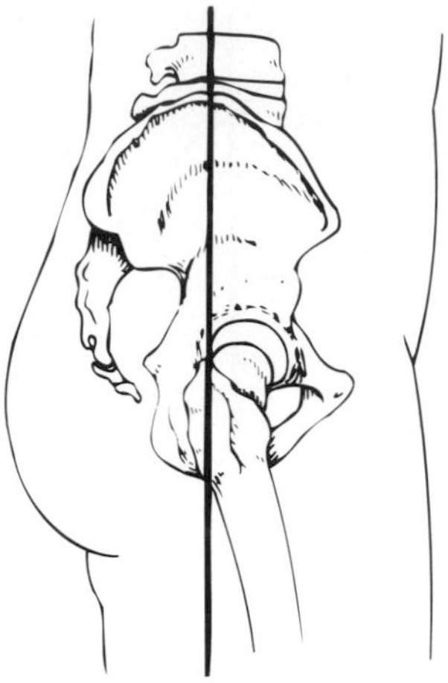

1. This section extends through the sacroiliac joints, rectosigmoid colon, seminal vesicles, and ischiorectal fossae.
2. The distal sigmoid colon and most proximal rectum are visualized on this section.
3. The seminal vesicles are bordered by low-signal intensity foci associated with the vesical venous plexus. The seminal vesicles are two lobulated membranous pouches between the fundus of the bladder and the rectum.
4. The vas deferens are seen medial and superior to the seminal vesicles. The vas deferens are the excretory ducts of the testes and are a continuation of the canal of the epididymis.
5. The anus is bordered laterally by the levator ani muscles. The anus is normally 2.5 to 4.0 cm long. It begins where the ampulla of the rectum narrows at about the level of the apex of the prostate in males.
6. The anterior recesses of the ischiorectal fossae are noted again.
7. The tendinous insertions of the piriformis, obturator internus, gemelli, and obturator externus muscles are noted on the right.

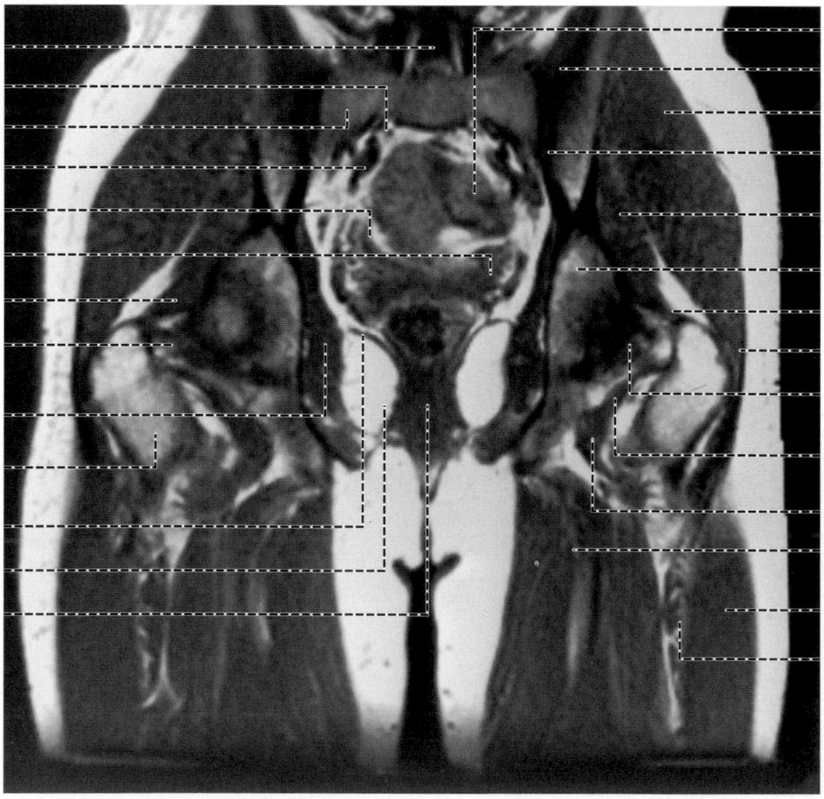
Thecal sac
S1 n. root
Sacrum
Internal iliac vessels
Vas deferens
Seminal vesicles
Piriformis tendon and m.
Obturator internus and gemelli tendons
Obturator internus m.
Femur
Levator ani m.
Ischiorectal fossa
Distal rectum and anus
Rectosigmoid colon
Iliacus m.
Gluteus medius m.
Sacroiliac joint
Gluteus minimus m.
Innominate bone
Piriformis tendon
Gluteus maximus m.
Obturator internus and gemelli mm.
Obturator externus m. and tendon
Quadratus femoris m.
Adductor magnus m.
Vastus lateralis m.
Gluteus maximus m.

1. This section extends through the S1 sacral foramina, sacroiliac joints, rectum, and ischial tuberosities.

2. The lumbosacral plexus is seen anterior to the sacrum. The S1 nerve roots can be identified with their foramina.

3. The tips of the seminal vesicles are noted and are separated from the rectum by the rectovesical fascia as are the rest of the seminal vesicles.

4. The ischiorectal fossae are seen bilaterally. They are limited laterally by the obturator internus muscle and ischial tuberosity and medially by the levator ani muscles and external anal sphincter.

5. The ischiorectal fossae contain fat, the inferior rectal vessels and nerves, and the internal pudendal vessels.

6. The quadratus femoris muscles are seen bilaterally. The quadratus femoris muscle belongs to the gluteal group of muscles and rotates the thigh laterally.

7. The semimembranosus tendon originates from the ischial tuberosity.

8. The distal insertions of the gluteus maximus muscles into the fasciae latae can be seen.

Figure 14.2.14

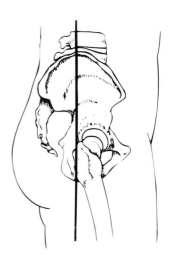

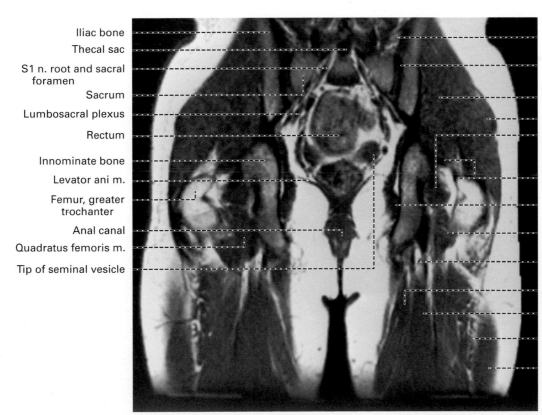

Figure 14.2.15

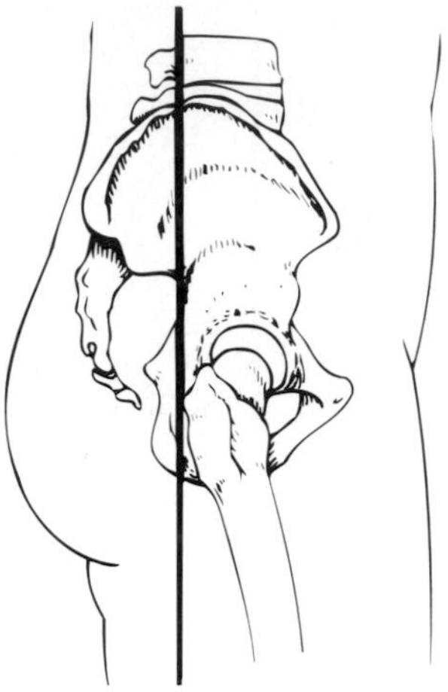

1. This section extends through the sacroiliac joints, rectum, anus, greater sciatic foramina, and ischial tuberosities.
2. The rectum is seen within the posterior pelvic cavity. The rectum begins at about S3. Peritoneum covers the ventral and lateral surfaces of the proximal two-thirds and the ventral surface of only the distal one-third.
3. Intermediate-signal intensity within the anterior inferior aspect of the sacroiliac joints corresponds to articular cartilage.
4. The sciatic nerve can be followed both within and distal to the greater sciatic foramen on the left. It shows intermediate-signal intensity on T1-weighted sections and lies lateral to the ischial tuberosity and common hamstring tendon.
5. The biceps femoris and semitendinosus muscles originate on the tuberosity of the ischium and contribute to extension of the hip and knee.
6. The quadratus femoris muscle, gemelli muscles, and obturator internus tendon are identified just lateral to the ischial ramus on the right.

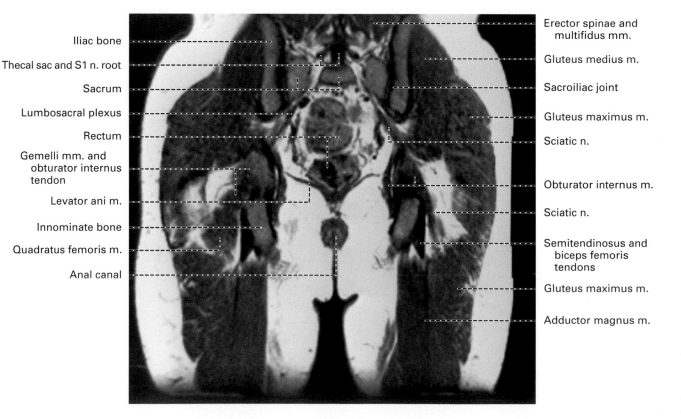

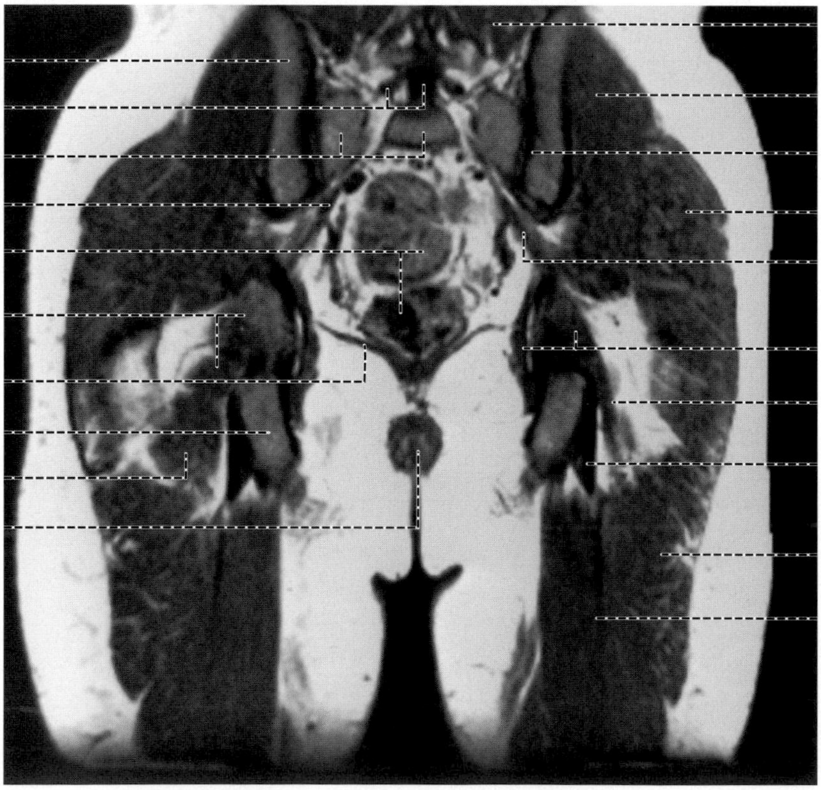
Iliac bone
Thecal sac and S1 n. root
Sacrum
Lumbosacral plexus
Rectum
Gemelli mm. and obturator internus tendon
Levator ani m.
Innominate bone
Quadratus femoris m.
Anal canal
Erector spinae and multifidus mm.
Gluteus medius m.
Sacroiliac joint
Gluteus maximus m.
Sciatic n.
Obturator internus m.
Sciatic n.
Semitendinosus and biceps femoris tendons
Gluteus maximus m.
Adductor magnus m.

1. This section extends through the sacroiliac joints, sciatic foramina, and ischial tuberosities.

2. The piriformis muscles are seen within the greater sciatic foramina. The inferior gluteal vessels can be seen exiting the pelvis just below the piriformis muscles.

3. The greater sciatic foramen is limited superiorly by the innominate bone, posteriorly by the sacrotuberous ligament, and inferiorly by the sacrospinous ligament. It contains the piriformis muscle, the superior and inferior gluteal vessels and nerves, the internal pudendal artery and nerve, the sciatic and posterior femoral cutaneous nerves, and the nerves to the obturator internus and quadratus femoris muscles.

4. The obturator internus muscles and tendons are visualized within the lesser sciatic foramen.

5. The lesser sciatic foramen is limited anteriorly by the tuberosity and body of the ischium, superiorly by the sacrospinous ligament, and posteriorly by the sacrotuberous ligament.

6. The gluteus maximus muscles are seen bilaterally.

7. The multifidus and erector spinae muscles of the deep back can be delineated on this section.

Figure 14.2.16

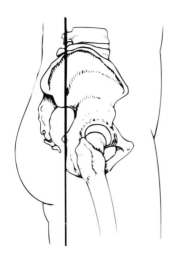

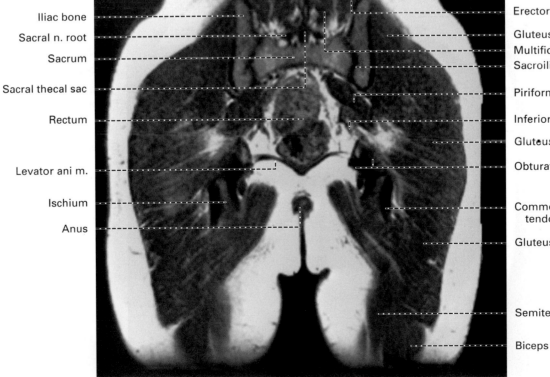

Iliac bone
Sacral n. root
Sacrum
Sacral thecal sac
Rectum
Levator ani m.
Ischium
Anus

Erector spinae m.
Gluteus medius m.
Multifidus m.
Sacroiliac joint
Piriformis m.
Inferior gluteal vessels
Gluteus maximus m.
Obturator internus m.
Common hamstring tendon
Gluteus maximus m.
Semitendinosus m.
Biceps femoris m.

Figure 14.3.3

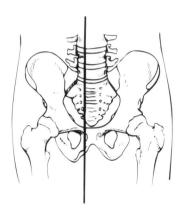

1. This paramedian sagittal section extends through the pelvic cavity.

2. The rectosigmoid colon, urinary bladder, seminal vesicle, and prostate gland are again noted.

3. The first and second sacral nerve roots are seen within their respective foramina.

4. The origin of the piriformis muscle from the anterior sacrum is seen from S2 through S4.

5. The common tendinous insertion of the erector spinae muscles is seen over the posterior aspect of the distal sacrum.

6. The rectus abdominis muscle and tendon are noted; they insert onto the pubic crest.

7. The distal aspect of the spermatic cord is seen in relation to the epididymis and testis within the scrotum.

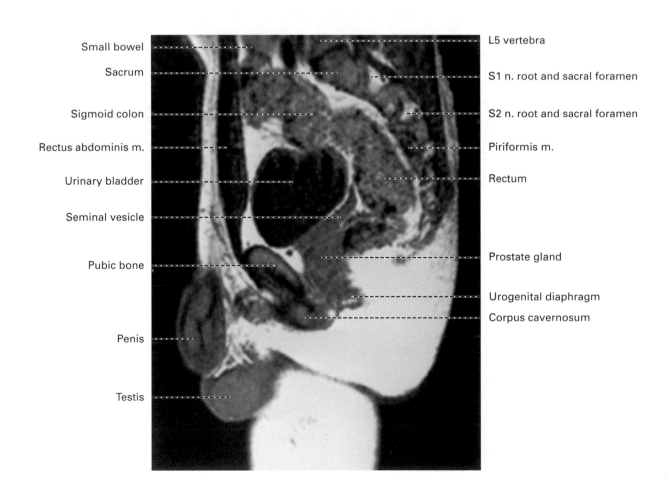

Small bowel — Sacrum — Sigmoid colon — Rectus abdominis m. — Urinary bladder — Seminal vesicle — Pubic bone — Penis — Testis

L5 vertebra — S1 n. root and sacral foramen — S2 n. root and sacral foramen — Piriformis m. — Rectum — Prostate gland — Urogenital diaphragm — Corpus cavernosum

1. This section extends through the pelvic cavity at the lateral margin of the pubis.

2. The pelvic diaphragm, composed of the levator ani and coccygeus muscles, is seen.

3. The ischiorectal fossa is limited superiorly and laterally by the pelvic diaphragm, posteriorly by the gluteus maximus muscle, and anteriorly by the transverse perinei profundus and superficialis muscles on this section.

4. The section extends obliquely through the urogenital diaphragm, corpus cavernosum, and ischiocavernosus muscle posterior and inferior to the ischial ramus.

5. The tendinous origin of the adductor longus muscle from the anterior pubis and the origins of the adductor brevis and obturator externus muscles from the inferior pubic ramus are seen.

6. The origins of the gluteus maximus muscle from the erector spinae aponeurosis and sacrum are noted.

7. The spermatic cord consists of the cremasteric muscles, the ductus deferens, the arteries of the ductus and testes, and the pampiniform plexus.

8. The sacral nerve roots are again seen within their respective foramina.

Figure 14.3.4

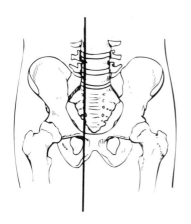

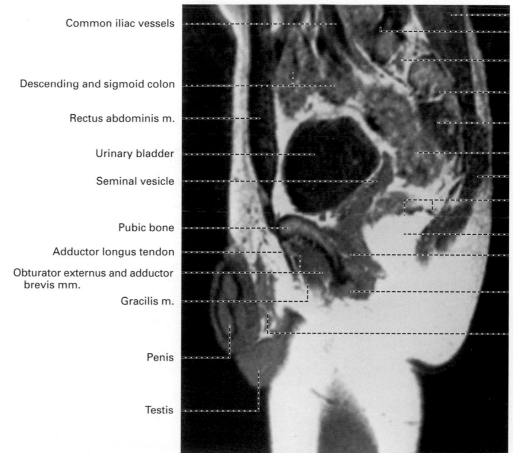

Common iliac vessels

Descending and sigmoid colon

Rectus abdominis m.

Urinary bladder

Seminal vesicle

Pubic bone

Adductor longus tendon

Obturator externus and adductor brevis mm.

Gracilis m.

Penis

Testis

Erector spinae mm.

L5 n. root and foramen

S1 n. root and foramen

S2 n. root and foramen

Piriformis m.

Rectum

Gluteus maximus m.

Levator ani and coccygeus mm.

Ischiorectal fossa

Obturator internus m.

Corpus cavernosum and ischiocavernosus m.

Spermatic cord

Figure 14.3.5

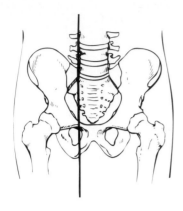

1. This paramedian sagittal section extends through the pelvic cavity and obturator foramen.

2. The sacral nerve roots and piriformis muscle are visualized anterior to the sacral ala.

3. The pelvic diaphragm and ischiorectal fossa are seen again.

4. This section extends through the tip of the seminal vesicle and illustrates part of the vas deferens. The vas deferens extends from the medial aspect of the seminal vesicle, along the pelvic sidewall and external iliac vessels, and through the inguinal canal to join the spermatic cord within the processus vaginalis.

5. The proximal obturator externus, adductor brevis, and adductor longus muscles are seen anterior to the obturator membrane.

6. The gracilis muscle is noted in the medial thigh.

7. The most anterior origin of the obturator internus muscle is seen between the obturator membrane and the levator ani muscle.

8. The spermatic cord is again noted over the anterior pelvis.

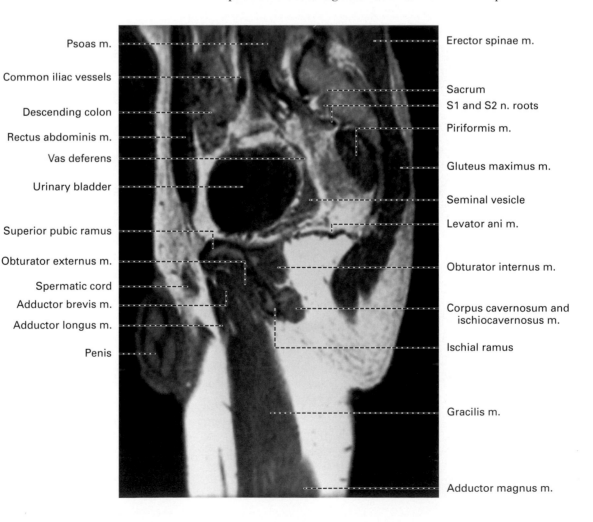

Psoas m.

Common iliac vessels

Descending colon

Rectus abdominis m.

Vas deferens

Urinary bladder

Superior pubic ramus

Obturator externus m.

Spermatic cord

Adductor brevis m.

Adductor longus m.

Penis

Erector spinae m.

Sacrum
S1 and S2 n. roots

Piriformis m.

Gluteus maximus m.

Seminal vesicle

Levator ani m.

Obturator internus m.

Corpus cavernosum and ischiocavernosus m.

Ischial ramus

Gracilis m.

Adductor magnus m.

1. This section includes the pelvic cavity, obturator foramen, sacroiliac joint, and medial thigh.

2. This section extends through the medial aspect of the psoas muscle. The external iliac vessels are visualized anterior to the psoas muscle and posterior to the internal iliac vessels.

3. Numerous vessels associated with the perivesical and periprostatic venous plexuses are seen around the tip of the seminal vesicle and lateral to the prostate (anterior and inferior to the seminal vesicle).

4. The vas deferens is noted over the anterior pelvis just external to the inguinal canal.

5. The medial femoral muscles include the pectineus, gracilis, adductor longus, adductor brevis, and adductor magnus muscles.

6. The descending colon lies within the anterior pararenal space of the retroperitoneum.

Figure 14.3.6

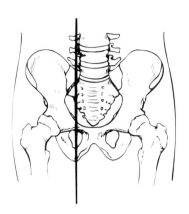

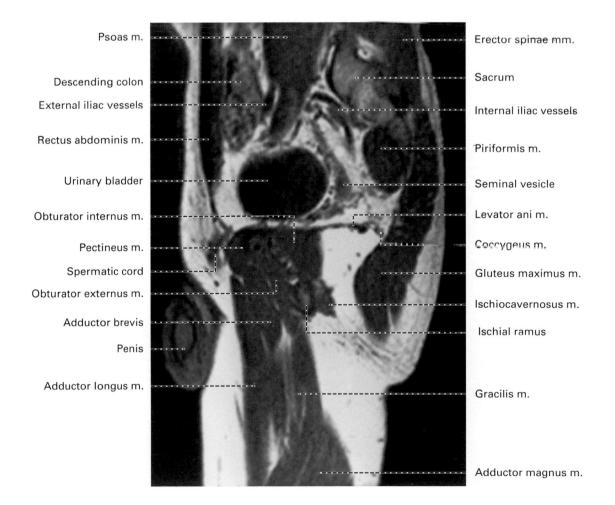

Psoas m.

Descending colon

External iliac vessels

Rectus abdominis m.

Urinary bladder

Obturator internus m.

Pectineus m.

Spermatic cord

Obturator externus m.

Adductor brevis

Penis

Adductor longus m.

Erector spinae mm.

Sacrum

Internal iliac vessels

Piriformis m.

Seminal vesicle

Levator ani m.

Coccygeus m.

Gluteus maximus m.

Ischiocavernosus m.

Ischial ramus

Gracilis m.

Adductor magnus m.

FIGURE 14.3.12?

Chapter 15

HIP AND THIGH

Musculature of the Hip

Ischiopubofemoral Muscles

The ischiopubofemoral muscles include obturator internus, the two gemelli, quadratus femoris, and obturator externus. They extend from the pubis and ischium across the back of the hip joint to the greater trochanter and nearby portions of the shaft of the femur. Obturator internus is a large, flat, somewhat triangular muscle that arises from the pubic surface of the innominate (hip) bone and from the obturator membrane and surrounding bone. Obturator internus joins the two gemelli (superior and inferior) at the lesser sciatic notch. The gemelli muscles arise from the bony projections that create the notch. The tendons of all three muscles join and insert into the trochanteric fossa. Quadratus femoris courses from the tuberosity of the ischium to insert onto the femur, somewhat behind and below the greater trochanter. These muscles are supplied by the anterior division of the sacral plexus.

The last muscle of this group, obturator externus, arises from the outer surface of the bones forming the obturator foramen and the obturator membrane and inserts by a tendon into the trochanteric fossa. Obturator externus is innervated by a branch from the obturator nerve.

These five muscles, as a group, are strong lateral rotators of the thigh. Obturator internus and gemelli abduct the thigh; obturator externus and quadratus femoris adduct the thigh.

Iliofemoral muscles

The iliofemoral muscles are divided by the iliac blade into an anterior and posterior group. The anterior group includes the iliopsoas, innervated by the lumbar plexus, and the posterior group includes the gluteal muscles, piriformis, and the tensor fasciae latae, innervated by the sacral plexus.

The anterior group of muscles includes the fan-shaped iliacus muscle, which arises from the iliac fossa. The fusiform psoas major muscle arises from the sides of the T12 and L5 vertebra. The muscle courses along the medial side of iliacus. These two muscles join and then insert, by a common tendon, onto the lesser trochanter of the femur. Together the two muscles form the iliopsoas muscle. A third muscle, the psoas minor, which is inconstant, small, flattened, and fusiform, arises from the T12 vertebra, crosses psoas major to its medial side, and inserts onto the iliopubic eminence.

Iliacus is innervated by the femoral nerve and psoas major by branches from the L2 to L4 nerves. Psoas minor, when present, receives its nerve supply from the L1 and L2 nerves.

Iliopsoas muscle flexes the thigh at the hip and the pelvis on the trunk. Psoas minor aids in flexing the pelvis on the trunk.

The posterior group of muscles arise from the ilium and sacrum. They cover the dorsolateral surface of the hip and are inserted onto the greater trochanter and shaft of the femur and into the iliotibial tract. The muscles form three layers. The first layer contains the flat, quadrilateral tensor fasciae latae, arising from the front part of the crest of the ilium and inserting into the iliotibial tract, and the thick rhomboid gluteus maximus, arising from the iliac ala, thoracolumbar fascia, sacrum and coccyx, and sacrotuberous ligament and inserting, in part, into the iliotibial tract and in part onto the back of the upper part of the shaft of the femur. The iliotibial tract is a flat tendon that is contained in the fascia lata and extends to the anterolateral part of the upper end of the tibia. The second layer is composed of the flat, thick, somewhat triangular gluteus medius and the piriformis muscles. Gluteus medius arises from the upper and posterior surface of the ala of the ilium. Piriformis arises from the ventral surface of the sacrum and the posterior border of the greater sciatic notch. Both muscles insert onto the top of the greater trochanter of the femur. The third layer is composed of the fan-shaped gluteus minimus. This muscle arises from the inferior ventral part of the outer surface of the ala of the ilium. The muscle inserts onto the front of the greater trochanter of the femur.

Gluteus maximus is innervated by the inferior gluteal nerve, the piriformis by the first or by the second sacral nerve or by both nerves; the gluteus medius and minimus are supplied by the superior gluteal nerve. The nerves all derive from the upper part of the dorsal aspect of the sacral plexus.

The muscles of the posterior group extend, flex, abduct, and rotate the thigh at the hip. Gluteus maximus and the posterior parts of gluteus medius and minimus are extensors of the hip joint; the anterior parts of gluteus medius and the tensor fasciae latae are flexors. All the muscles serve to abduct; the gluteus maximus also acts in a similar way only when the hip is flexed. When the thigh is extended, the inferior part of gluteus maximus is also an adductor. Gluteus maximus, the posterior part of gluteus medius, and piriformis are lateral rotators of the thigh. The anterior parts of gluteus medius and minimus and the tensor fasciae latae act as medial rotators. Gluteus maximus and the tensor fasciae latae are also medial rotators of the thigh. Finally, gluteus maximus and the tensor fasciae latae acting through the iliotibial tract can maintain extension of the knee joint.

Table 15-1. Ischiopubofemoral Musculature of the Hip

Muscle	Origin	Insertion	Nerve Supply	Arterial Supply
Obturator internus	Pelvic surface of the pubic rami near obturator foramen, pelvic surface of ischium between foramen and greater sciatic notch, deep surface of obturator internus fascia, the fibrous arch that surrounds foramen for obturator vessels and nerve, most of the pelvic surface of obturator membrane except lower part	Medial side of greater trochanter in front of the trochanteric fossa of femur	Nerve to obturator internus, from lumbosacral trunk, and 1st and 2nd sacral nerves	Superior gluteal, deep inferior branch
Gemellus superior	Outer surface of ischial spine and edge of lesser sciatic notch	After union with the tendon of obturator internus, inserts into the medial side of the greater trochanter in front of the trochanteric fossa	By a small nerve, branch of nerve to obturator internus or of that to quadratus femoris	Superior gluteal, deep inferior branch
Gemellus inferior	Upper part of inner border of tuberosity of the ischium, sacrotuberous ligament, and edge of lesser sciatic notch	By union with tendon of obturator internus or by a tendon onto the greater trochanter below the obturator internus muscle	By a small nerve, branch of the nerve to the quadratus femoris	Superior gluteal, deep inferior branch
Quadratus femoris	Upper part of the outer border of tuberosity of the ischium	Onto the inferodorsal angle of the greater trochanter	Lumbosacral trunk and 1st sacral nerve	Medial femoral circumflex
Obturator externus	Lateral surface of pubic and ischial rami, where they surround the obturator membrane, lateral surface of the obturator membrane	The trochanteric fossa	Obturator	Obturator artery, anterior branch

557

Table 15-2. Iliofemoral Musculature of the Hip

Muscle	Origin	Insertion	Nerve Supply	Arterial Supply
Anterior group				
Psoas major	By a series of thick fasciculi from the intervertebral disks and bodies between T12 and L5, from the bodies of L1 to L4, and from slender fascicles from the ventral surfaces of the transverse processes of the lumbar vertebrae	Arises deep within the muscle, becomes free above the inguinal ligament; on its medial side, fibers join the tendon until it inserts into the lesser trochanter of the femur; iliacus is attached to the lateral side of the tendon from the iliopathic eminence distally	Branches from L1 (often), L2, L3, and L4	External iliac and its deep circumflex iliac branch, the iliolumbar lumbar branch, and the lateral femoral circumflex
Iliacus	Iliac crest, iliolumbar ligament, iliac fossa, anterior sacroiliac ligaments, often from ala of the sacrum, and from the ventral border of the ilium between the two anterior spines	Lateral surface of the psoas tendon (above the inguinal ligament) and onto the femur immediately distal to the lesser trochanter; the lateral portion arises from the ventral border of the ilium and is attached to the tendon of rectus femoris and the capsule of the hip joint	Femoral and L1 to L4	External iliac and its deep circumflex iliac branch, superficial circumflex iliac, and lateral femoral circumflex
Posterior group, first layer				
Tensor fasciae latae	External lip of iliac crest, notch between anterior superior and anterior iliac spines, and gluteus medius	Muscle fibers pass distally in parallel array, unite with tendon, and join the iliotibial tract about one-third of the way down the thigh	Superior gluteal	Superior gluteal, inferior branch; lateral femoral circumflex, ascending branch
Gluteus maximus	Dorsal fifth of outer lip of the iliac crest, ilium dorsal to posterior gluteal line, thoracolumbar fascia between the posterior superior spine of ilium and side of sacrum, lateral parts of S4, S5, and coccygeal vertebrae, and from back of sacrotuberous ligament	Into iliotibial tract, gluteal tuberosity of femur, adjacent part of tendinous origin of vastus lateralis	Inferior gluteal by two branches from sacral plexus (separately or as a united nerve)	Superior gluteal, superficial branch; inferior gluteal; internal pudendal; lateral femoral circumflex, transverse branch; deep femoral, first perforating artery
Posterior group, second layer				
Gluteus medius	Ventral three-fourths of iliac crest, outer surface of ilium between anterior and posterior gluteal lines, and from investing fascia	Onto the posterosuperior angle and the external surface of greater trochanter	Superior gluteal (L4, L5, S1)	Superior gluteal, deep inferior branches
Piriformis	Lateral part of the ventral surface of S2, S3, and S4, posterior border of the greater sciatic notch, from the sacrotuberous ligament near the sacrum	Onto the anterior and inner parts of the upper border of the greater trochanter	S1 or S2 or from a loop between S1 or S2	Superior gluteal, deep inferior branch

Continues

558

Table 15-2. *(Continued)*

Muscle	Origin	Insertion	Nerve Supply	Arterial Supply
Posterior group, third layer				
Gluteus minimus	Outer surface of ilium between the anterior and inferior gluteal lines, from the septum between it and gluteus medius near the anterior superior iliac spine, and capsule of the hip joint	Onto the anterior border of the greater trochanter of the femur	Superior gluteal nerve from a branch that supplies the tensor fasciae latae	Superior gluteal, deep inferior and superior branches
Posterior (hamstring) group				
Biceps femoris, long head	Medial facet on posterior surface of ischial tuberosity and sacro-tuberous ligament	By a tendon that extends to the lateral condyle of the femur	Tibial part of sciatic	Medial femoral circumflex, muscular branches
Biceps femoris, short head	From the lateral lip of the linea aspera of the femur, from the middle of the shaft to the bifurcation of the linea aspera, proximal two-thirds of supra-condylar ridge, and lateral intermuscular septum	Head of the fibula in front of the apex, partially onto the lateral condyle of the tibia, and into the fascia of the leg	Peroneal part of sciatic	Medial femoral circumflex, muscular branches; popliteal muscular branch
Semitendinosus	Distal margin of ischial tuberosity and from the tendon common to it and the long head of biceps femoris	By a triangular tendinous expansion into the proximal part of the medial surface of the tibia behind and distal to the insertion of gracilis	Sciatic nerve or directly from the lumbosacral plexus by two nerves: from S1 and S2 and from L5 and S1	First and second perforating artery; deep femoral
Semimembranosus	Lateral facet on posterior surface of ischial tuberosity	By a tendon onto the back of the medial condyle of the tibia, by aponeurotic expansions into the capsule of the joint, onto the lateral condyle of the femur, into the tibial collateral ligament, and into fascia of popliteus muscle	Sciatic nerve branch (also supplies adductor magnus)	First and second perforating artery; popliteal, muscular branch; deep femoral

Musculature of the Thigh

The thigh is composed of three groups of muscles: the anterior or extensor group, the medial or adductor group, and the posterior or flexor group.

In the proximal part of the thigh, the anterior group of muscles is separated from the medial group by the iliopsoas muscle and by the femoral blood vessels and nerve. The posterior group is separated from the anterior group by the gluteus maximus muscle. Distally, the anterior group is separated from the medial group by the medial intermuscular septum and from the posterior group by the lateral intermuscular septum.

The anterior group of muscles includes sartorius and quadriceps femoris. Sartorius is a long, ribbonlike muscle that arises from the anterior superior iliac spine and courses along the medial border of quadriceps, having crossed obliquely the upper part of the thigh. It descends to the dorsomedial side of the knee. Its tendon curves forward and inserts onto the ventromedial surface of the superior (proximal) edge of the tibia.

Quadriceps femoris is composed of four muscles. Rectus femoris, arising from the ventrolateral margin of the ileum by two tendons, is the most completely differentiated of the four. Vastus lateralis arises from the superior end of the ventral surface of the shaft of the femur and from the lateral lip of the linea aspera; vastus medialis arises from the medial lip of the linea aspera and from the intertrochanteric line; and the vastus intermedius arises between these two and beneath the rectus from the anterior surface of the femur. The three vastus muscles are not always clearly differentiated. The vastus intermedius and vastus lateralis may be partially fused at their insertion and the vastus intermedius and vastus medialis at their origin. All four muscles contribute to a tendon that is inserted onto the tuberosity of the tibia and contains the largest sesamoid bone in the body, the patella.

The sartorius and the quadriceps muscles are innervated by the femoral nerve. This nerve also supplies iliacus and the pectineus muscles.

The sartorius flexes, abducts, and rotates the thigh laterally; it flexes and medially rotates the leg. Quadriceps extends the leg; rectus femoris also flexes the thigh.

The medial or adductor group of muscles includes gracilis; pectineus; adductor brevis, longus, and magnus; and obturator externus. The most superficial muscle of this group is gracilis. Gracilis is a straplike muscle that arises from the inferior ischial and pubic rami. The muscle extends along the medial aspect of the thigh; it gives rise to a tendon that curves forward from behind the medial condyle of the femur to be inserted beneath the tendon of sartorius onto the medial side of the proximal end of the tibia.

Pectineus arises from the superior ramus of the pubis. Adductor longus, triangular in shape, also arises from the superior ramus of the pubis but medial to pectineus. Pectineus inserts onto the pectineal line of the femur. Adductor longus inserts onto the middle third of the linea aspera. Adductor brevis, also triangular in shape, arises from the inferior pubic ramus below adductor longus. Adductor brevis inserts onto the pectinal line and the upper third of the linea aspera. Adductor magnus, the large triangular muscle, arises from the inferior ramus and the tuberosity of the ischium. It is inserted behind the long and short adductors onto the entire length of the linea aspera and by a special tendon onto the adductor tubercle of the femur. The deepest muscle is obturator externus. It arises from the outer surface of the bones surrounding the ventral two-thirds of the obturator foramen. This muscle inserts by a tendon into the trochanteric fossa of the femur.

The muscles of this group receive their innervation from the obturator nerve, except pectineus, which is usually supplied by the femoral nerve. Adductor magnus receives a part of its supply from the sciatic nerve.

All of the muscles of this group adduct the thigh. Those attached to the pubis flex the thigh. The distal part of adductor magnus extends the thigh. The adductor muscles and pectineus also rotate the thigh. Adductor longus, pectineus, and distal posterior part of adductor magnus normally rotate the thigh medially. Adductor brevis and the proximal part of adductor magnus rotate the thigh laterally.

The posterior or hamstring group of muscles includes semitendinosus, semimembranosus, and biceps femoris. Semitendinosus and the long head of biceps femoris arise by a common tendon from the tuberosity of the ischium. The fusiform semitendinosus becomes tendinous in the lower half of the thigh. The tendon curves forward behind the knee and inserts, deep to sartorius, onto the medial side of the tibia. The penniform short head of the biceps arises from the linea aspera in the lower part of the thigh. The short head inserts, along with long head, by a tendon that crosses the lateral side of the knee and is attached to the head of the fibula. Semimembranosus arises from the tuber ischii by a long triangular tendon. The muscle increases in thickness distally and inserts, by a strong tendon, onto the medial condyle of the tibia. The tendons of all the hamstring muscles contribute to the crural fascia.

The muscles of this group are supplied by the tibial part of the sciatic nerve except for the short head of biceps femoris, which is supplied from the peroneal part of the sciatic nerve.

Table 15-3. Musculature of the Thigh

Muscle	Origin	Insertion	Nerve Supply	Arterial Supply
Anterior group Sartorius	Anterior superior iliac spines and adjacent area below	Medial surface of the tibia, near tuberosity and neighboring fascia	Femoral	Deep circumflex iliac; lateral femoral circumflex, descending branch; descending genicular, saphenous branch
Quadriceps femoris, rectus femoris	Anterior inferior iliac spine, posterior tendon, posterosuperior surface of the rim of the acetabulum	Through patellar ligament to tibial tuberosity	Femoral	Medial and lateral femoral circumflex, descending branches
Quadriceps femoris, vastus lateralis	Shaft of femur along anteroinferior margin of greater trochanter, above gluteal tuberosity, and upper half of linea aspera	Proximal border of patella, front of lateral condyle of tibia and fascia of leg	Femoral	Lateral femoral circumflex, descending branch, all perforating arteries
Quadriceps femoris, vastus medialis	The medial lip of linea aspera and distal half of intertrochanteric line, and the aponeurosis of tendons of insertion of adductor muscles	Upper two-thirds of the medial margin and proximal margin of the patella, medial condyle of tibia, and investing deep fascia of the leg with the tendons of vastus intermedius, lateralis, and rectus and through patellar ligament onto the front of the tibial tuberosity	Femoral	Deep femoral, lateral femoral circumflex branch; descending genicular, articular branch
Quadriceps femoris, vastus intermedius	The distal half of the lateral margin of linea aspera and its lateral bifurcation and from anterolateral part of the shaft of the femur	Proximal margin and deep surface of patella, aponeurosis of vastus lateralis, medially and laterally to the tendons of vastus medialis and lateralis, to patellar ligament and onto the tibial tuberosity	Femoral	Deep femoral, lateral, transverse, and descending branches
Medial (adductor) group Gracilis	Medial margin of inferior ramus of pubis and pubic end of inferior ramus of ischium	By an expanded tendinous process onto the tibia below the medial condyle	Anterior division of obturator	Deep femoral; medial femoral; circumflex deep external, pudendal branch
Pectineus	Pectin of the pubic bone, bone anterior to the pectin, pectineal fascia, anterior margin of obturator sulcus, and from pubofemoral ligament	Upper half of pectineal line behind lesser trochanter	Femoral, also from accessory obturator and/or obturator	Deep femoral; medial femoral; circumflex deep external, pudendal branch
Adductor longus	Pubic tubercle to symphysis pubis	Middle third of linea aspera	Anterior division of obturator, also occasionally branch from femoral	Medial femoral circumflex, deep external pudendal and muscular branches
Adductor brevis	Medial part of the outer surface of the inferior ramus of the pubis	Distal two-thirds of the pectineal line and the upper one-third of linea aspera	Anterior (or posterior) branch of the obturator	Medial femoral circumflex, muscular branch
Adductor magnus	Inferior ramus of the pubis	Medial side of gluteal ridge and superior part of linea aspera by a tendon from distal three-fourths of linea aspera and adductor tubercle at distal end of the medial supracondylar ridge	Posterior branch of obturator and a branch from the sciatic	Medial femoral circumflex, muscular branch; fourth perforating artery

Figure 15.1.1

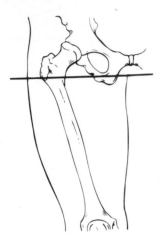

1. The common tendon of the hamstrings originates from the ischial tuberosity.

2. The adductor group is composed of the adductor longus, brevis, and magnus muscles. This order as seen from anterior to posterior is preserved as the adductors course inferiorly until the adductor brevis inserts into the linea aspera.

3. The sciatic nerve courses between the short external rotators of the hip and the gluteus maximus.

4. The vastus intermedius originates from the anterolateral portion of the femur, deep to vastus lateralis.

5. The femoral vessels lie within the femoral triangle. The floor of the femoral triangle is composed of pectineus and iliopsoas.

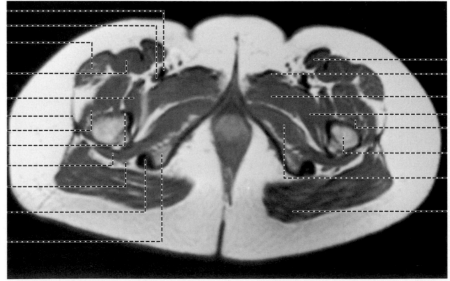

Femoral v.
Femoral a.
Tensor fasciae latae m.
Rectus femoris m.
Iliopsoas m.
Iliotibial tract
Vastus lateralis m.
Lesser trochanter
Quadratus femoris m.
Sciatic n.
Hamstrings, common tendon
Ischium

Sartorius m.
Adductor longus m.
Adductor brevis m.
Pectineus m.
Vastus intermedius m.
Femur
Adductor magnus m.
Gluteus maximus m.

1. Note the origin of vastus lateralis from the lateral lip of the linea aspera at this level.

2. In the right thigh, the common tendon of origin of the hamstring muscles has divided into the more anterior tendon of the semimembranosus and the more posterior conjoint tendon of biceps femoris and semitendinosus.

3. Iliopsoas is inserting on the lesser trochanter.

Figure 15.1.2

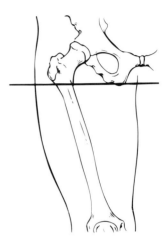

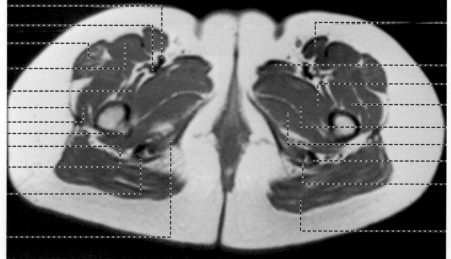

Femoral v.
Femoral a.
Tensor fasciae latae m.
Rectus femoris m.
Iliopsoas tendon
Iliotibial tract
Vastus lateralis m.
Lesser trochanter
Quadratus femoris m.
Sciatic n.
Biceps femoris and semitendinosus tendons
Ischium

Sartorius m.
Adductor longus m.
Pectineus m.
Vastus intermedius m.
Adductor brevis m.
Adductor magnus m.
Semimembranosus tendon
Semitendinosus and biceps femoris tendons
Gluteus maximus m.

Figure 15.1.3

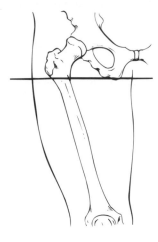

1. A portion of the gluteus maximus inserts into the iliotibial tract. The remainder inserts on the posterior aspect of the femur.

2. Semitendinousus is becoming muscular at this level. The other two hamstrings (semimembranosus and biceps femoris) remain tendinous.

3. Semimembranosus, semitendinosus, and biceps femoris originate from the ischial tuberosity.

4. The adductor muscle group originates primarily from the inferior pubic ramus.

5. A portion of the adductor magnus originates from the ischium and functions as a hamstring muscle. This portion of the adductor magnus receives its innervation from the sciatic nerve.

Rectus femoris m.

Tensor fasciae latae m.

Femoral vessels

Deep femoral vessels

Iliotibial tract

Vastus lateralis m.

Sciatic n.

Biceps femoris tendon

Gracilis m.

Sartorius m.

Adductor longus m.

Adductor brevis m.

Vastus intermedius m.

Femur

Adductor magnus m.

Semitendinosus m.

Gluteus maximus m.

Semimembranosus tendon

1. The majority of the gluteus maximus inserts on the posterior aspect of the femur. A small portion inserts in the iliotibial tract.

2. At this level, the sciatic nerve courses on the posterior surface of adductor magnus.

3. The most medial muscle of the thigh is gracilis. It originates from the inferior pubic ramus.

Figure 15.1.4

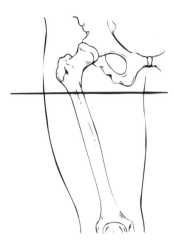

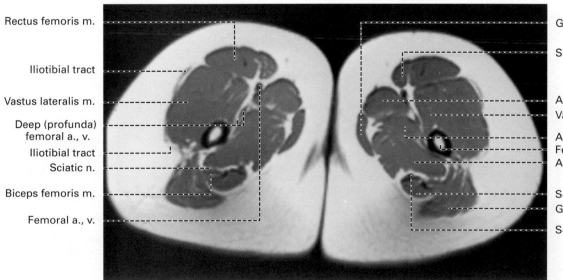

Rectus femoris m.

Iliotibial tract

Vastus lateralis m.

Deep (profunda) femoral a., v.

Iliotibial tract

Sciatic n.

Biceps femoris m.

Femoral a., v.

Gracilis m.

Sartorius m.

Adductor longus m.

Vastus intermedius m.

Adductor brevis m.

Femur

Adductor magnus m.

Semitendinosus m.

Gluteus maximus m.

Semimembranosus m.

Figure 15.1.5

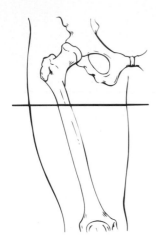

1. Rectus femoris is distinct from the muscle mass of the vastus group.

2. The profunda femoris (deep femoral) artery, the largest branch of the femoral artery, courses deep into the thigh and lies between the adductor magnus and vastus intermedius.

3. Note that the gluteus maximus contains more fat (marbling) than the hamstring muscles.

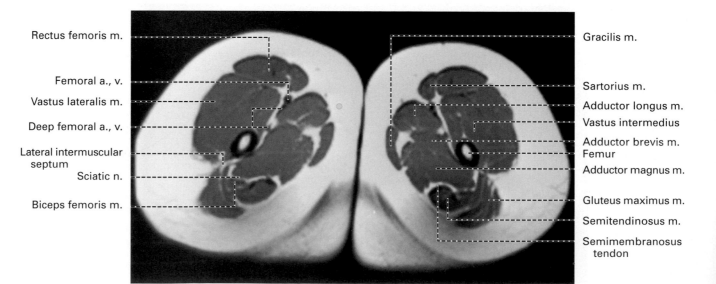

1. The femoral artery and vein course in the adductor canal of Hunter, formed by the sartorius anteriorly, the adductor longus medially, and the quadriceps group laterally.

2. The quadriceps muscle group is composed of the rectus femoris, vastus intermedius, vastus lateralis, and vastus medialis. The vastus medialis becomes visible in lower sections.

3. The hamstring muscle group is composed of semimembranosus, semitendinosus, and biceps femoris.

4. The muscular portion of the long head of biceps femoris is situated medial to gluteus maximus and lateral to semitendinosus.

Figure 15.1.6

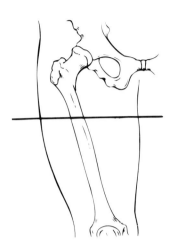

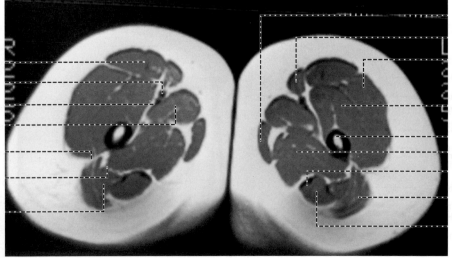

Rectus femoris m.
Femoral a.
Femoral v.
Adductor longus m.
Lateral intermuscular septum
Sciatic n.
Biceps femoris m.

Gracilis m.
Sartorius m.
Vastus lateralis m.
Vastus intermedius m.
Femur
Adductor magnus m.
Semimembranosus tendon
Gluteus maximus m.
Semitendinosus m.

Figure 15.1.9

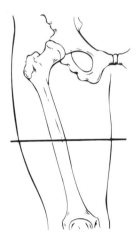

1. The femoral artery and vein lie within the fat of the medial intermuscular septum that separates the adductors from the quadriceps group. Sartorius covers these vascular structures.

2. Note the four components of the quadriceps group with vastus lateralis being the largest at this level.

3. Biceps femoris now has two heads: its larger, long head originating from the ischial tuberosity, and its smaller, short head originating from the postero-lateral distal femur.

4. The sciatic nerve is surrounded by biceps femoris and adductor magnus.

5. In successive sections, the sartorius is seen coursing from its origin on the anterior superior iliac spine to its insertion on the anteromedial proximal tibia.

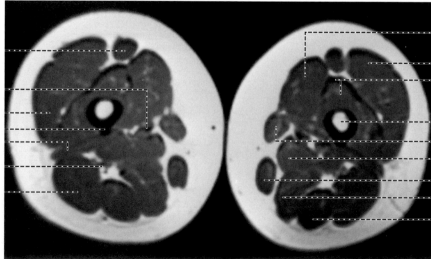

Rectus femoris m.

Femoral a., v.

Vastus lateralis m.
Linea aspera
Biceps femoris m., short head
Sciatic n.

Biceps femoris m., long head

Vastus medialis m.

Vastus lateralis m.
Vastus intermedius m. and tendon

Femur

Sartorius m.
Adductor magnus m.

Gracilis m.
Semimembranosus m.

Semitendinosus m.

1. Note the transformation of the rectus femoris muscle into the rectus femoris tendon.

2. The short head of biceps femoris maintains a rectangular configuration compared with the more oval appearance of the long head.

3. The size of the adductor magnus decreases as the sections proceed inferiorly.

4. The linea aspera is the rough linear area on the posterior aspect of the femur providing an attachment site for vastus medialis, vastus lateralis, adductor longus, adductor brevis, adductor magnus, and the short head of biceps.

5. At this level, the sciatic nerve has divided into the tibial and common peroneal nerves.

Figure 15.1.10

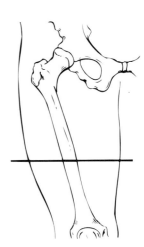

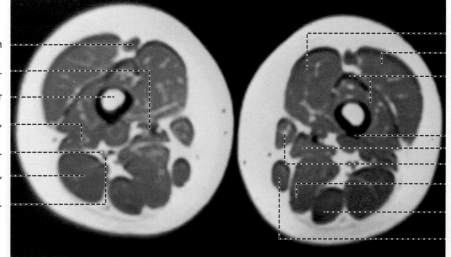

Rectus femoris tendon

Femoral a., v.

Femur

Biceps femoris m., short head

Common peroneal n.

Biceps femoris m., long head

Tibial n.

Vastus medialis m.

Vastus lateralis m.

Vastus intermedius m. and tendon

Linea aspera
Adductor magnus m.

Sartorius m.

Semimembranosus m.

Semitendinosus m.

Gracilis m.

Figure 15.1.13

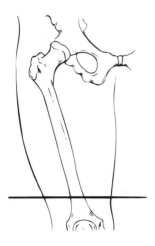

1. This section is at the level of the superior aspect of the popliteal space.

2. Note that the popliteal artery courses medial and anterior to the popliteal vein.

3. From this level down to the knee, the vastus medialis remains the most prominent member of the quadriceps group.

4. Gracilis and semitendinosus are tendinous from this level to their insertion on the proximal aspect of the anteromedial tibia.

5. At this level, the short head of biceps femoris is larger than the long head.

6. The tendons of vastus intermedius and rectus femoris are starting to fuse, forming the proximal portion of the quadriceps tendon.

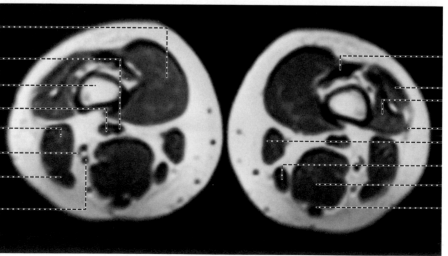

Vastus medialis m.

Popliteal a.

Femur

Popliteal v.

Biceps femoris m., short head

Common peroneal n.

Biceps femoris m., long head

Tibial n.

Quadriceps femoris tendon

Vastus lateralis m.

Vastus intermedius m.

Iliotibial tract

Sartorius m.

Gracilis m.

Semimembranosus m.

Semitendinosus m.

1. The quadriceps tendon is now clearly identifiable.

2. Vastus lateralis inserts into the lateral patellar retinaculum.

3. The iliotibial tract, which lies adjacent to vastus lateralis, is coursing toward its insertion on the anterolateral tibia.

4. The common peroneal nerve is adjacent to the medial surface of the short head of biceps femoris. The tendon of biceps femoris will insert on the head of the fibula.

5. The neurovascular bundle is seen posterior to the distal femur. At the level of the popliteal space, the artery is the most anterior, followed by the vein and the tibial nerve as the most posterior. The more lateral common peroneal nerve is deep to biceps femoris posterolaterally.

6. The three muscles that constitute the pes anserinus (sartorius, gracilis, and semitendinosus) will insert on the anteromedial upper tibia. The semimembranosus will insert on the posteromedial upper tibia, closer to the joint than the pes anserinus.

Figure 15.1.14

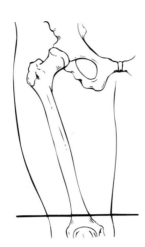

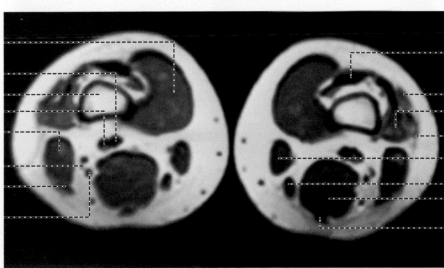

Vastus medialis m.

Popliteal a.

Femur

Popliteal v.

Biceps femoris m., short head

Common peroneal n.

Biceps femoris m., long head

Tibial n.

Quadriceps femoris tendon

Vastus lateralis m.

Vastus intermedius m.

Iliotibial tract

Sartorius m.

Gracilis m.

Semimembranosus m.

Semitendinosus m.

Figure 15.2.1

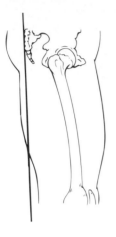

1. This section passes through the posterior aspect of the buttocks.

2. Gluteus maximus originates from the posterior aspect of the ilium, dorsal sacrum, and coccyx. It covers the origin of the hamstring group on the ischial tuberosity.

3. From medial to lateral, the proximal portion of the hamstring group consists of semimembranosus, semitendinosus, and long head of biceps femoris.

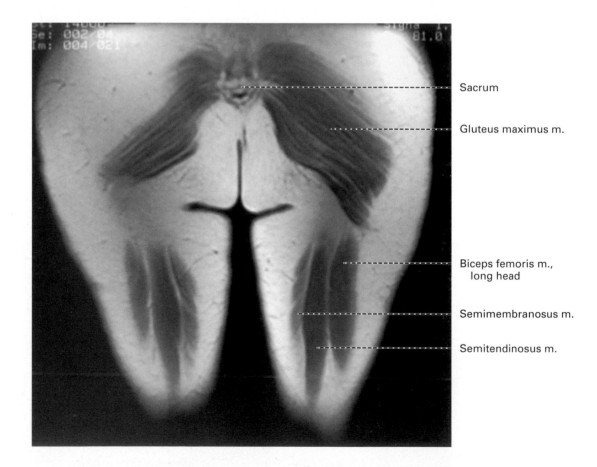

Sacrum

Gluteus maximus m.

Biceps femoris m., long head

Semimembranosus m.

Semitendinosus m.

1. Gluteus maximus originates from the posterior ilium, dorsolateral sacrum, and coccyx.

2. The long head of the biceps femoris originates from the ischial tuberosity. The short head originates from the posterior aspect of the distal femur.

Figure 15.2.2

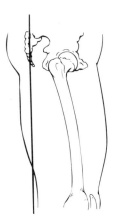

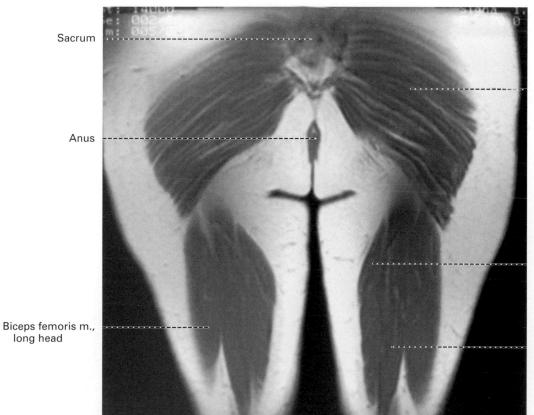

Sacrum

Gluteus maximus m.

Anus

Semimembranosus m.

Biceps femoris m., long head

Semitendinosus m.

Figure 15.2.3

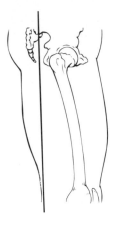

1. The external anal sphincter is noted around the anus.

2. Gracilis is partially visualized on this image.

3. Gracilis originates from the inferior pubic ramus near the symphysis and inserts on the proximal anteromedial tibia as part of the pes anserinus (goose's foot).

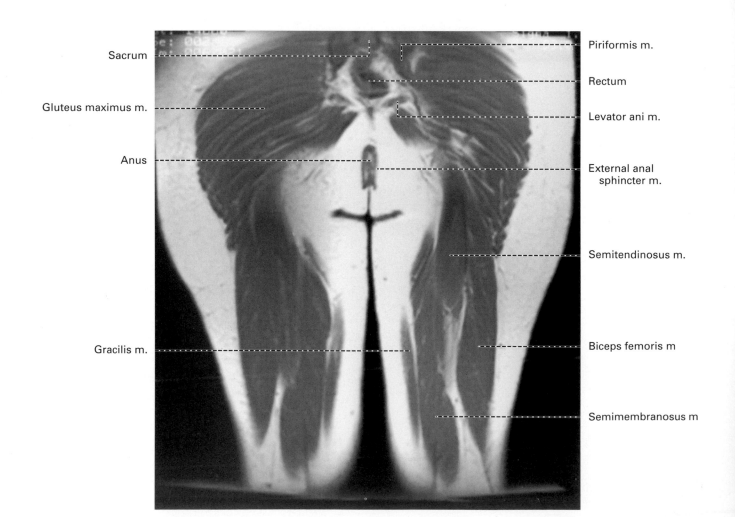

1. The conjoint tendon of the hamstring group arises from the ischium and is composed of semitendinosus and biceps femoris.

2. The fat of the ischiorectal fossa is in continuity with the medial subcutaneous fat of the proximal thigh.

3. The sciatic nerve exits the pelvis beneath the piriformis and above the superior gemellus.

4. Note that on the left side the sciatic nerve has divided into its two components, the tibial and peroneal nerves.

Figure 15.2.4

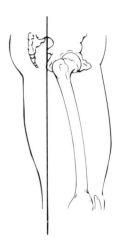

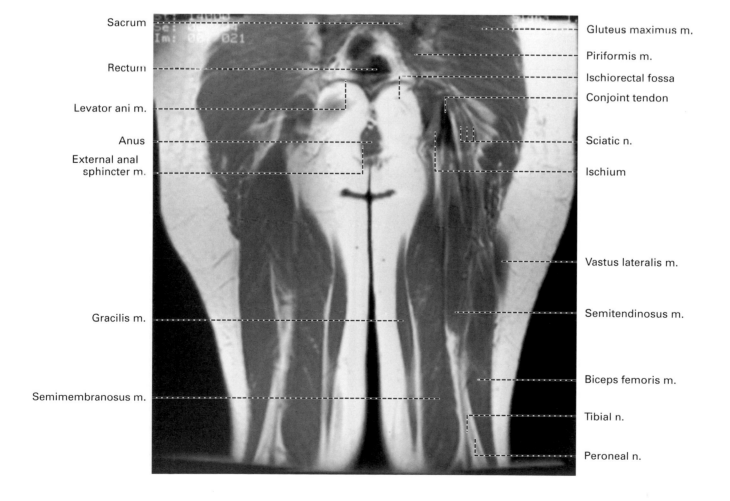

Figure 15.2.11

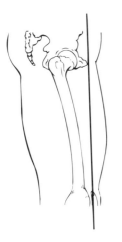

1. The common femoral vessels can be seen superiorly at the level of the groin; the artery is lateral to the vein.

2. The rectus femoris is seen coursing from its origins on the anterior superior iliac spine and posterolateral supra-acetabular region to its insertion in the quadriceps tendon.

3. Pectineus and adductor longus are seen arising from the superior pubic ramus and pubic bone near the symphysis, respectively.

4. Vastus medialis is seen lateral to sartorius; it arises from the posteromedial femur.

5. A portion of the femoral circumflex circulation can be seen at this level.

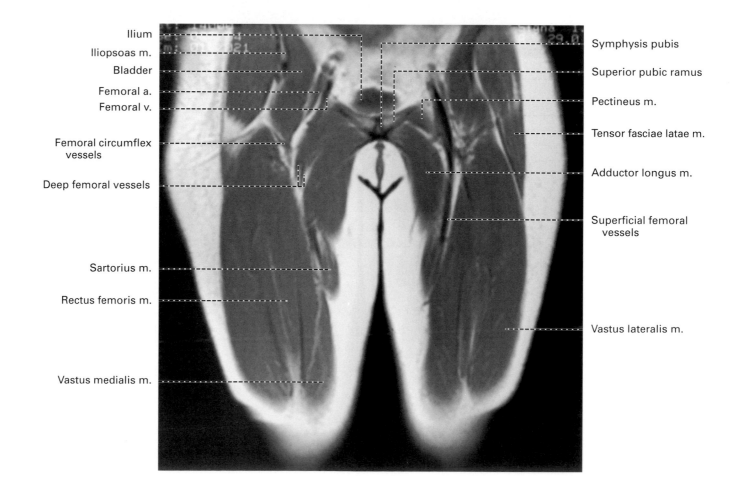

1. Tensor fasciae latae arises from the anterior iliac crest and is well visualized at this level.

2. The great saphenous vein is seen draining into the femoral vein.

3. The linea alba is the anterior midline aponeurosis between the two rectus abdominus muscles.

Figure 15.2.12

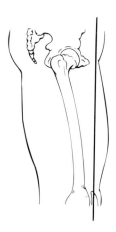

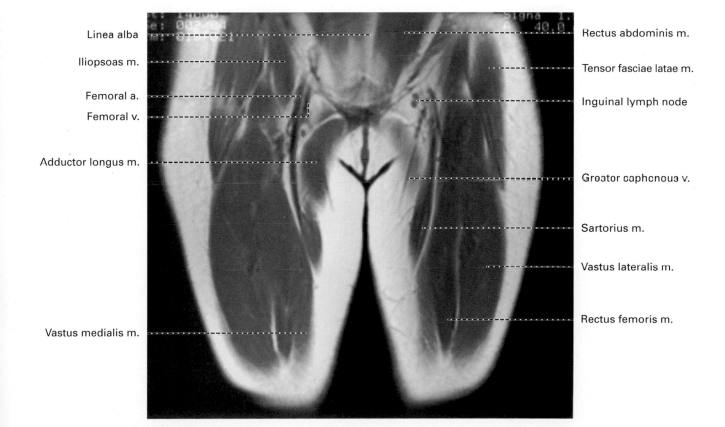

Linea alba

Iliopsoas m.

Femoral a.

Femoral v.

Adductor longus m.

Vastus medialis m.

Rectus abdominis m.

Tensor fasciae latae m.

Inguinal lymph node

Greater saphenous v.

Sartorius m.

Vastus lateralis m.

Rectus femoris m.

Figure 15.2.13

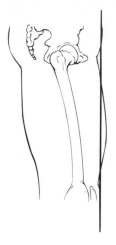

1. Note sartorius coursing inferiorly from its origin at the anterior superior iliac spine.

2. Rectus femoris is coursing inferiorly from its origin at the anterior inferior iliac spine and posterolateral supra-acetabular region.

3. Note inguinal lymph nodes bilaterally.

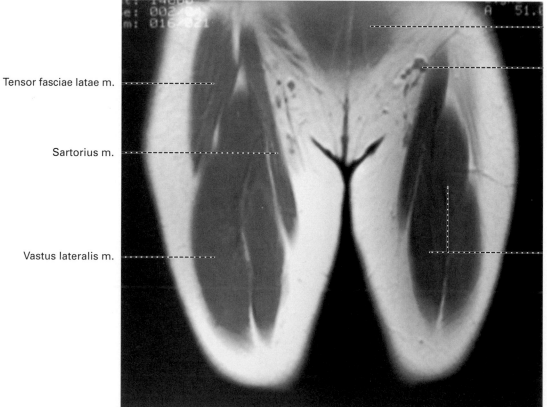

Tensor fasciae latae m.

Sartorius m.

Vastus lateralis m.

Rectus abdominis m.

Inguinal lymph nodes

Rectus femoris m.

1. This section passes through the anterior aspect of the thigh.

Figure 15.2.14

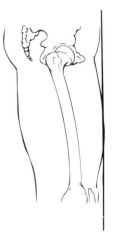

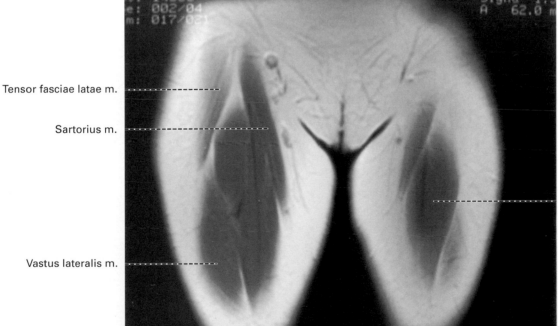

Tensor fasciae latae m.

Sartorius m.

Rectus femoris m.

Vastus lateralis m.

SAGITTAL

Figure 15.3.1

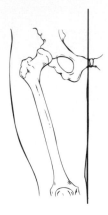

1. This section passes sagittally through the most medial aspect of the thigh.

2. Gracilis is partially demonstrated arising from the pubic ramus near the symphysis.

3. Gluteus maximus arises from the dorsomedial aspect of the ilium, sacrum, and coccyx.

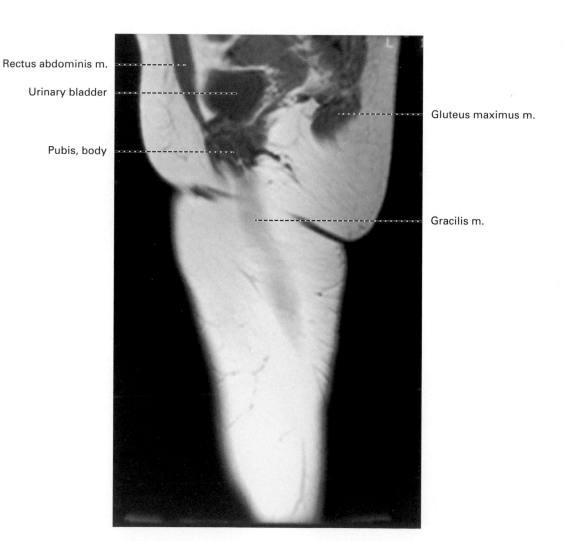

Rectus abdominis m.

Urinary bladder

Pubis, body

Gluteus maximus m.

Gracilis m.

1. Gracilis arises from the inferior pubic ramus near the symphysis.

2. Vastus medialis and sartorius are seen anterior to the gracilis.

3. The pectineus and adductor brevis are arising from the superior and inferior pubic rami, respectively.

Figure 15.3.2

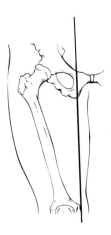

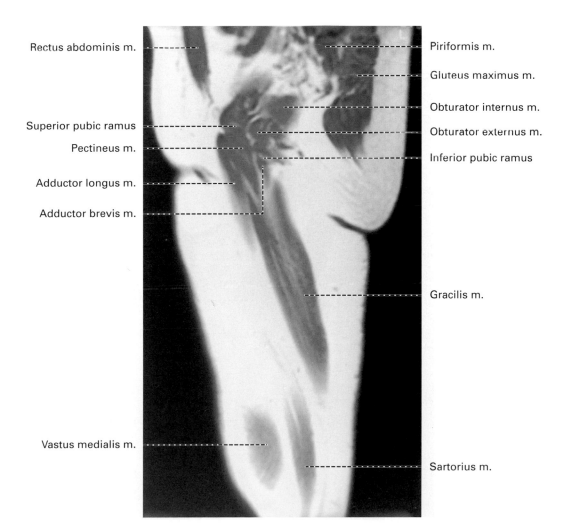

Rectus abdominis m.

Superior pubic ramus

Pectineus m.

Adductor longus m.

Adductor brevis m.

Vastus medialis m.

Piriformis m.

Gluteus maximus m.

Obturator internus m.

Obturator externus m.

Inferior pubic ramus

Gracilis m.

Sartorius m.

Figure 15.3.5

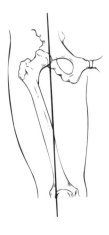

1. The pectineus arises from the pecten (edge) of the superior pubic ramus and courses posterolaterally to insert on the pectineal line of the femur. It forms the medial floor of the femoral triangle.

2. The iliopsoas courses anterior to the femoral head. It turns nearly 90 degrees posteriorly to insert on the lesser trochanter. It forms the lateral floor of the femoral triangle.

3. The semitendinosus muscle courses distally posterior to the semimembranosus muscle. It forms the posterior component of the pes anserinus complex (sartorius, gracilis, and semitendinosus), which inserts on the anteromedial aspect of the proximal tibia.

4. Note the superficial femoral vessels coursing distally underneath the sartorius in the adductor canal.

5. As the superficial femoral vessels exit the adductor hiatus, distal to the muscular portion of the adductor magnus, they become the popliteal vessels.

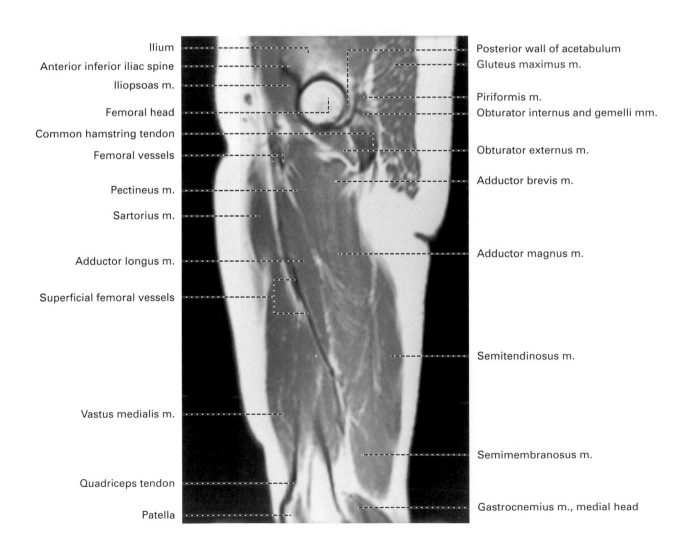

Ilium
Anterior inferior iliac spine
Iliopsoas m.
Femoral head
Common hamstring tendon
Femoral vessels
Pectineus m.
Sartorius m.
Adductor longus m.
Superficial femoral vessels
Vastus medialis m.
Quadriceps tendon
Patella

Posterior wall of acetabulum
Gluteus maximus m.
Piriformis m.
Obturator internus and gemelli mm.
Obturator externus m.
Adductor brevis m.
Adductor magnus m.
Semitendinosus m.
Semimembranosus m.
Gastrocnemius m., medial head

1. Note the sciatic nerve exiting the pelvis inferior to the piriformis and superior to the obturator internus and gemelli muscles.

2. The deep femoral artery (profunda femoris artery) is seen coursing posterior to the adductor longus.

3. Rectus femoris is seen merging into the quadriceps tendon. The quadriceps tendon is formed from the insertion of the rectus femoris, vastus medialis, vastus lateralis, and vastus intermedius.

4. The semimembranosus tendon is seen at its origin from the ischial tuberosity. The semitendinosus tendon and muscle are posterior to the origin of the semimembranosus tendon.

5. The sciatic nerve courses distally on the posterior surface of the adductor magnus.

Figure 15.3.6

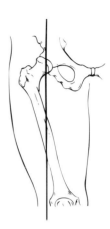

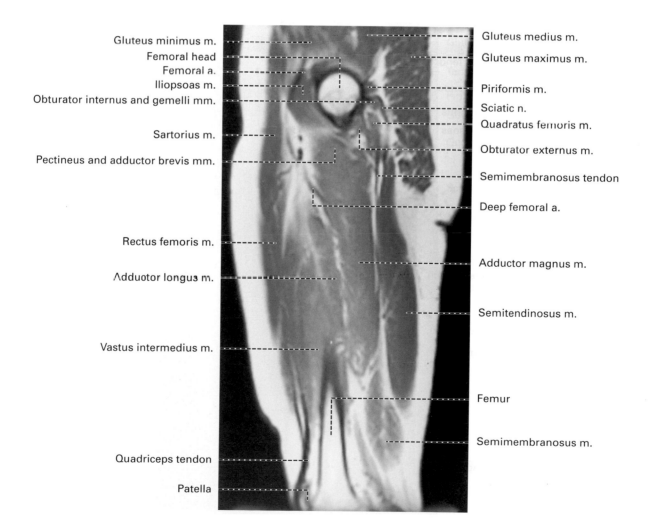

Figure 15.3.9

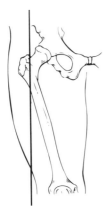

1. Vastus lateralis is partially demonstrated as the sections move more laterally.

2. The long and short heads of the biceps femoris merge in the distal thigh to insert on the fibular head.

3. Adductor magnus inserts on the medial supracondylar line of the femur.

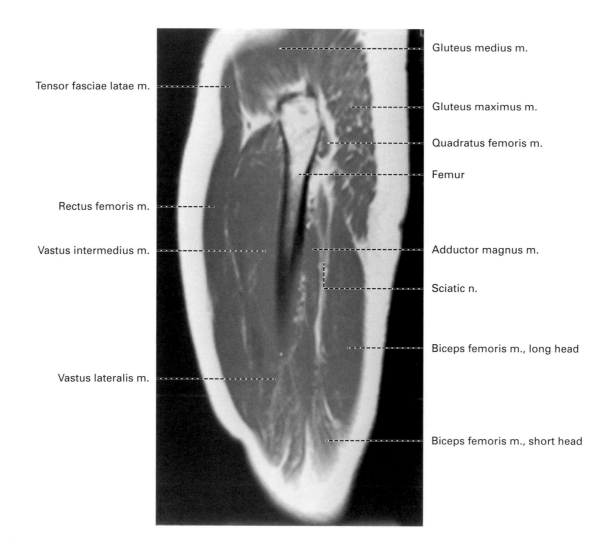

1. Gluteus medius is identified close to its insertion on the greater trochanter.

2. Tensor fasciae latae is partially demonstrated in the proximal anterolateral thigh. It extends distally as the iliotibial band and inserts on a prominence on the anterolateral tibia known as Gerdy's tubercle.

3. Rectus femoris originates deep to tensor fasciae latae from the anterior inferior iliac spine (straight head) and the posterolateral supra-acetabular region (reflected head).

Figure 15.3.10

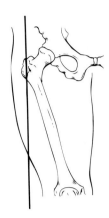

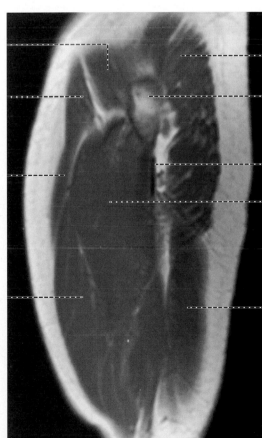

Gluteus medius m.

Tensor fasciae latae m.

Rectus femoris m.

Vastus lateralis m.

Gluteus maximus m.

Greater trochanter

Iliotibial tract

Vastus intermedius m.

Biceps femoris m., long head

Figure 15.3.11

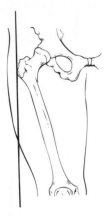

1. The superficial fibers of gluteus maximus insert into the iliotibial tract. The deeper fibers insert on the posterolateral femur below the intertrochanteric line.

2. The tensor fascia lata muscle originates from the anterior iliac crest.

3. Vastus lateralis makes up the majority of the lateral musculature of the thigh.

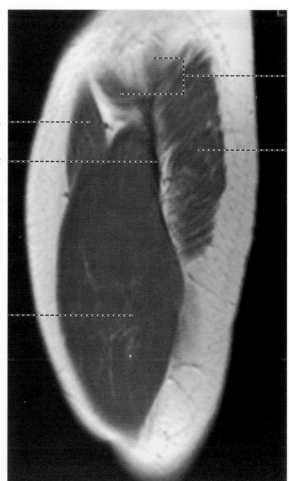

Tensor fasciae latae m.

Iliotibial tract

Vastus lateralis m.

Gluteus medius m.

Gluteus maximus m.

1. Gluteus maximus inserts on the posterolateral femur and the iliotibial tract.

2. Vastus lateralis originates from the posterolateral femur along the lateral portion of the linea aspera. Its most superior origin is from the anterior and lateral surface of the proximal femur at the level of the mid- and lower portions of the greater trochanter.

Figure 15.3.12

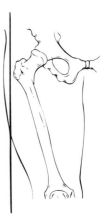

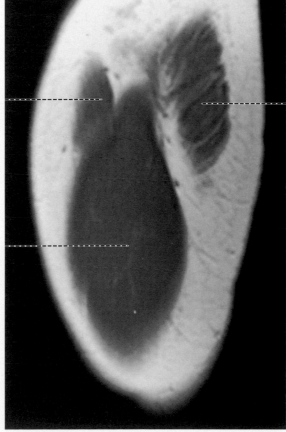

Tensor fasciae latae m.   Gluteus maximus m.

Vastus lateralis m.

Figure 15.3.13

1. This section cuts through the most lateral aspect of the thigh, passing through vastus lateralis and gluteus maximus.

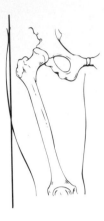

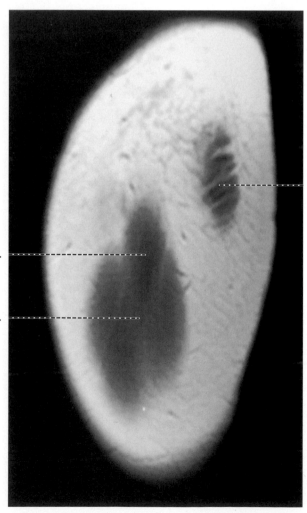

Gluteus maximus m.

Tensor fasciae latae m.

Vastus lateralis m.

Chapter 16

KNEE

Figure 16.1.1

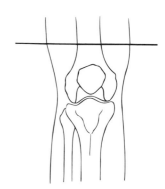

1. Semitendinosus is tendinous at this level and lies posterior to semimembranosus.

2. Gracilis is nearly completely tendinous at this level.

3. The popliteal artery is anterior and medial to the popliteal vein in the superior popliteal fossa.

4. The tendinous continuation of adductor magnus lies posterior to vastus medialis.

5. Quadriceps tendon is well defined, and the superior portion of the lateral patellar retinaculum is visualized.

6. The sciatic nerve, having already divided into the tibial and common peroneal nerves, lies adjacent to the biceps femoris (short head).

7. The communicating peroneal nerve branches from the common peroneal nerve and courses posteromedially as it extends inferiorly to join the sural nerve.

8. The popliteal fossa is a diamond-shaped space defined superiorly by the biceps femoris laterally and the semitendinosus and semimembranosus medially. Its inferior borders are the respective medial and lateral heads of the gastrocnemius.

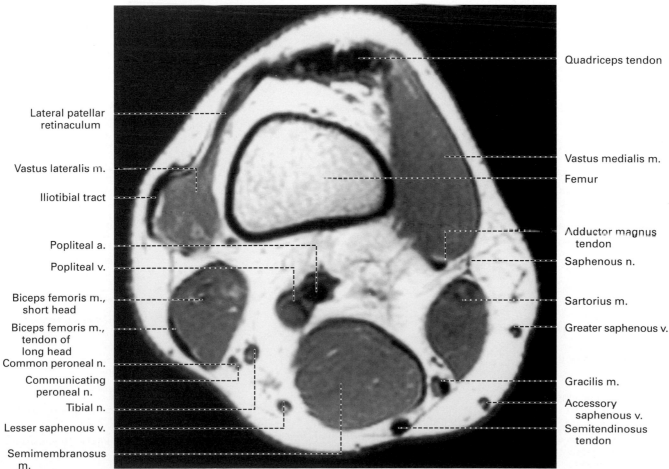

Quadriceps tendon

Lateral patellar retinaculum

Vastus lateralis m.

Iliotibial tract

Vastus medialis m.

Femur

Popliteal a.

Popliteal v.

Adductor magnus tendon

Saphenous n.

Biceps femoris m., short head

Biceps femoris m., tendon of long head

Common peroneal n.

Communicating peroneal n.

Tibial n.

Lesser saphenous v.

Semimembranosus m.

Sartorius m.

Greater saphenous v.

Gracilis m.

Accessory saphenous v.

Semitendinosus tendon

Figure 16.1.2

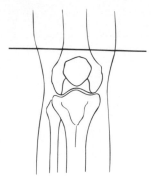

1. Iliotibial tract is superficial to the last vestiges of vastus lateralis muscle.

2. Lesser saphenous vein is nearly midline posteriorly. This individual has a pair of veins in place of one prominent greater saphenous vein. The posterior branch is probably part of the accessory saphenous vein, which joins the greater saphenous vein in the thigh at a variable level. The anterior branch is the greater saphenous vein.

3. Posterior femoral cutaneous nerve lies immediately adjacent to the lesser saphenous vein.

4. Gracilis has become tendinous at this level.

5. The synovial space of the suprapatellar bursa is discernible. Note the extent of the bursa around the anterolateral margin of the femur.

6. The vertical "grooves" in the quadriceps tendon are its very superior insertion into the superior pole of the patella.

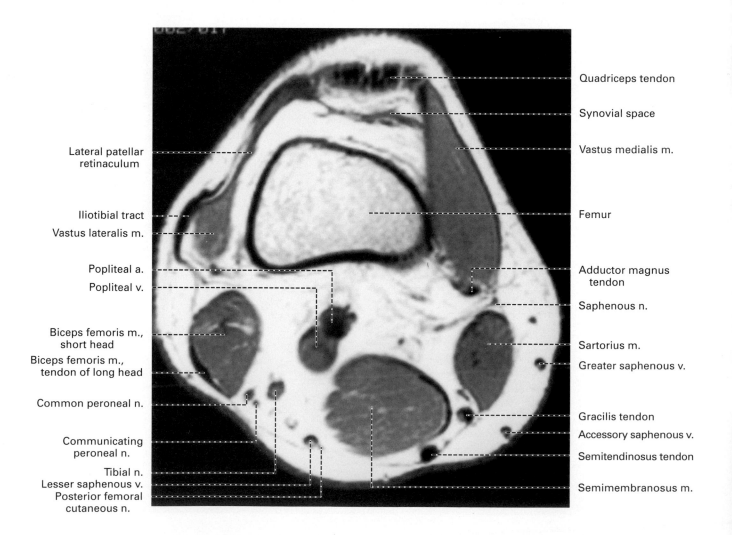

1. The iliotibial tract blends with the lateral patellar retinaculum anterolaterally.

2. The tendinous portion of the semimembranosus is crescentic and continues thus until its insertion on the posterior medial aspect of the tibial condyle.

3. The tendon of adductor magnus is near its insertion on the adductor tubercle of the medial femoral condyle.

4. The superior genicular artery (medial and lateral branches) arises at this level.

5. A medial patellar retinaculum can now be identified.

Figure 16.1.3

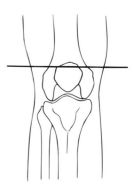

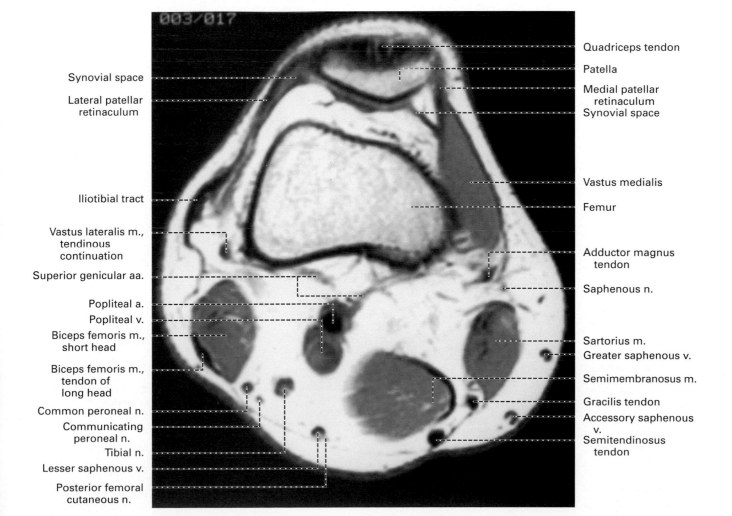

Figure 16.1.4

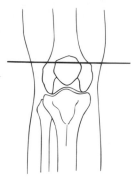

1. At this level, the lateral patellar retinaculum, iliotibial tract, and fascia of biceps femoris are continuous.

2. Plantaris and gastrocnemius (lateral head) arise in close proximity and may be difficult to differentiate as in this section. Plantaris will be deep and medial to the lateral head gastrocnemius.

3. Tendon of adductor magnus inserts on the superior medial femoral condyle known as the adductor tubercle.

4. In the extended knee, the patellar articular cartilage is partially superior to the articular cartilage of the anterior patellar surface of the femur.

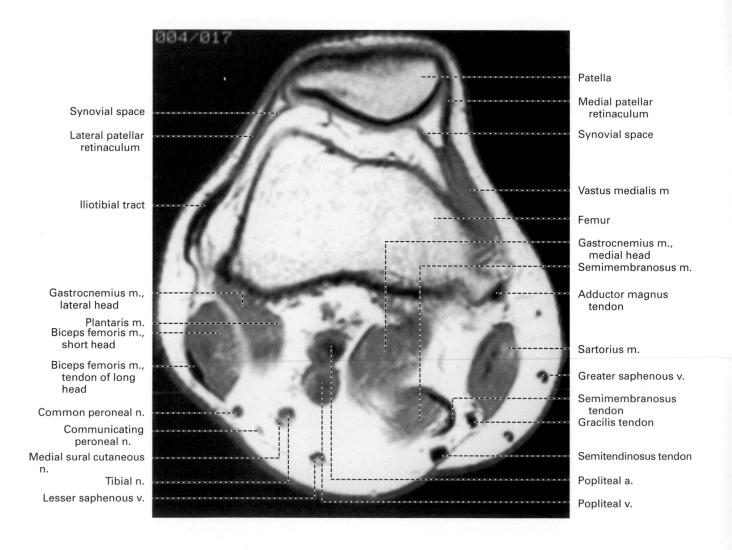

004/017

Synovial space
Lateral patellar retinaculum
Iliotibial tract
Gastrocnemius m., lateral head
Plantaris m.
Biceps femoris m., short head
Biceps femoris m., tendon of long head
Common peroneal n.
Communicating peroneal n.
Medial sural cutaneous n.
Tibial n.
Lesser saphenous v.

Patella
Medial patellar retinaculum
Synovial space
Vastus medialis m
Femur
Gastrocnemius m., medial head
Semimembranosus m.
Adductor magnus tendon
Sartorius m.
Greater saphenous v.
Semimembranosus tendon
Gracilis tendon
Semitendinosus tendon
Popliteal a.
Popliteal v.

1. The popliteal vessels have an anterior-posterior relation at this level; the artery is anterior.

2. This section is at the level of the patellar "equator" in the extended knee.

3. The two heads of gastrocnemius remain "separated" by the major popliteal vessels.

4. The medial sural cutaneous nerve has originated from the tibial nerve. It will join the communicating branch of the peroneal nerve before the next (distal) image.

5. Tibial (medial) collateral ligament originates from this superior portion of the medial femoral condyle.

6. Semimembranous persists solely as a crescentic tendon from this level to its insertion on the posterior medial tibial condyle.

7. Common peroneal nerve migrates laterally, continuing to follow the biceps femoris muscle and tendon.

8. Tibial nerve migrates toward the popliteal vessels.

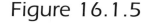

Figure 16.1.5

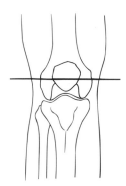

Articular cartilage

005/017

Patella

Lateral patellar retinaculum

Medial patellar retinaculum

Lateral femoral condyle

Synovial space

Iliotibial tract

Femur

Tibial collateral lig.

Biceps femoris m., short head

Popliteal a.

Gastrocnemius m., lateral head

Sartorius m.

Biceps femoris m., tendon of long head

Greater saphenous v.

Medial sural cutaneous n.

Semimembranosus tendon

Common peroneal n.

Gracilis tendon

Communicating peroneal n.

Semitendinosus tendon

Tibial n.

Gastrocnemius m., medial head

Lesser saphenous v.

Popliteal v.

Figure 16.1.6

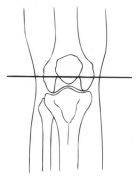

1. The superior articular cartilage of the patellar surface of the femur is more prominent laterally.

2. At this level of the intercondylar notch, the anterior cruciate ligament arises from the lateral femoral condyle.

3. At this level, the lateral patellar retinaculum is thicker than the medial patellar retinaculum.

4. Sartorius remains muscular at this level. It is the most anterior of the pes anserinus (sartorius, gracilis, semitendinosus), a tendon complex that inserts on the anteromedial tibia.

5. Middle genicular artery branches supply the anterior and posterior cruciate ligaments as well as their investing synovium.

6. The bursa between the semimembranosus tendon and the medial head of gastrocnemius is also insinuated between the articular cartilage of the posterior medial femoral condyle and the medial head of gastrocnemius.

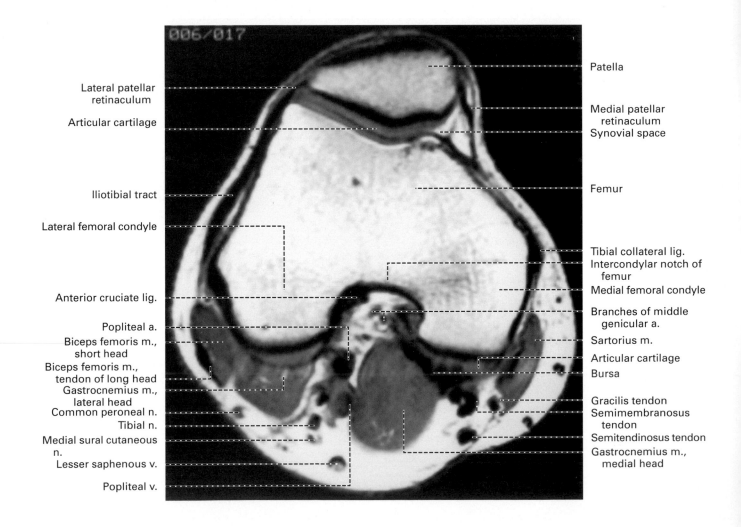

1. At this level, the iliotibial tract and the fibular (lateral) collateral ligament are difficult to distinguish, although the former is more anterior.

2. Note the bursa identifiable between the tendon of semimembranosus and the medial head of gastrocnemius. This is a common finding. The bursa may communicate with that of the knee joint.

3. The fibular collateral ligament arises from a prominence on the lateral femoral condyle.

4. Note that the patellar retinaculum and, laterally, the iliotibial tract are the structures that attach the patella to the collateral ligaments.

Figure 16.1.7

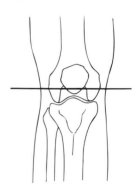

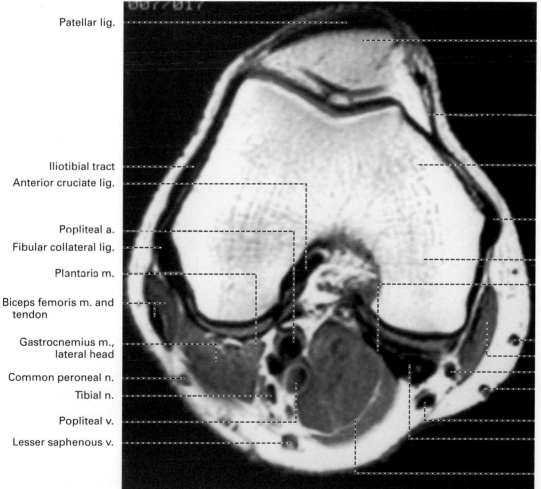

Patellar lig.

Iliotibial tract
Anterior cruciate lig.

Popliteal a.
Fibular collateral lig.

Plantaris m.

Biceps femoris m. and
tendon

Gastrocnemius m.,
lateral head

Common peroneal n.
Tibial n.

Popliteal v.

Lesser saphenous v.

Patella

Medial patellar
retinaculum

Femur

Tibial collateral lig.

Medial femoral condyle

Bursa between
gastrocnemius m. and
tendon of
semimembranosus m.

Greater saphenous v.
Sartorius m.
Gracilis tendon
Accessory saphenous v.

Semitendinosus tendon
Semimembranosus
tendon

Gastrocnemius m.,
medial head

Figure 16.1.8

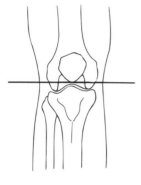

1. This level is at the lower pole of the patella, where the proximal portion of the patellar ligament (also referred to as the patellar tendon) is visualized anterior to the infrapatellar fat pad.

2. The posterior cruciate ligament arises from the inner surface of the medial femoral condyle at this level.

3. The most superior aspect of the popliteus tendon inserts into the popliteus groove or recess. It is deep to and separate from the fibular collateral ligament.

4. The tibial nerve remains between the two heads of the gastrocnemius and posterior to the popliteal vessels.

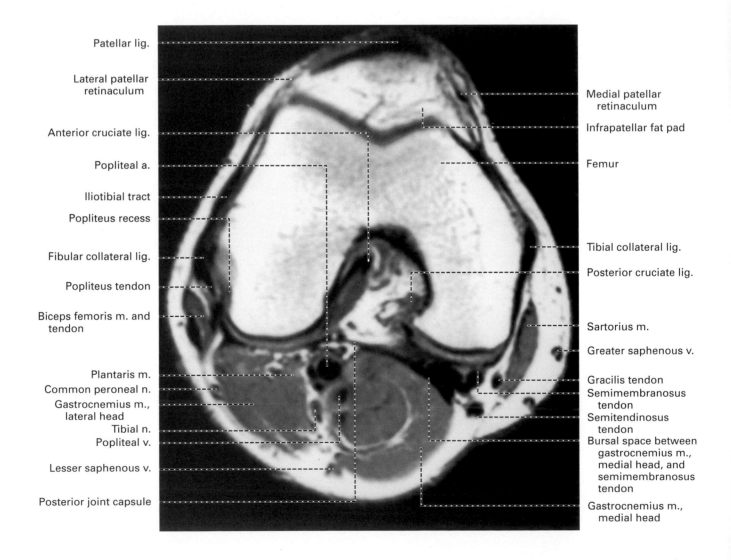

Patellar lig.

Lateral patellar retinaculum

Anterior cruciate lig.

Popliteal a.

Iliotibial tract

Popliteus recess

Fibular collateral lig.

Popliteus tendon

Biceps femoris m. and tendon

Plantaris m.
Common peroneal n.
Gastrocnemius m., lateral head
Tibial n.
Popliteal v.

Lesser saphenous v.

Posterior joint capsule

Medial patellar retinaculum

Infrapatellar fat pad

Femur

Tibial collateral lig.

Posterior cruciate lig.

Sartorius m.

Greater saphenous v.

Gracilis tendon
Semimembranosus tendon
Semitendinosus tendon
Bursal space between gastrocnemius m., medial head, and semimembranosus tendon

Gastrocnemius m., medial head

1. A well-defined, thin posterior joint capsule is identifiable just above the tibiofemoral joint.

2. Sartorius still has a muscular component in addition to a tendinous component.

3. The common peroneal nerve lies deep to the investing fascia between the tendon of biceps femoris and the lateral head of gastrocnemius.

4. The lesser saphenous vein occupies the cleft between the two heads of gastrocnemius.

Figure 16.1.9

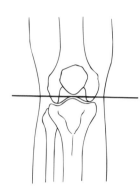

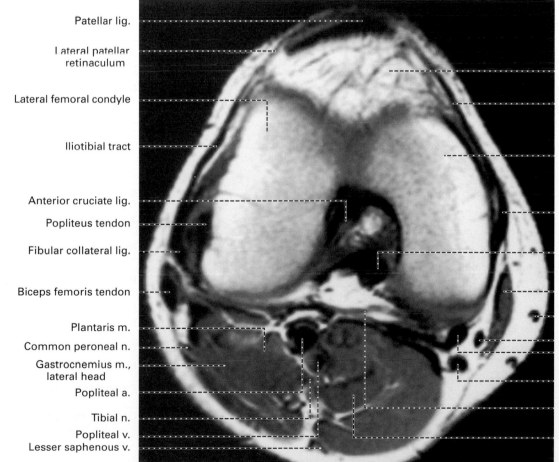

Patellar lig.

Lateral patellar retinaculum

Lateral femoral condyle

Iliotibial tract

Anterior cruciate lig.

Popliteus tendon

Fibular collateral lig.

Biceps femoris tendon

Plantaris m.

Common peroneal n.

Gastrocnemius m., lateral head

Popliteal a.

Tibial n.

Popliteal v.
Lesser saphenous v.

Infrapatellar fat

Medial patellar retinaculum

Medial femoral condyle

Tibial collateral lig.

Posterior cruciate lig.

Sartorius m. and tendon

Greater saphenous v.

Gracilis tendon
Semimembranosus tendon

Semitendinosus tendon

Posterior joint capsule

Gastrocnemius m., medial head

Figure 16.1.10

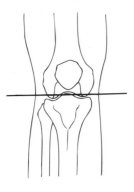

1. This image is at the level of the joint line.

2. The anterior cruciate ligament inserts on the tibia anterior to the anterior intercondylar eminence. It has an anteromedial portion as well as a posterolateral bundle of fibers. The anteromedial portion crosses over the posterolateral bundle when the knee flexes.

3. The posterior cruciate ligament attaches to a depression on the posterior intercondylar region of the tibia behind the posterior intercondylar tubercle.

4. Biceps femoris tendon and the fibular collateral ligament approach one another as they progress inferiorly, becoming essentially conjoint at their attachment on the fibular head.

5. Note that the greater saphenous vein courses with sartorius.

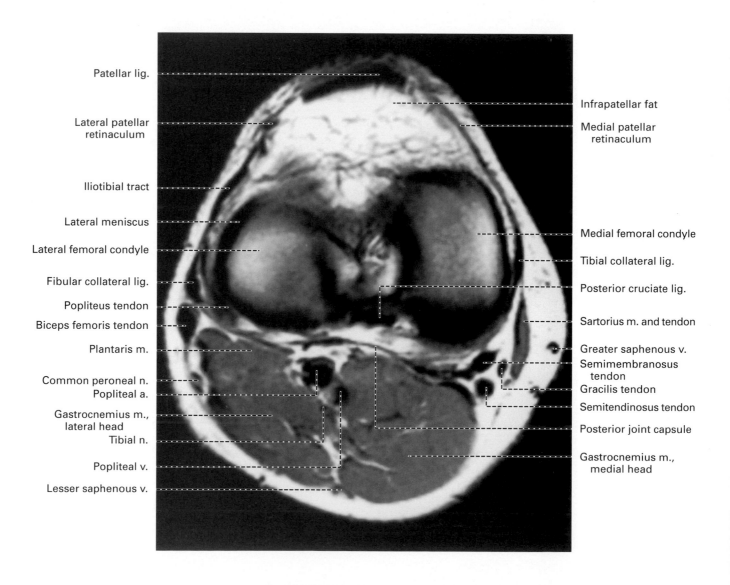

1. This section is through the joint line.

2. At the level of the proximal tibia, the popliteus tendon is adjacent and slightly inferior to the lateral meniscus. At the posterolateral margin of the joint the tendon is an intra-articular structure.

3. The superior edge of popliteus is noted between the popliteal artery and the tibia. Popliteus is a prominent muscle separating the popliteal vessels and tibial nerve from the proximal tibia. This muscle becomes very important in exophytic tumors of the proximal tibia. If its integrity is preserved limb salvage is usually possible.

4. The deep veins of the proximal calf course within the substance of the heads of gastrocnemius. Deep venous thrombosis can sometimes be seen in these veins.

5. The lateral sural cutaneous nerve, carrying sensation from the posterior and lateral surfaces of the leg, has branched posteriorly from the common peroneal nerve. It is difficult to visualize inferiorly.

6. A prominent inferior lateral genicular artery branch is seen between popliteus tendon and the fibular collateral ligament.

Figure 16.1.11

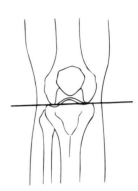

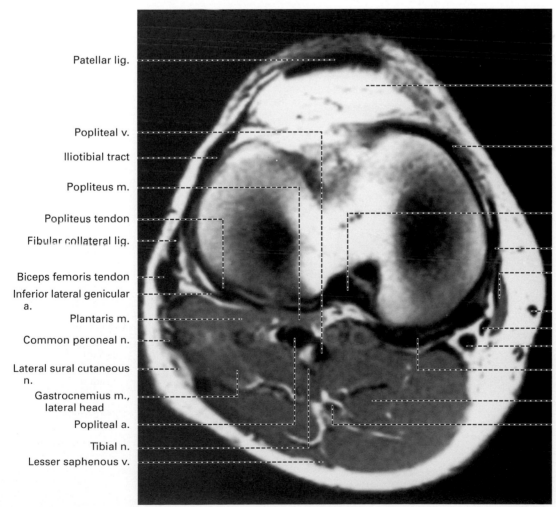

Patellar lig.

Infrapatellar fat pad

Popliteal v.

Iliotibial tract

Coronary lig.

Popliteus m.

Popliteus tendon

Posterior cruciate lig.

Fibular collateral lig.

Tibial collateral lig.

Biceps femoris tendon

Sartorius m. and tendon

Inferior lateral genicular a.

Plantaris m.

Greater saphenous v.

Gracilis tendon

Common peroneal n.

Semitendinosus tendon

Lateral sural cutaneous n.

Semimembranosus tendon

Gastrocnemius m., lateral head

Gastrocnemius m., medial head

Popliteal a.

Deep veins of calf

Tibial n.

Lesser saphenous v.

Figure 16.1.12

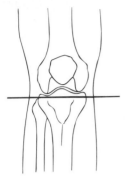

1. The fibular collateral ligament and biceps femoris tendon have become conjoined at their attachment to the proximal fibula.

2. The tibial collateral ligament is attached to the tibia; however, some fibers will continue with the pes anserinus (goose's foot tendon complex).

3. The pes anserinus (the tendons of insertion of sartorius, gracilis, and semi-tendinosus) is identifiable on the medial border of the proximal tibia, just prior to its migration anteriorly. Sartorius is now primarily tendinous.

4. As the patellar ligament extends inferiorly it becomes slightly thicker but narrower.

5. The common peroneal nerve is seen posterior to the biceps femoris tendon.

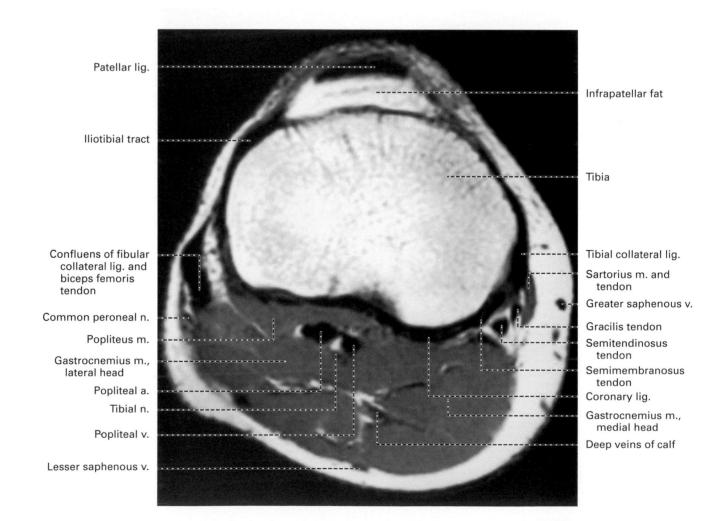

Patellar lig.

Iliotibial tract

Confluens of fibular collateral lig. and biceps femoris tendon

Common peroneal n.

Popliteus m.

Gastrocnemius m., lateral head

Popliteal a.

Tibial n.

Popliteal v.

Lesser saphenous v.

Infrapatellar fat

Tibia

Tibial collateral lig.

Sartorius m. and tendon

Greater saphenous v.

Gracilis tendon

Semitendinosus tendon

Semimembranosus tendon

Coronary lig.

Gastrocnemius m., medial head

Deep veins of calf

1. This section is through the tip of the fibular head. Note that the conjoint biceps tendon and fibular collateral ligament are extending anterolaterally.

2. The proximal tibiofibular joint is visualized. This joint has variable obliquity.

3. The prominence on the anterolateral surface of the tibia is known as Gerdy's tubercle. It serves as the insertion site of the iliotibial tract (also known as the iliotibial band).

4. At this level, the greater saphenous vein divides into a smaller persistent greater saphenous vein adjacent to sartorius and into a smaller posterior branch that is part of the accessory saphenous system.

Figure 16.1.13

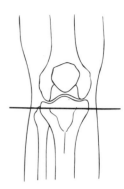

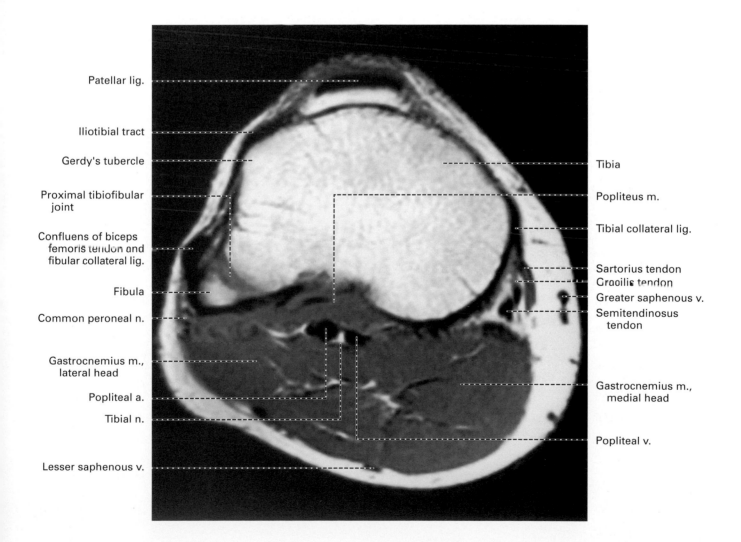

Figure 16.1.14

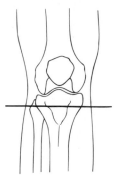

1. The soleus can be appreciated as it arises from the proximal fibula posteriorly.

2. Gerdy's tubercle, the insertion site of the iliotibial tract, is noted.

3. Just posterior and lateral to Gerdy's tubercle is the origin of the most superior fibers of tibialis anterior.

4. The tendons forming pes anserinus (sartorius, gracilis, and semitendinosus) are no longer round but are now ovoid or flattened as they begin to course anteriorly.

5. Patellar ligament is seen inserting on the tibial tuberosity, which is not in the middle of the tibia but more lateral.

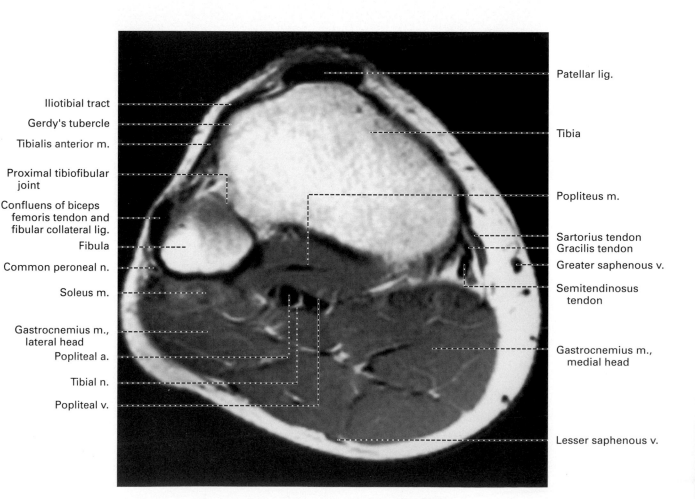

1. Note at this level that the superficial group of muscles of the posterior compartment (gastrocnemius, soleus, and plantaris) are separated from the only muscle of the deep group (popliteus) by the popliteal vessels.

2. The popliteal vessels are now oriented side by side with the popliteal artery being lateral to the vein.

3. The vessels remain as "popliteal" vessels until they reach the inferior border of popliteus.

4. Note that the common peroneal nerve is beginning to migrate anteriorly around the lateral aspect of the proximal fibular head and neck.

5. The superior origin of the long extensor of the toes is seen as this muscle gains fibers from the anterior border of the fibula as well as the proximal tibia.

Figure 16.1.15

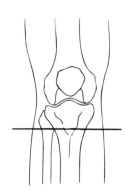

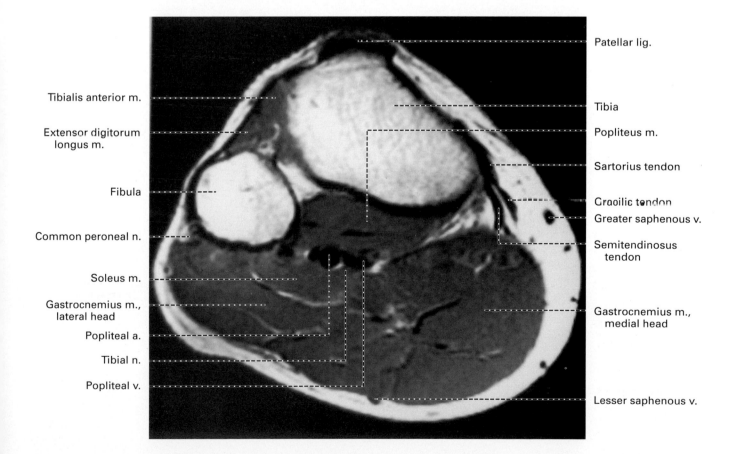

Patellar lig.

Tibialis anterior m.

Tibia

Extensor digitorum longus m.

Popliteus m.

Sartorius tendon

Fibula

Gracilis tendon

Greater saphenous v.

Common peroneal n.

Semitendinosus tendon

Soleus m.

Gastrocnemius m., lateral head

Gastrocnemius m., medial head

Popliteal a.

Tibial n.

Popliteal v.

Lesser saphenous v.

Figure 16.1.16

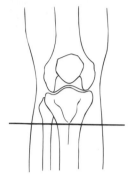

1. This image is at the lower border of popliteus. A portion of the anterior tibial artery is visualized.

2. Tibialis posterior is seen arising from the posterior surface of the interosseous membrane.

3. Peroneus longus is arising from the anterolateral metaphyseal flare of the fibula. Immediately behind is the common peroneal nerve.

4. The tibial nerve remains adjacent but posterior to the popliteal vessels.

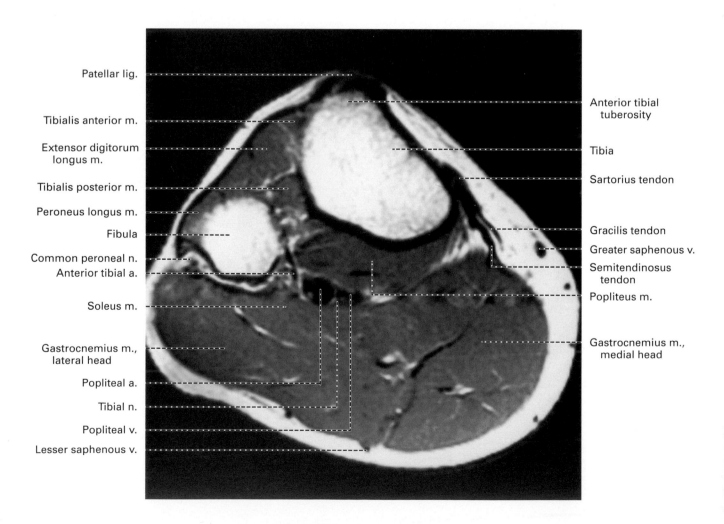

1. This level is at the inferior border of popliteus. The branching of the popliteal artery into anterior and posterior tibial arteries is noted.

2. The image is still too superior to include the other two muscles of the deep group of the posterior compartment (flexor hallucis longus and flexor digitorum longus).

3. The common peroneal nerve is now lateral to the fibular neck and under partial cover of peroneus longus.

4. The pes anserinus now appears as a confluent tendon complex along the surface of the anteromedial aspect of the tibia.

Figure 16.1.17

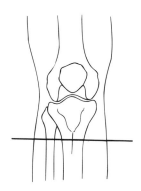

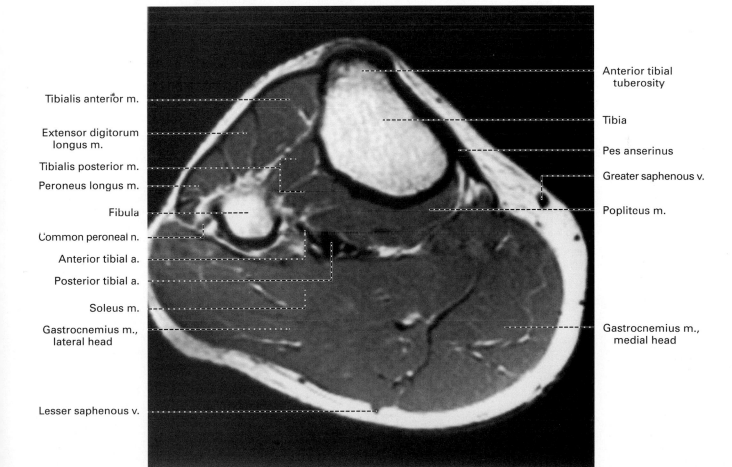

Anterior tibial tuberosity

Tibialis anterior m.

Extensor digitorum longus m.

Tibialis posterior m.

Peroneus longus m.

Fibula

Common peroneal n.

Anterior tibial a.

Posterior tibial a.

Soleus m.

Gastrocnemius m., lateral head

Lesser saphenous v.

Tibia

Pes anserinus

Greater saphenous v.

Popliteus m.

Gastrocnemius m., medial head

Figure 16.2.1

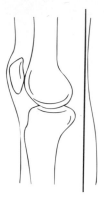

1. The lesser saphenous vein is posterior to the cleft formed by the two heads of gastrocnemius.

2. In this image, the tibial nerve is visualized superior to the two heads of gastrocnemius.

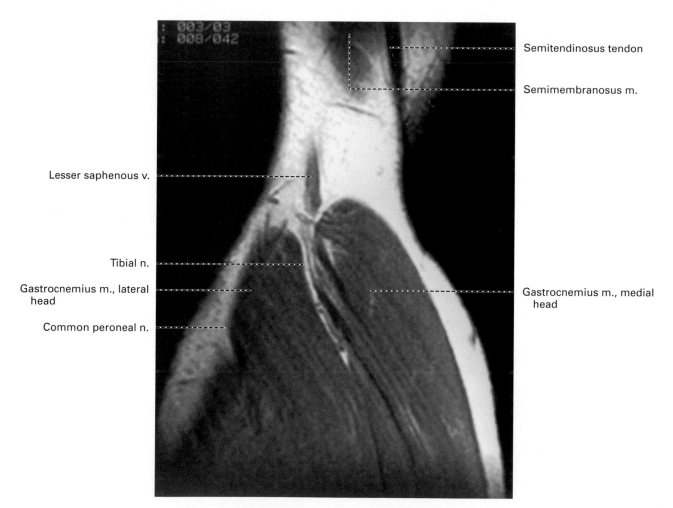

Semitendinosus tendon

Semimembranosus m.

Lesser saphenous v.

Tibial n.

Gastrocnemius m., lateral head

Common peroneal n.

Gastrocnemius m., medial head

1. The communicating peroneal nerve is identified. It is posterior to the common peroneal nerve, having branched from it superiorly. It is a communicating branch to the sural cutaneous nerve.

2. Soleus is identifiably separate from gastrocnemius.

3. The common peroneal nerve is within the investing fascia of the lateral head of gastrocnemius. It is easily identifiable because of its accompanying fat.

4. The descent of the tibial nerve in the cleft between the two heads of gastrocnemius is demonstrated in this posterior image.

Figure 16.2.2

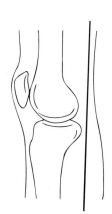

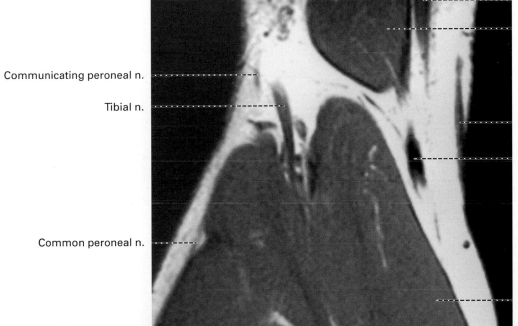

Communicating peroneal n.

Tibial n.

Common peroneal n.

Soleus m.

Gastrocnemius m., lateral head

Gracilis m.

Semimembranosus m.

Accessory saphenous v.

Semitendinosus tendon

Gastrocnemius m., medial head

Figure 16.2.3

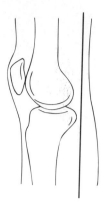

1. Semimembranosus has formed a dense prominent tendon.

2. Adjacent to semimembranosus are the three muscle tendons composing the pes anserinus (goose's foot tendon of insertion): sartorius, gracilis, and semitendinosus. There is still some muscular component of the sartorius at the knee joint.

3. A long segment of the common peroneal nerve is seen in this image.

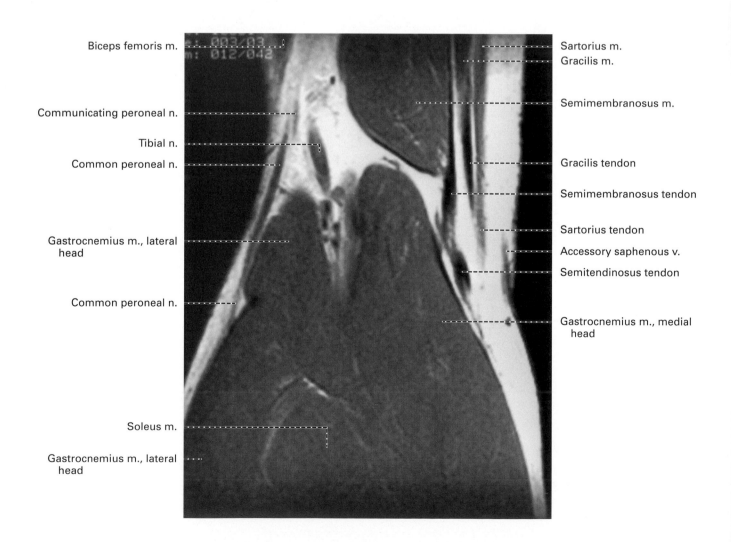

1. The tibial nerve diverges from the more lateral peroneal nerve as the sciatic nerve divides. The tibial nerve courses toward the popliteal vessels between the two heads of gastrocnemius.

2. The large soleus muscle can be seen in this image between and deep to the two heads of gastrocnemius.

3. The peroneal vein is more superficial than the popliteal vein and noted here close to the origin of the posterior tibial vein.

Figure 16.2.4

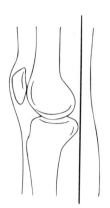

Biceps femoris m.

Common peroneal n.

Tibial n.

Gastrocnemius m., lateral head

Peroneal v.

Semimembranosus tendon

Common peroneal n.

Soleus m.

Gastrocnemius m., lateral head

Sartorius m.

Gracilis m.

Semimembranosus m.

Gastrocnemius m., medial head

Bursa between semimembranosus tendon and gastrocnemius m., medial head

Gracilis tendon

Sartorius tendon

Semitendinosus tendon

Posterior tibial tendon

Gastrocnemius m., medial head

Figure 16.2.5

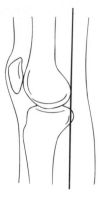

1. The sciatic nerve is closely approximated to the medial border of the short head of biceps femoris.

2. As the biceps femoris tendon courses inferiorly to approach the fibular head, it lies next to the common peroneal nerve.

3. The three tendons of the pes anserinus are identifiable: sartorius, gracilis, and semitendinosus.

4. Semimembranosus tendon is thick at this level just proximal to its insertion on the posterior medial condyle.

5. A portion of popliteus is visible. This muscle marks the inferior margin of the popliteal space. It is usually at the level of this muscle that the popliteal artery branches into the anterior and posterior tibial arteries. This muscle also provides an important buffer between the tibia and the popliteal and the tibial vessels.

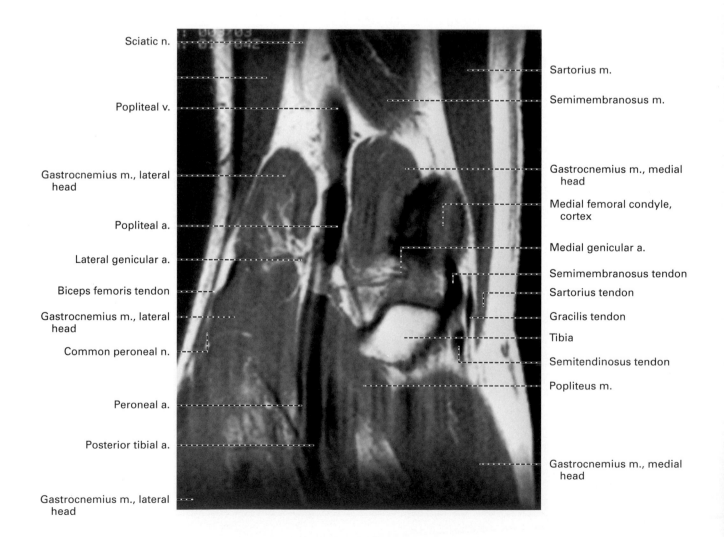

1. This level is at the insertion of semimembranosus tendon.

2. The proximal fibula sustains the insertion of biceps femoris tendon and the inferior attachment of the fibular (lateral) collateral ligament.

3. There is some variation in the level of the origin of the genicular arteries. Usually there are paired superior medial and lateral genicular branches, a single middle genicular artery, and paired inferior medial and lateral genicular arteries. The meniscal supply is usually from these last two branches; the middle genicular artery supplies the synovium and ligaments in the intercondylar notch.

Figure 16.2.6

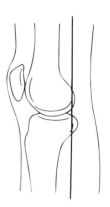

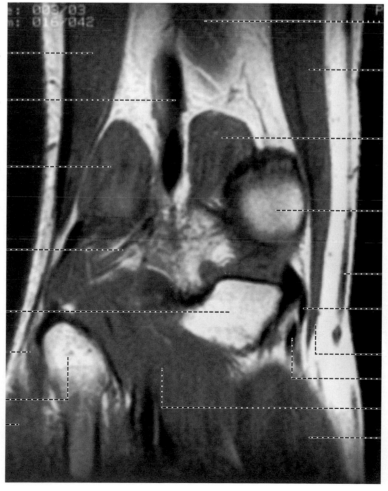

Biceps femoris m.

Popliteal a.

Gastrocnemius m., lateral head

Inferior lateral genicular a.

Tibia

Common peroneal n.

Fibular head

Gastrocnemius m., lateral head

Semimembranosus m.

Sartorius m.

Gastrocnemius m., medial head

Medial femoral condyle

Greater saphenous v.

Gracilis tendon

Sartorius tendon

Semitendinosus tendon

Popliteus m.

Gastrocnemius m., medial head

Figure 16.2.13

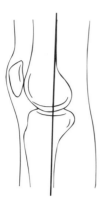

1. The posterior cruciate ligament has an ovoid shape in coronal section because of its nearly horizontal component in the extended knee. Its attachment to the lateral side of the medial femoral condyle is noted in this image.

2. The popliteus tendon is inserting on the femur in the recess for the popliteal tendon in this section.

3. The tibial collateral ligament is closely attached to the medial meniscus but as the image planes move anteriorly the meniscus will be seen to be more loosely attached to the ligament.

4. The pes anserinus tendon of insertion crosses over the distal portion of the tibial collateral ligament.

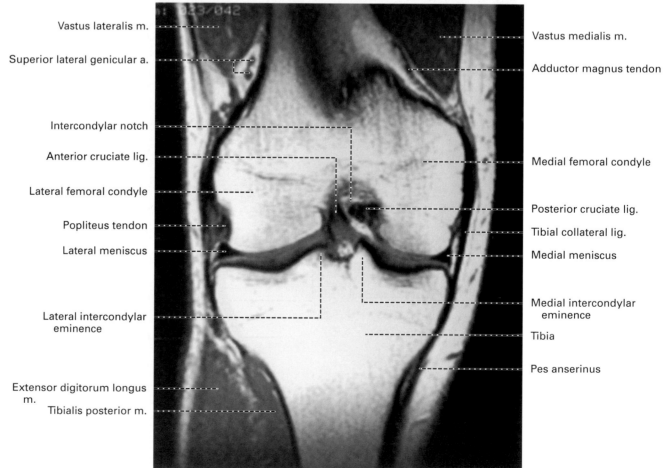

Vastus lateralis m.

Superior lateral genicular a.

Intercondylar notch

Anterior cruciate lig.

Lateral femoral condyle

Popliteus tendon

Lateral meniscus

Lateral intercondylar eminence

Extensor digitorum longus m.

Tibialis posterior m.

Vastus medialis m.

Adductor magnus tendon

Medial femoral condyle

Posterior cruciate lig.

Tibial collateral lig.

Medial meniscus

Medial intercondylar eminence

Tibia

Pes anserinus

1. The anterior cruciate ligament attaches to the area anterior to the medial intercondylar eminence.

2. In this section, the midportions of the menisci appear as dense, dark triangles.

3. The vascular structures between the tibial collateral ligament and the mid-portion of the medial meniscus are branches of the inferior medial genicular vessels.

4. The superior genicular vessel branches are located between vastus lateralis and the femur and vastus medialis and the femur.

5. The iliotibial tract (or band) becomes more prominent as the imaging plane moves more anteriorly.

Figure 16.2.14

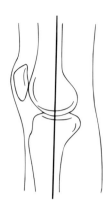

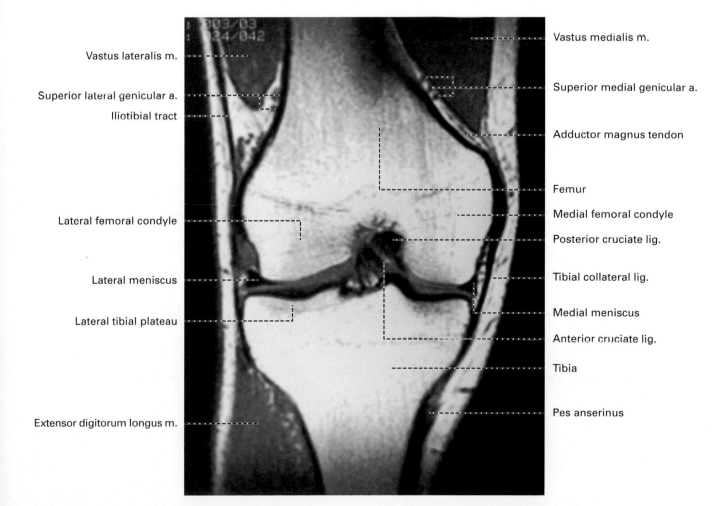

Vastus lateralis m.

Superior lateral genicular a.

Iliotibial tract

Lateral femoral condyle

Lateral meniscus

Lateral tibial plateau

Extensor digitorum longus m.

Vastus medialis m.

Superior medial genicular a.

Adductor magnus tendon

Femur

Medial femoral condyle

Posterior cruciate lig.

Tibial collateral lig.

Medial meniscus

Anterior cruciate lig.

Tibia

Pes anserinus

Figure 16.2.15

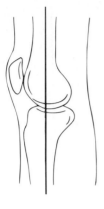

1. The origin of extensor digitorum longus is complex. It includes the lateral condyle of the tibia, the anterior surface of the proximal fibula, and the anterior surface of the interosseous membrane.

2. The pes anserinus inserts on the anterior medial aspect of the proximal tibia.

3. In this anterior section, the tibial collateral ligament has no attachment to the medial meniscus.

4. A very small part of tibialis anterior is seen in this image. It arises from the lateral condyle and lateral surface of the proximal tibia. It is the most medial of the anterior compartment muscles, which include tibialis anterior, extensor hallucis longus, extensor digitorum longus, and peroneus tertius.

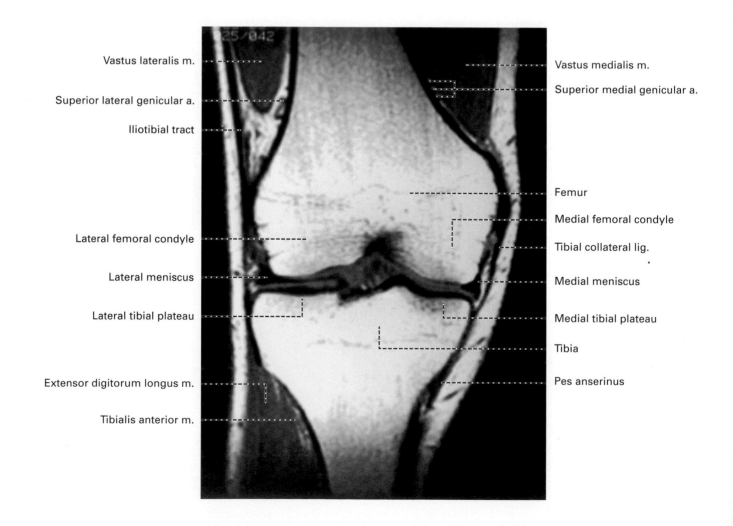

Vastus lateralis m.

Superior lateral genicular a.

Iliotibial tract

Lateral femoral condyle

Lateral meniscus

Lateral tibial plateau

Extensor digitorum longus m.

Tibialis anterior m.

Vastus medialis m.

Superior medial genicular a.

Femur

Medial femoral condyle

Tibial collateral lig.

Medial meniscus

Medial tibial plateau

Tibia

Pes anserinus

1. The anterior horn of the lateral meniscus is demonstrated in this coronal image. Part of this anterior horn continues to the anterior horn of the medial meniscus. This thickened bundle of fibers is called the transverse ligament. Its size and presence are variable.

2. The inferior lateral genicular branches are noted in the space between the anterolateral body of the lateral meniscus and the iliotibial tract.

Figure 16.2.16

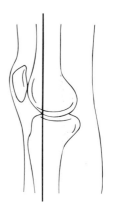

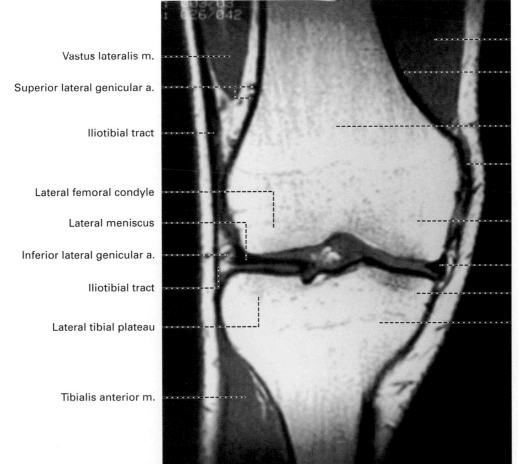

Vastus lateralis m.

Superior lateral genicular a.

Iliotibial tract

Lateral femoral condyle

Lateral meniscus

Inferior lateral genicular a.

Iliotibial tract

Lateral tibial plateau

Tibialis anterior m.

Vastus medialis m.

Superior medial genicular a.

Femur

Tibial collateral lig.

Medial femoral condyle

Medial meniscus

Medial tibial plateau

Tibia

Figure 16.2.17

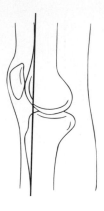

1. Note that the inferior lateral genicular vessels continue to follow the anterior margin of the lateral meniscus.

2. The anterior horn of the medial meniscus is demonstrated.

3. Vastus lateralis diminishes anteriorly while vastus medialis remains prominent.

4. The prominent iliotibial tract inserts on an anterolateral bony prominence of the proximal tibia known as Gerdy's tubercle.

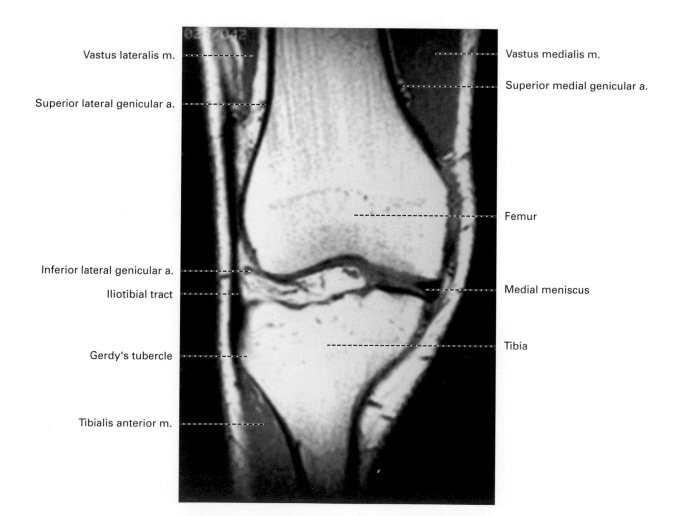

1. The patellar ligament inserts on and around the tibial tuberosity. This structure is frequently termed the "patellar tendon," but since it extends between two bones (patella and tibia) it is more appropriately called the patellar ligament.

2. The medial and lateral retinacula attach to the patellar ligament inferiorly.

3. The infrapatellar fat pad is present between the anterior margin of the proximal tibia and the posterior edge of the patellar ligament.

4. The superior genicular branches extend along the anterior surface of the distal femur and supply portions of the femur with short perforating branches, some of which are immediately proximal to the anterior femoral articular cartilage. This is better demonstrated on axial images.

Figure 16.2.18

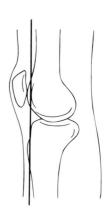

Vastus medialis m.

Vastus lateralis m.

Superior lateral genicular a.

Superior medial genicular a.

Iliotibial tract

Femur

Lateral patellar retinaculum

Medial patellar retinaculum

Infrapatellar fat

Tibial tuberosity

Figure 16.2.19

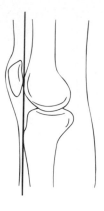

1. The synovial space of the suprapatellar bursa nearly always communications with the rest of the synovial spaces of the knee joint.

2. The iliotibial tract is contiguous with the lateral margin of the lateral femoral condyle anteriorly.

3. Note that the medial patellar retinaculum is continuous with part of vastus medialis.

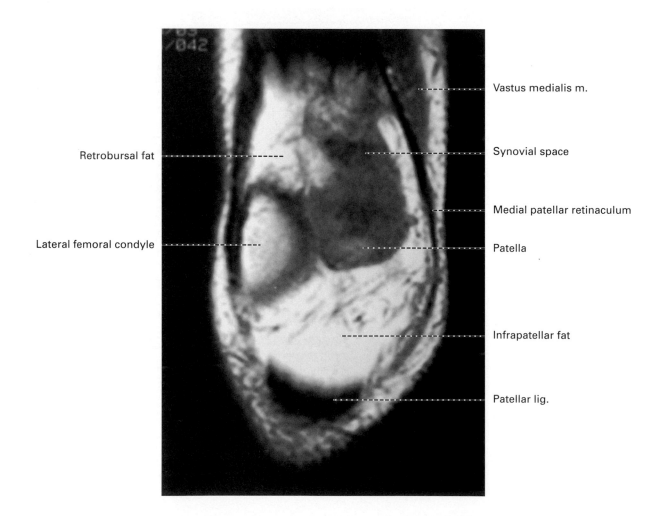

Retrobursal fat

Lateral femoral condyle

Vastus medialis m.

Synovial space

Medial patellar retinaculum

Patella

Infrapatellar fat

Patellar lig.

1. The quadriceps muscles (vastus lateralis, vastus intermedialis, vastus medialis, and rectus femoris) have condensed into a thick, frequently multilayered tendon called the quadriceps tendon.

2. The articular surface of the patella has two facets. Here the medial and lateral articulations of the patellofemoral joint are demonstrated.

3. The iliotibial tract is continuous with a portion of the lateral retinaculum at the level of the patella.

Figure 16.2.20

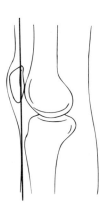

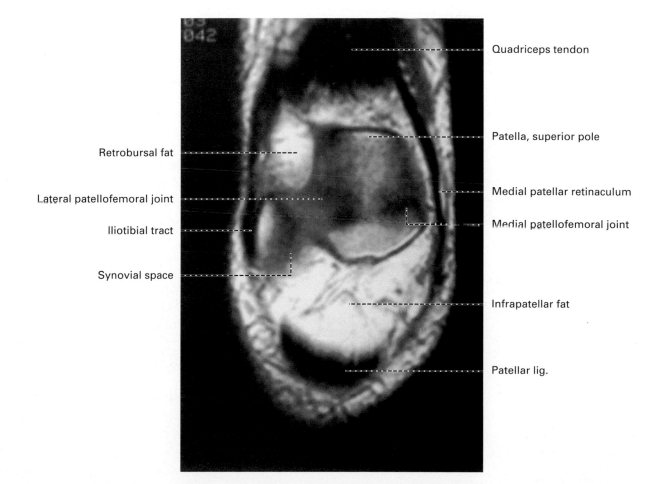

Quadriceps tendon

Patella, superior pole

Retrobursal fat

Medial patellar retinaculum

Lateral patellofemoral joint

Iliotibial tract

Medial patellofemoral joint

Synovial space

Infrapatellar fat

Patellar lig.

Figure 16.2.21

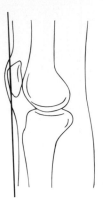

1. The prominent lateral and medial poles of the patella are noted. The lateral and medial retinacula attach here, respectively.

2. The inferior pole of the patella gives rise to the patellar ligament. This junction is where the abnormalities of "jumper's knee" occur.

3. Quadriceps tendon inserts on the anterior surface of the superior pole of the patella.

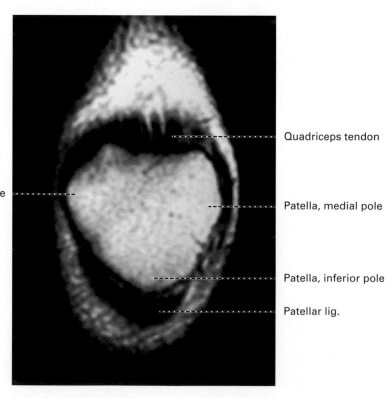

Quadriceps tendon

Patella, lateral pole

Patella, medial pole

Patella, inferior pole

Patellar lig.

1. This is the most medial section of the calf. A portion of the tibial collateral ligament is noted.

2. The greater saphenous vein is demonstrated in the calf and distal thigh. The structure posterior to the sartorius is another prominent superficial vein and not the tendon of the gracilis muscle.

Figure 16.3.1

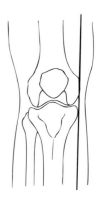

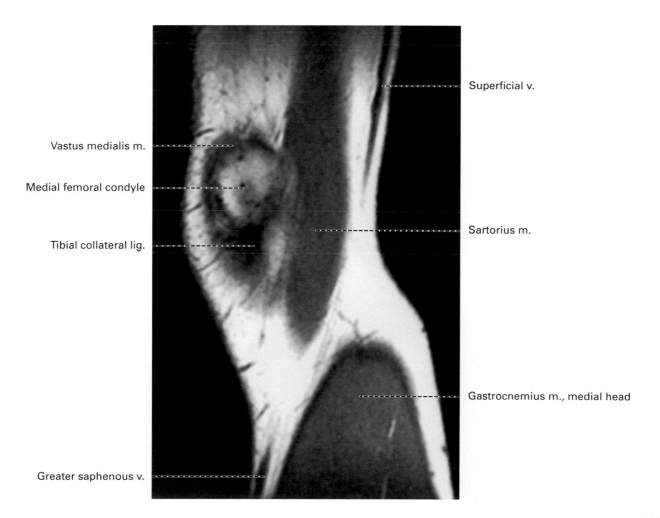

Superficial v.

Vastus medialis m.

Medial femoral condyle

Tibial collateral lig.

Sartorius m.

Gastrocnemius m., medial head

Greater saphenous v.

Figure 16.3.12

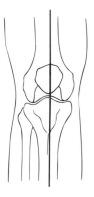

1. The oblique portion of posterior cruciate ligament (PCL) is visualized in this image. PCL has a slightly curved appearance when the knee is in extension. It becomes straight when the knee is flexed.

2. The transverse ligament is imaged in cross section and appears as a prominent "dot" in the infrapatellar fat.

3. The patellar ligament appears as a straight structure extending from the inferior pole of the patella to the tibial tubercle.

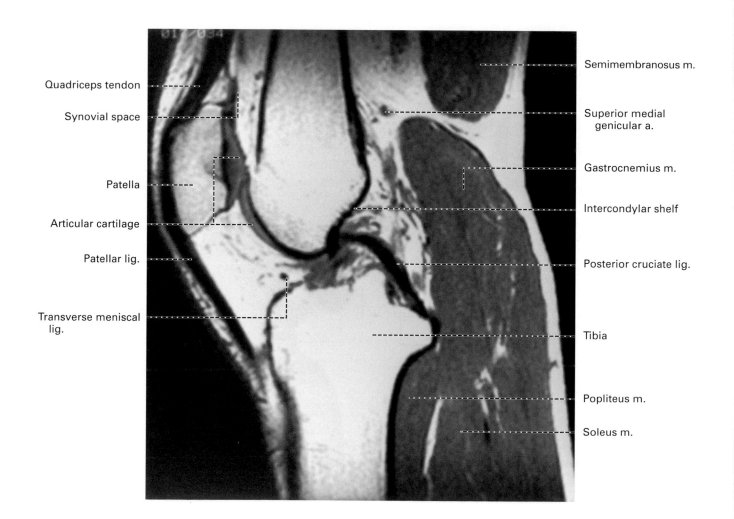

Quadriceps tendon
Synovial space
Patella
Articular cartilage
Patellar lig.
Transverse meniscal lig.

Semimembranosus m.
Superior medial genicular a.
Gastrocnemius m.
Intercondylar shelf
Posterior cruciate lig.
Tibia
Popliteus m.
Soleus m.

1. The anterior cruciate ligament (ACL) is smaller in diameter than the posterior cruciate ligament (PCL). The ACL also has a more heterogeneous signal intensity than that of PCL.

2. At this level, the continuity of the quadriceps tendon with the patellar ligament can be appreciated. The patella is truly a sesamoid bone.

3. The patella, patellar ligament, infrapatellar fat pad, and tibial tubercle are all seen on this section.

Figure 16.3.13

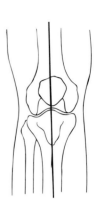

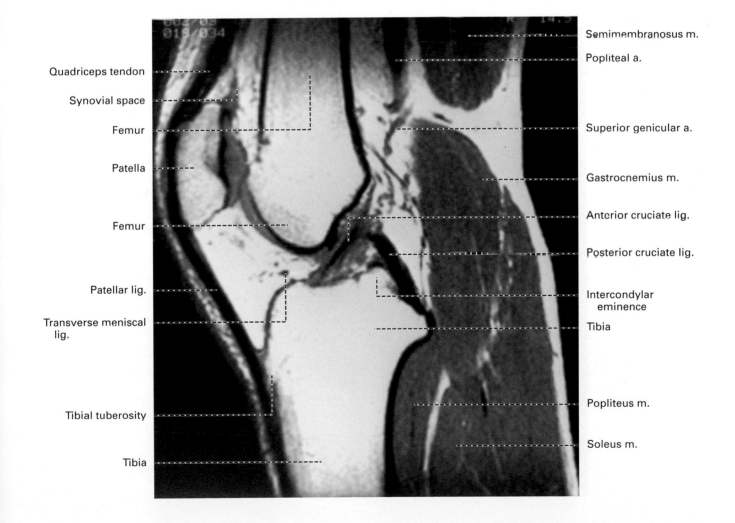

Figure 16.3.14

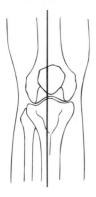

1. The popliteal artery enters the popliteal fossa anterior to semimembranosus. It lies medial and anterior to the popliteal vein.

2. The thin posterior joint capsule extends from the posterior surface of the femur above the condyles to the posterior edge of the posterior intercondylar fossa.

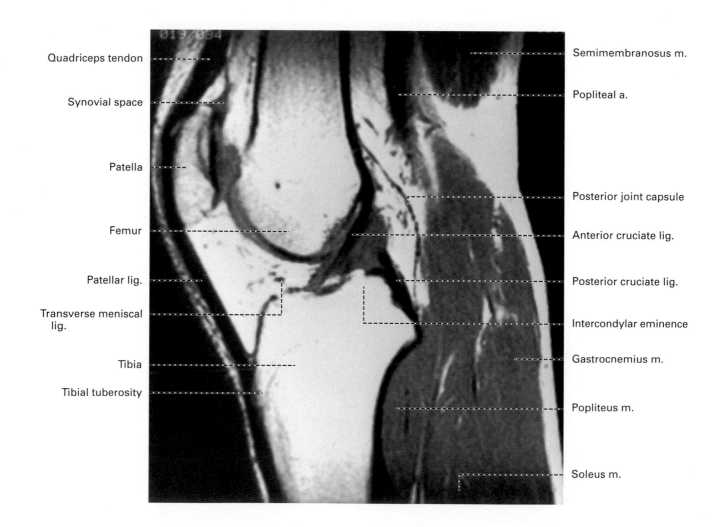

Quadriceps tendon

Synovial space

Patella

Femur

Patellar lig.

Transverse meniscal lig.

Tibia

Tibial tuberosity

Semimembranosus m.

Popliteal a.

Posterior joint capsule

Anterior cruciate lig.

Posterior cruciate lig.

Intercondylar eminence

Gastrocnemius m.

Popliteus m.

Soleus m.

1. At the level of the femoral condyles the popliteal vein lies posterior to the popliteal artery.

2. The posterior capsule appears thicker as the images move laterally, away from midline.

Figure 16.3.15

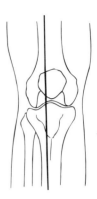

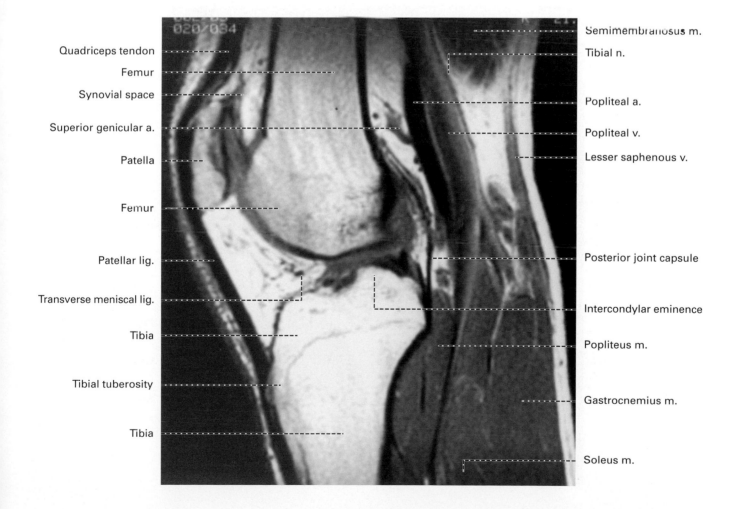

Quadriceps tendon

Femur

Synovial space

Superior genicular a.

Patella

Femur

Patellar lig.

Transverse meniscal lig.

Tibia

Tibial tuberosity

Tibia

Semimembranosus m.

Tibial n.

Popliteal a.

Popliteal v.

Lesser saphenous v.

Posterior joint capsule

Intercondylar eminence

Popliteus m.

Gastrocnemius m.

Soleus m.

Figure 16.3.16

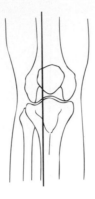

1. The popliteal vessels course distal to the knee on the surface of the popliteus muscle where the popliteal artery trifurcates, with some variation, into the anterior tibial, posterior tibial, and peroneal arteries.

2. The relation of the popliteus muscle to the vessels becomes very important in exophytic sarcomas of the proximal tibia. The popliteus muscle frequently provides protection from contamination of the popliteal neurovascular structures so that limb salvage remains a surgical option.

3. The posterior horn of the lateral meniscus is now visible. Its most central portion frequently has heterogeneous signals.

4. The deep veins of the calf join the popliteal vein after passing through the medial and lateral heads of the gastrocnemius muscle.

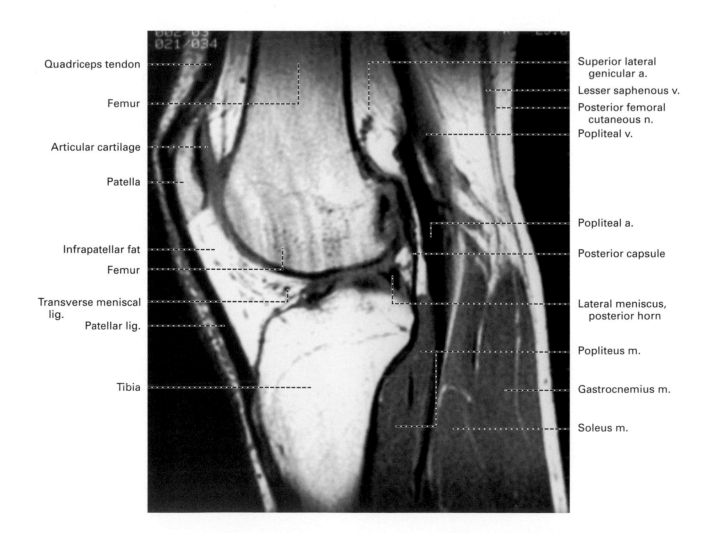

1. Note the relation of the popliteal artery to the popliteus muscle. The popliteal artery crosses over the posterior surface of the popliteus muscle.

2. The origin of the anterior tibial artery is demonstrated. In this image, it resides within the posterior compartment, not yet having passed across the upper edge of the interosseous membrane to enter the anterior compartment.

Figure 16.3.17

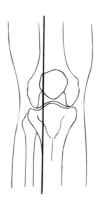

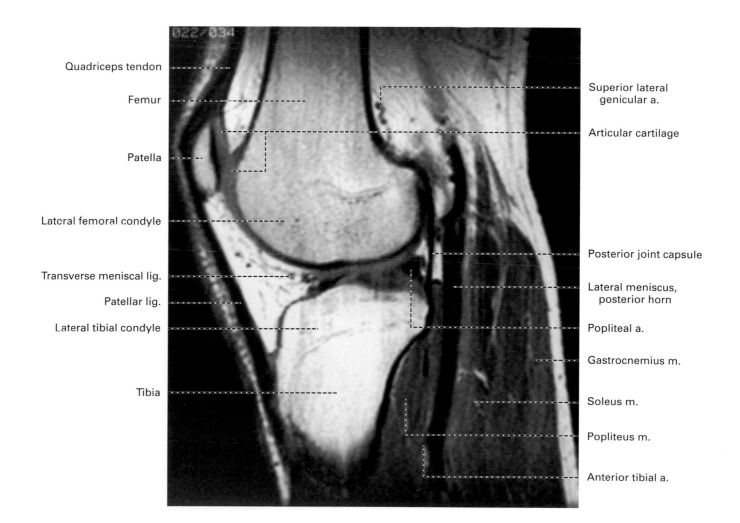

Quadriceps tendon

Femur

Patella

Lateral femoral condyle

Transverse meniscal lig.

Patellar lig.

Lateral tibial condyle

Tibia

Superior lateral genicular a.

Articular cartilage

Posterior joint capsule

Lateral meniscus, posterior horn

Popliteal a.

Gastrocnemius m.

Soleus m.

Popliteus m.

Anterior tibial a.

Figure 16.3.24

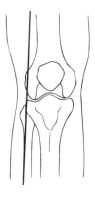

1. The popliteus tendon inserts on the lateral femoral condyle in this image.

2. The soleus arises from the proximal fibular head in this image. More laterally, its origin includes the proximal one-third of the fibula.

3. The tendinous origin of the lateral head of the gastrocnemius muscle is demonstrated here.

4. Observe the common peroneal nerve making its way toward the fibular head and neck.

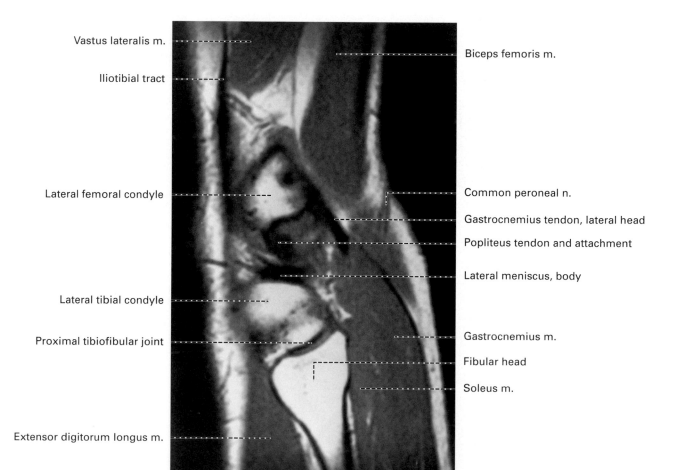

1. The inferior genicular artery is demonstrated in this image. Observe that it is superficial to the popliteus tendon but deep to the fibular collateral ligament.

2. The common peroneal nerve is passing obliquely toward the fibular head.

3. The peroneus longus muscle is seen at this level.

Figure 16.3.25

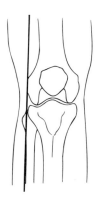

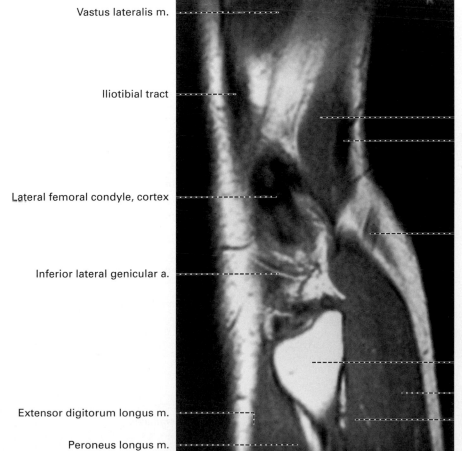

Vastus lateralis m.

Iliotibial tract

Biceps femoris m., short head

Biceps femoris tendon, long head

Lateral femoral condyle, cortex

Common peroneal n.

Inferior lateral genicular a.

Fibular head

Gastrocnemius m.

Extensor digitorum longus m.

Soleus m.

Peroneus longus m.

Figure 16.3.26

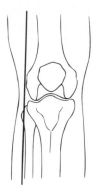

1. Laterally, the fibular collateral ligament is demonstrated. It has an oblique course, but may be indistinguishable from the tendon of the biceps femoris muscle as it inserts on the posterior aspect of the fibular head.

2. The biceps femoris muscle condenses to a thick tendon prior to inserting on the posterior apex of the fibular head. It runs more vertically than the fibular collateral ligament.

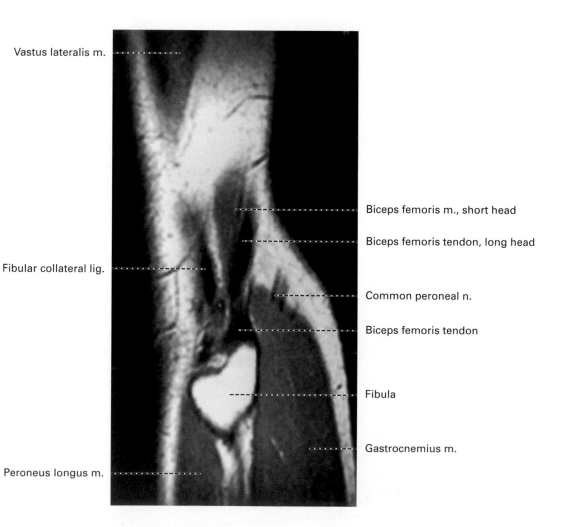

Vastus lateralis m.

Biceps femoris m., short head

Biceps femoris tendon, long head

Fibular collateral lig.

Common peroneal n.

Biceps femoris tendon

Fibula

Gastrocnemius m.

Peroneus longus m.

Chapter 17

LEG

Musculature

The musculature of the leg arises in part from the distal end of the femur and primarily from the tibia and fibula. The muscle bellies are best developed in the proximal part of the leg; the muscle gives rise to tendons distally that attach these muscles to the bones of the foot.

The musculature is divisible into an anterior, lateral, and posterior group. The anterior and lateral groups are separated by an intermuscular septum. The anterolateral groups are separated from the posterior group by the tibia and fibula, the interosseus membrane, and an intermuscular septum that extends from the lateral crest of the shaft of the fibula to the fascia enveloping the leg. Medially, the separation is provided by the broad medial surface of the tibia. Laterally, the line of division is not clearly marked externally. In the proximal part of the leg, the dorsal musculature protrudes somewhat ventrally; in the distal part, the lateral musculature passes dorsal to the lower end of the fibula. The posterior group is divided into superficial and deep divisions by the septum.

In general, the anterior group of muscles flexes the ankle dorsally, inverts the foot, and extends the toes. The lateral group plantar-flexes the ankle and everts the foot. The posterior group flexes the knee, plantar-flexes the ankle, inverts the foot, and flexes the toes.

The anterior and lateral groups develop from the primitive dorsal musculature of the limb and are innervated by the peroneal nerve; the posterior group is ventral in origin and receives innervation from the tibial nerve.

The anterior group consists of four muscles: tibialis anterior, extensor digitorum longus, peroneus tertius, and extensor hallucis longus. Tibialis anterior has a somewhat quadrangular belly that arises from the lateral surface of the tibia and adjacent interosseus membrane in the proximal half of the leg. Its tendon passes over the front of the tibia to the first metatarsal. Extensor digitorum longus is a transversely flattened, fusiform muscle that arises from the anterior surface of the fibula and the adjacent interosseus membrane; it gives rise to a tendon that passes over the front of the distal extremity of the tibia and sends tendons to the terminal phalanges of the four lateral toes. Peroneus tertius represents a differentiated or specialized portion of extensor digitorum longus. Its tendon passes laterally through the same osteofibrous canal in the same synoveal sheath but terminates on the fifth metatarsal. Extensor hallucis longus is a narrow muscle that arises from the distal half of the anterior surface of the fibula and the interosseus membrane. Its tendon extends over the ankle to the distal phalanx of the great toe. The tendons of these muscles are held in place by the superior and inferior extensor retinacula.

All the muscles of this group dorsiflex the foot. The extensors extend the toes; peroneus tertius and the extensor digitorum longus also evert the foot; the tibialis anterior inverts it. They are supplied by the deep peroneal nerve.

The lateral muscles consist of peroneus longus and peroneus brevis. The two muscles plantar-flex and evert the foot. The thick, angular belly of peroneus longus arises from the proximal half of the lateral surface of the fibula and from neighboring structures; the small peroneus brevis arises from the middle third of the lateral surface of the fibula. Peroneus longus partially covers peroneus brevis. The tendons of these two muscles pass around and behind the lateral malleolus. The tendons are held in place by the superior and inferior peroneal retinacula. The tendon of peroneus longus lies lateral to and then crosses behind that of peroneus brevis and curves around the lateral side of the calcaneus and then across the sole (plantar surface) of the foot. The tendon of peroneus longus lies against the cuboid and the tarsometatarsal articulations and terminates on the base of the first metatarsal. The tendon of peroneus brevis lies on the lateral side of the dorsum of the foot on the base of the fifth metatarsal. These two muscles are supplied by the superficial peroneal nerve.

The muscles at the back of the leg consist of a superficial and a deep group. The superficial group includes the gastrocnemius, soleus, and plantaris muscles. These muscles plantar-flex the foot and flex the leg. The two ovoid heads of gastrocnemius arise, one on each side, from above the medial and lateral condyles of the femur. The bellies of the muscle extend to about the middle of the back of the leg. The muscle inserts into the deep side of the calcaneal (Achilles) tendon and by this tendon onto the dorsal surface of the calcaneus.

The soleus is flat and oval, and deep to gastrocnemius. Soleus arises from the tibia and fibula and is inserted as far distally as the ankle into the deep surface of the calcaneal (Achilles) tendon, along with gastrocnemius. The two muscles, soleus and gastrocnemius, form a "three-headed muscle" commonly referred to as triceps surae. Plantaris is a slender muscle that passes along the medial edge of the lateral head of gastrocnemius. The muscle gives rise to a slender tendon that runs between gastrocnemius and soleus and along the medial margin of the calcaneal tendon and inserts onto the calcaneus. These three muscles are supplied by the tibial nerve.

The deep group, separated from the superficial group by the transverse septum, includes popliteus, flexor digitorum longus, and tibialis posterior muscles. Popliteus arises from the lateral condyle of the femur and inserts onto the popliteal line of the tibia. This small muscle flexes the leg and rotates the leg medially when the knee is flexed. Flexor digitorum longus arises from the popliteal line and the dorsal surface of the tibia. Its tendon passes around the medial malleolus and enters the sole of the foot. At this point, the tendon divides into four slips, which insert onto the base of the terminal phalanx of the second to fifth toes. Flexor hallucis longus arises from the distal two-thirds of the fibula and the intermuscular septum between it and tibialis posterior, passes behind the medial malleolus, enters the sole of the foot, and inserts onto the terminal phalanx of the great toe. Tibialis posterior arises from the lateral portion of the tibia and the interosseus membrane and

passes behind the medial malleolus to an extensive insertion on the plantar surface of the foot. The muscle is attached primarily to the tubercle of the navicular bone but spreads to attach to the cuneiforms and other structures.

The muscles of this group plantar-flex and invert the foot. Flexor hallucis flexes the great toe, and flexor digitorum flexes the remaining four toes. Tibialis posterior, tibialis anterior, and the peroneal muscles support and adjust movements of the foot. These muscles are innervated by the tibial nerve.

Table 17-1. Musculature of the Leg

Muscle	Origin	Insertion	Nerve Supply	Arterial Supply
Anterior group				
Tibialis anterior	Distal part of lateral condyle of the tibia, lateral surface of proximal half of the shaft of the tibia, adjacent interosseus membrane, overlying fascia near condyle of tibia, and intermuscular septum between it and extensor digitorum longus	Medial surface of the first cuneiform and the base of the first metatarsal	Branch from common peroneal and another from deep peroneal	Anterior tibial
Extensor digitorum longus	Lateral condyle of the tibia, anterior crest of the fibula, intermuscular membrane between it and tibialis anterior, lateral margin of the interosseous membrane, the septum between it and peroneus longus, and the fascia of the leg near the tibial origin	Each tendon, located on the dorsal surface of the toe to which it goes, divides into three fasciculi: the intermediate, attached to the dorsum of the base of the middle phalanx, and two lateral, which converge to the dorsum of the base on the distal phalanx. The margins of each tendon are bound to the sides of the back of the proximal phalanx.	By two branches of the deep peroneal	Anterior tibial
Peroneus tertius	Distal one-third of the anterior surface of fibula, neighboring interosseous membrane, anterior intermuscular septum	Onto the base of the fifth metatarsal and often onto the base of the fourth	The more distal nerve to extensor digitorum supplies this muscle (deep peroneal)	Anterior tibial
Extensor hallucis longus	Middle half of the anterior surface of the fibula near interosseous crest, and distal half of interosseous membrane	Onto the base of the distal phalanx of the great toe. On the back of the proximal phalanx the margins of the tendon are attached to the bone by bands of fibers.	Deep peroneal	Anterior tibial

Continues

Table 17-1. (Continued)

Muscle	Origin	Insertion	Nerve Supply	Arterial Supply
Lateral group				
Peroneus longus	Arterial head: anterior capitular ligament, neighboring lateral condyle of tibia, head of the fibula, proximal third of anterior intermuscular septum, and the crural fascia; posterior head: proximal half of lateral surface of shaft of fibula and posterior intermuscular septum	Inferior surface of first cuneiform and on the adjacent part of the inferolateral border and base of first metatarsal	Usually the common peroneal, sometimes partially by superficial peroneal	Posterior tibial, peroneal branch
Peroneus brevis	Middle one-third of lateral surface of fibula, from the septa that separates it from the anterior and posterior groups of muscles	Dorsal aspect of tuberosity of fifth metatarsal	Superficial peroneal or a branch to peroneus longus	Peroneal branch
Deeply placed posterior group				
Popliteus	Facet at the anterior end of the groove on the lateral aspect of the femoral condyle	Proximal lip of the popliteal line of the tibia and the shaft of the tibia proximal to this line	Tibial, a branch that arises independently, or with the nerve to the posterior tibial muscle	Inferior lateral and inferior medial genicular branch
Flexor digitorum longus	Popliteal line, medial side of the second quarter of the dorsal surface of the tibia, the fibrous septum between the muscle and tibialis posterior, and the fascia covering its proximal extremity	Onto the bases of the terminal phalanx of the second to fourth toes	Tibial, in company with nerves to other muscles of this group	Posterior tibial
Flexor hallucis longus	Distal two-thirds of posterior surface of the fibula, the septa between it and the tibialis posterior and peroneal muscles	Onto the base of the terminal phalanx of the great toe	Tibial, often in company with the nerve to flexor digitorum longus or the other muscles of this group	Peroneal
Tibialis posterior	Lateral half of the popliteal line and lateral half of the middle one-third of the posterior surface of the tibia, medial side of the head and part of the body of the fibula next to the interosseous membrane in the proximal two-thirds, the entire proximal and lateral portion of the lateral part of the posterior surface of the interosseous membrane, and the septa between its proximal portion and the long flexor muscles	The tendon divides into two parts: the deep part becomes attached primarily to the tubercle of the navicular bone, and usually to the first cuneiform; the superficial part attaches to the third cuneiform and base of the fourth metatarsal, and also, in part, to the second cuneiform, to the capsule of the naviculo-cuneiform joint, to the sulcus of the cuboid, and usually also to the origin of the short flexor of the big toe and base of the second metatarsal; slip may extend to other structures.	Tibial, in company with nerves to other muscles of this group	Peroneal

Continues

Table 17-1. (*Continued*)

Muscle	Origin	Insertion	Nerve Supply	Arterial Supply
Superficially placed posterior group				
Gastrocnemius	Medial head: back of medial condyle of femur above articular surface, back of femur supralateral to first origin, and the femoral margin of capsule of knee joint; lateral head: a facet on proximal part of posterolateral surface of lateral condyle of femur and an area extending medially and proximally from this, above the lateral condyle	Via the calcaneal tendon onto the posterior surface of calcaneus	Sciatic, tibial part	Sural
Soleus	By a fibular head from the back of the head and the proximal one-third of the posterior surface of the shaft of the fibula; intermuscular septum between it and peroneus longus, by a tibial head from the popliteal line and the middle one-third of the medial border of the tibia	Via the calcaneal tendon onto the posterior surface of calcaneus	Sciatic, tibial part	Popliteal, sural
Plantaris	Distal part of the lateral line of bifurcation of the linea aspera, in close association with the lateral head of gastocnemius	Via a flat narrow tendon running along the medial edge of the calcaneal tendon to posterior surface of calcaneus	Sciatic, tibial part	Popliteal, sural

Figure 17.1.1

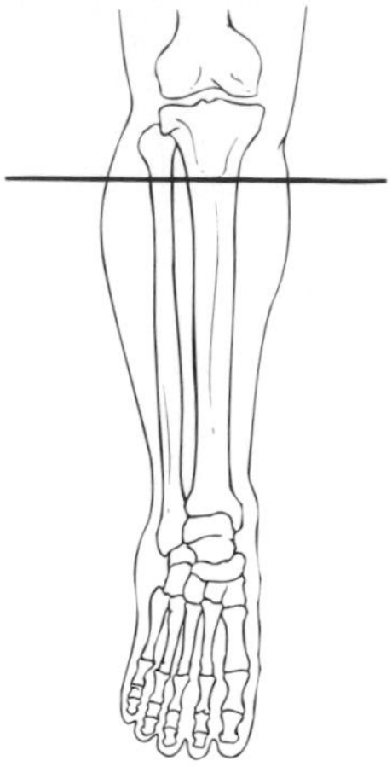

1. This image is below the trifurcation of the popliteal artery. Separate branches of the anterior tibial artery, peroneal artery, and posterior tibial artery are identifiable.

2. The anterior tibial artery lies on the anterior surface of the interosseous membrane.

3. At this level, both the peroneal and posterior tibial arteries lie in the space between the superficial and deep parts of the posterior compartment of the leg.

4. Plantaris tendon lies between the medial head of gastrocnemius and soleus muscles. It inserts on the medial side of the tuberosity of the calcaneus, just anterior to the insertion of the Achilles tendon.

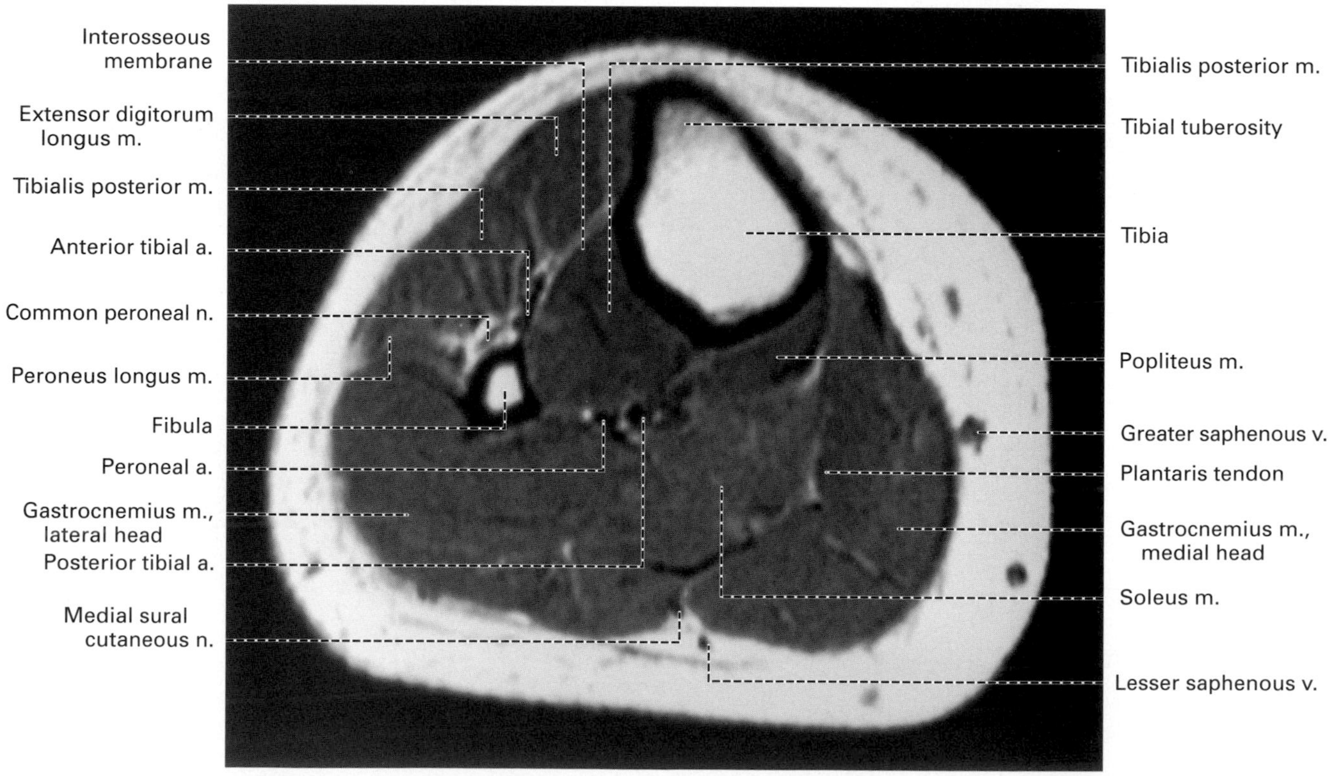
Interosseous membrane
Extensor digitorum longus m.
Tibialis posterior m.
Anterior tibial a.
Common peroneal n.
Peroneus longus m.
Fibula
Peroneal a.
Gastrocnemius m., lateral head
Posterior tibial a.
Medial sural cutaneous n.
Tibialis posterior m.
Tibial tuberosity
Tibia
Popliteus m.
Greater saphenous v.
Plantaris tendon
Gastrocnemius m., medial head
Soleus m.
Lesser saphenous v.

1. The anterior compartment muscles are distinguishable as tibialis anterior, extensor hallucis longus, and extensor digitorum longus.

2. This image is near the inferior edge of the popliteus muscle.

3. The large nutrient artery that courses obliquely through the posterior proximal tibial cortex can be seen at the outer edge of the cortex in this image. In the next few inferior images it will be seen coursing through the cortex until it becomes intramedullary.

4. The peroneal nerve courses down the anterior surface of the fibula deep to supply peroneus longus and brevis. These structures are in the lateral compartment. Peroneus brevis originates distal to peroneus longus.

Figure 17.1.2

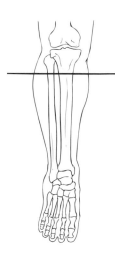

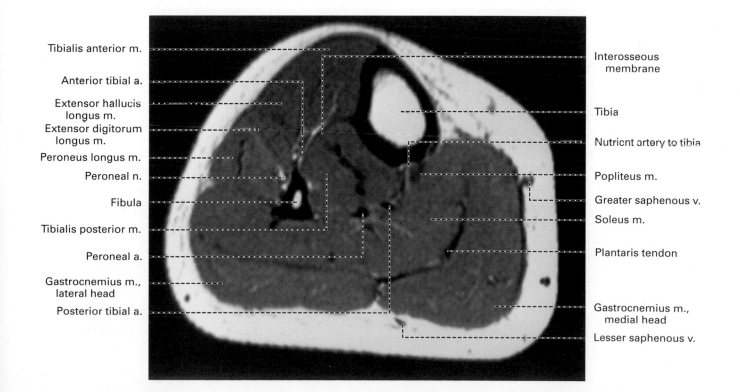

Tibialis anterior m.

Anterior tibial a.

Extensor hallucis longus m.
Extensor digitorum longus m.

Peroneus longus m.

Peroneal n.

Fibula

Tibialis posterior m.

Peroneal a.

Gastrocnemius m., lateral head

Posterior tibial a.

Interosseous membrane

Tibia

Nutrient artery to tibia

Popliteus m.

Greater saphenous v.

Soleus m.

Plantaris tendon

Gastrocnemius m., medial head

Lesser saphenous v.

Figure 17.1.3

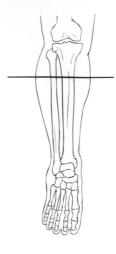

1. Peroneus brevis can now be clearly identified within the lateral compartment.

2. The intermuscular septa between the anterior and lateral compartments and between the lateral and posterior compartments are not as well defined as in the thigh.

3. At about this level, the common peroneal nerve has divided into its superficial and deep branches. The deep peroneal nerve descends with the anterior tibial artery. The superficial peroneal nerve courses between the peronei and the extensor digitorum longus to pierce the investing fascia and become subcutaneous.

4. The interosseous membrane is well identified and has a prominent anterior bow.

5. The nutrient artery of the tibia is in the midcortex in this image.

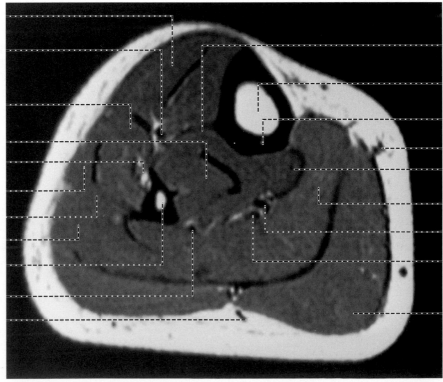

Tibialis anterior m.

Anterior tibial a., v., and deep peroneal n.

Extensor hallucis longus and extensor digitorum longus mm.

Tibialis posterior m.

Superficial peroneal n.

Peroneus longus m.

Peroneus brevis m.

Gastrocnemius m., lateral head

Fibula

Peroneal a.

Lesser saphenous v.

Interosseous membrane

Tibia

Nutrient a.

Greater saphenous v.

Flexor digitorum longus m.

Soleus m.

Posterior tibial a.

Tibial n.

Gastrocnemius m., medial head

1. The tibial nutrient artery is entering the medullary bone at this level.

2. The medial head of gastrocnemius extends more inferiorly than the lateral head. This produces asymmetry in the muscles in the calf.

3. Plantaris tendon flattens and becomes difficult to identify below this point.

4. The tibial nerve continues with the posterior tibial artery. They remain between the soleus and the muscles of the deep posterior compartment.

Figure 17.1.4

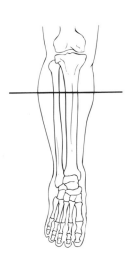

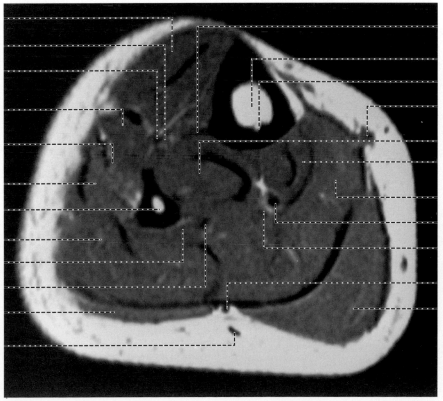

Tibialis anterior m.

Anterior tibial a., v.

Deep peroneal n.
Extensor hallucis longus and extensor digitorum longus mm.

Superficial peroneal n.

Peroneus longus and brevis mm.

Fibula

Soleus m.

Flexor hallucis longus m.

Peroneal a.

Gastrocnemius m., lateral head

Lesser saphenous v.

Interosseous membrane

Tibia

Nutrient a.

Greater saphenous v.

Tibialis posterior m.

Flexor digitorum longus m.

Soleus m.

Posterior tibial a.

Tibial n.

Medial sural cutaneous n.

Gastrocnemius m., medial head

Figure 17.1.5

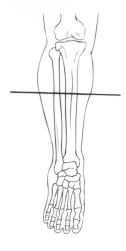

1. Flexor hallucis longus now joins flexor digitorum longus and tibialis posterior to make up the three long flexors of the foot.

2. The medial sural cutaneous nerve pierces the deep fascia and becomes subcutaneous. At this level, the communicating branch from the lateral sural cutaneous nerve joins it, creating the sural nerve.

3. The greater saphenous vein remains adjacent to the medial border of soleus.

4. The lateral head of gastrocnemius has inserted into the gastrocnemius tendon, but the medial head remains muscular.

5. Note that the gastrocnemius tendon becomes more prominent as the imaging planes move distally

6. The nutrient artery is clearly within medullary bone. Distal to this point it branches and becomes difficult to identify.

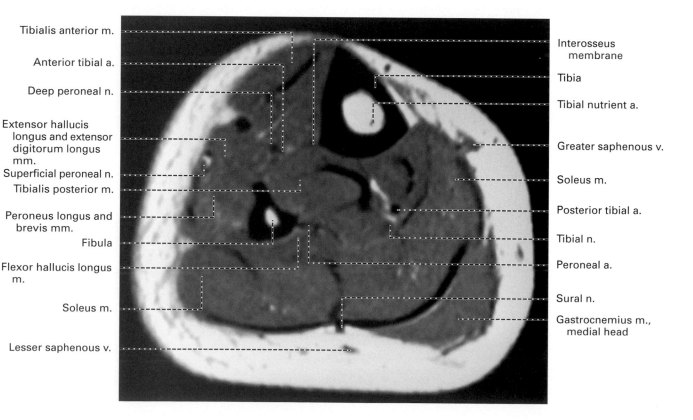

1. Note the relative triangular shape of the tibia near its midshaft.

2. The deep peroneal nerve and anterior tibial artery continue to descend together on the anterior surface of the interosseous membrane deep to the long extensors of the foot.

3. The peroneal artery is adjacent to the medial border of the fibula, between tibialis posterior and flexor hallucis longus muscles.

4. The tibial nerve and the posterior tibial artery lie between flexor digitorum longus and flexor hallucis longus, a relationship they maintain into the foot. They remain deep to soleus at this level.

Figure 17.1.6

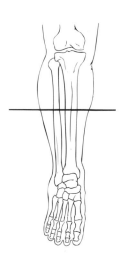

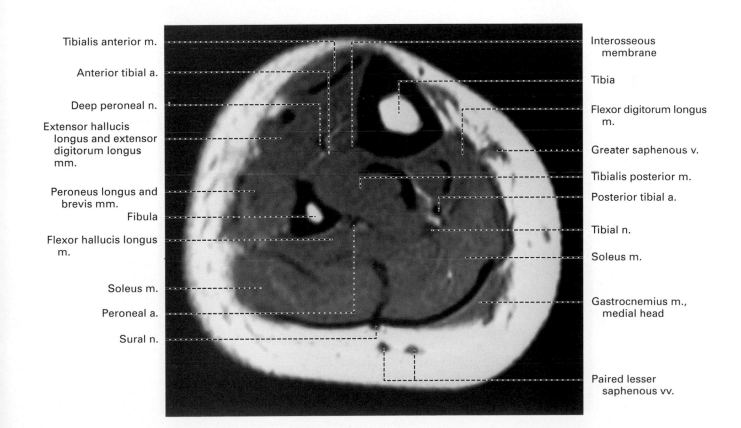

Tibialis anterior m.

Anterior tibial a.

Deep peroneal n.

Extensor hallucis longus and extensor digitorum longus mm.

Peroneus longus and brevis mm.

Fibula

Flexor hallucis longus m.

Soleus m.

Peroneal a.

Sural n.

Interosseous membrane

Tibia

Flexor digitorum longus m.

Greater saphenous v.

Tibialis posterior m.

Posterior tibial a.

Tibial n.

Soleus m.

Gastrocnemius m., medial head

Paired lesser saphenous vv.

Figure 17.1.7

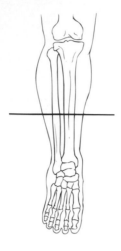

1. All of the gastrocnemius muscle fibers have inserted into the increasingly prominent tendon of gastrocnemius, which forms the posterior border of the soleus.

2. The long extensors of the foot are forming dense tendons. These include tibialis anterior, extensor hallucis longus, and extensor digitorum longus.

3. Peroneus longus lies posterior and lateral to peroneus brevis. It develops a prominent tendinous portion more proximal than peroneus brevis.

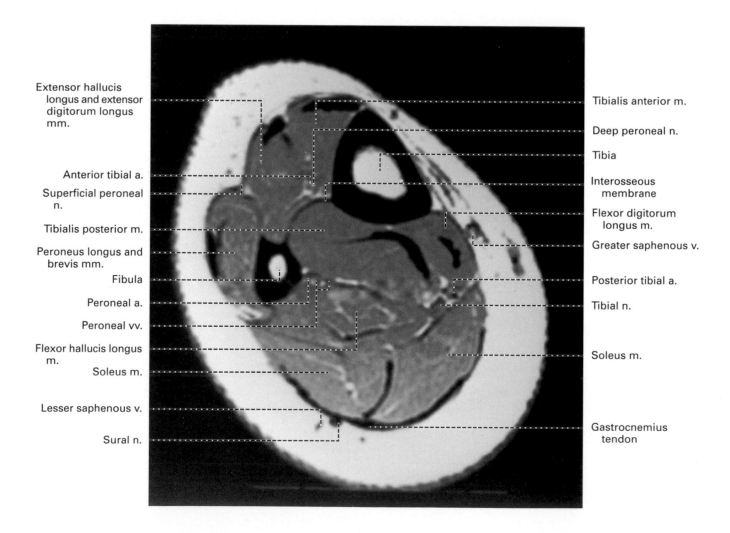

Extensor hallucis longus and extensor digitorum longus mm.

Anterior tibial a.

Superficial peroneal n.

Tibialis posterior m.

Peroneus longus and brevis mm.

Fibula

Peroneal a.

Peroneal vv.

Flexor hallucis longus m.

Soleus m.

Lesser saphenous v.

Sural n.

Tibialis anterior m.

Deep peroneal n.

Tibia

Interosseous membrane

Flexor digitorum longus m.

Greater saphenous v.

Posterior tibial a.

Tibial n.

Soleus m.

Gastrocnemius tendon

1. The peroneal vessels are immediately medial to the fibula and reside between flexor hallucis longus and the deeper tibialis posterior muscles.

2. The posterior tibial vessels lie under the medial cover of the soleus at the junction of the three deep posterior compartment muscles (tibialis posterior, flexor digitorum longus, and flexor hallucis longus).

3. The greater saphenous vein lies adjacent to the medial border of flexor digitorum longus.

4. The lesser saphenous vein and the sural nerve remain posterior structures superficial to the investing fascia.

Figure 17.1.8

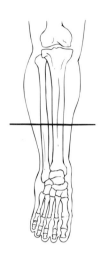

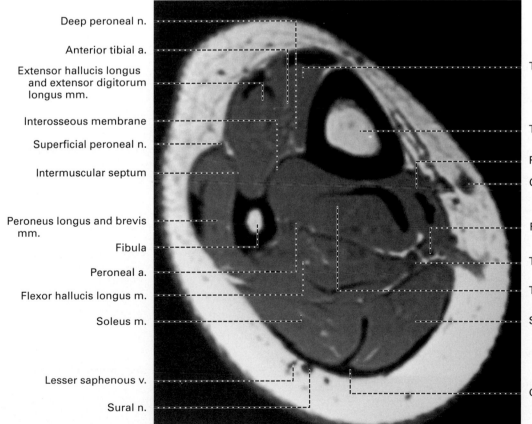

Deep peroneal n.

Anterior tibial a.

Extensor hallucis longus and extensor digitorum longus mm.

Interosseous membrane

Superficial peroneal n.

Intermuscular septum

Peroneus longus and brevis mm.

Fibula

Peroneal a.

Flexor hallucis longus m.

Soleus m.

Lesser saphenous v.

Sural n.

Tibialis anterior m.

Tibia

Flexor digitorum longus m.

Greater saphenous v.

Posterior tibial a.

Tibial n.

Tibialis posterior m.

Soleus m.

Gastrocnemius tendon

Figure 17.1.9

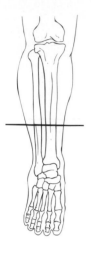

1. The superficial peroneal nerve descends in the junction between the anterior and lateral compartments. It will subsequently divide into the medial and intermediate dorsal cutaneous nerves. Once the superficial peroneal nerve penetrates the deep fascia it is a cutaneous nerve with no subsequent significant motor branches.

2. As soleus becomes smaller, the tendon of gastrocnemius thickens.

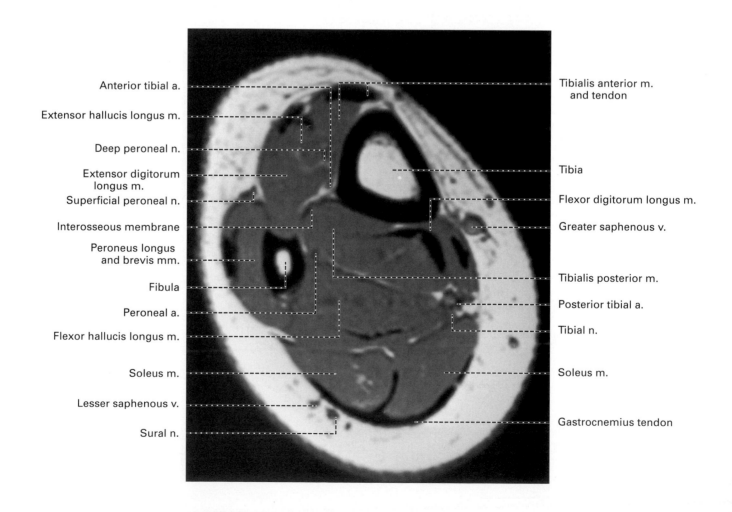

Anterior tibial a.
Extensor hallucis longus m.
Deep peroneal n.
Extensor digitorum longus m.
Superficial peroneal n.
Interosseous membrane
Peroneus longus and brevis mm.
Fibula
Peroneal a.
Flexor hallucis longus m.
Soleus m.
Lesser saphenous v.
Sural n.

Tibialis anterior m. and tendon
Tibia
Flexor digitorum longus m.
Greater saphenous v.
Tibialis posterior m.
Posterior tibial a.
Tibial n.
Soleus m.
Gastrocnemius tendon

1. Extensor hallucis is almost tendinous at this level.

2. The lesser saphenous vein is associated with other prominent branches, which accompany the sural nerve.

3. The tibial diameter begins to enlarge and the cortex thins as the imaging plane moves inferiorly.

Figure 17.1.10

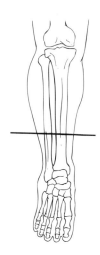

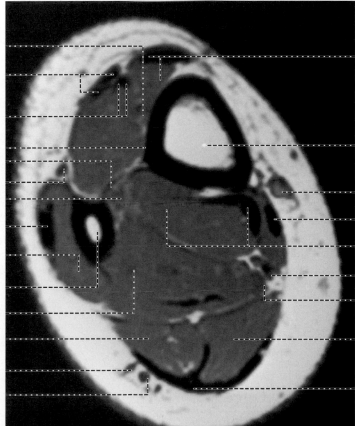

Deep peroneal n.

Extensor hallucis longus m. and tendon

Extensor digitorum longus m. and tendon

Anterior tibial a.
Interosseous membrane

Superficial peroneal n.

Peroneal a.

Peroneus longus and brevis tendons

Peroneus longus and brevis mm.

Fibula

Flexor hallucis longus m.

Soleus m.

Lesser saphenous v.

Sural n.

Tibialis anterior m. and tendon

Tibia

Greater saphenous v.

Flexor digitorum longus tendon

Tibialis posterior m. and tendon

Posterior tibial a.

Tibial n.

Soleus m.

Gastrocnemius tendon

Figure 17.1.11

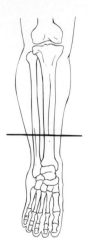

1. Note that the anterior tibial artery has migrated anteromedially and is adjacent to the tibial cortex and tibialis anterior muscle.

2. Peroneus longus is nearly all tendinous at this level.

3. Of the deep posterior compartment muscles, flexor hallucis longus is the most prominent.

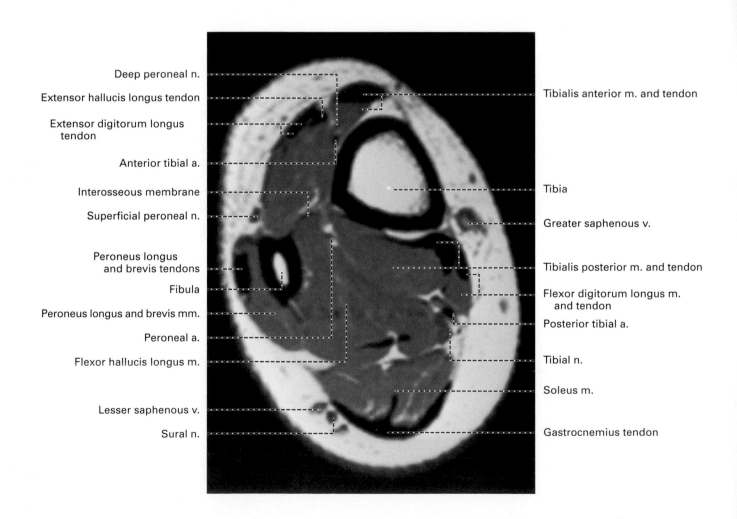

Deep peroneal n.

Extensor hallucis longus tendon

Extensor digitorum longus tendon

Anterior tibial a.

Interosseous membrane

Superficial peroneal n.

Peroneus longus and brevis tendons

Fibula

Peroneus longus and brevis mm.

Peroneal a.

Flexor hallucis longus m.

Lesser saphenous v.

Sural n.

Tibialis anterior m. and tendon

Tibia

Greater saphenous v.

Tibialis posterior m. and tendon

Flexor digitorum longus m. and tendon

Posterior tibial a.

Tibial n.

Soleus m.

Gastrocnemius tendon

1. The greater saphenous vein is now adjacent to the posteromedial cortex of the tibia.

2. The peroneal artery has migrated anteriorly to reside between the tibial cortex and flexor hallucis longus, just posterior to the interosseous membrane.

3. The tibial nerve is on the medial edge of flexor hallucis longus.

4. Peroneus longus is entirely tendinous here and is adjacent to peroneus brevis tendon. Peroneus brevis muscle persists, posterior to peroneus longus and brevis tendons.

Figure 17.1.12

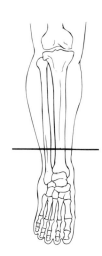

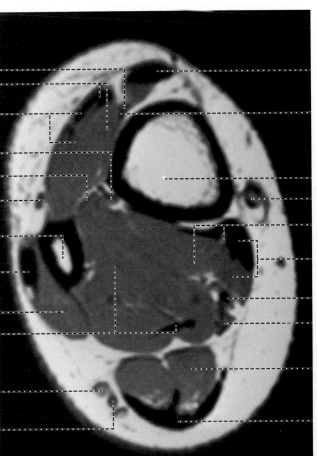

Deep peroneal n.
Extensor hallucis longus m. and tendon
Extensor digitorum longus m. and tendon
Peroneal a.
Interosseous membrane
Superficial peroneal n.
Fibula
Peroneus longus and brevis tendons
Peroneus longus and brevis mm.
Flexor hallucis longus m. and tendon
Lesser saphenous v.
Sural n.

Tibialis anterior tendon
Anterior tibial a.
Tibia
Greater saphenous v.
Tibialis posterior m. and tendon
Flexor digitorum longus m. and tendon
Posterior tibial a.
Tibial n.
Soleus m.
Gastrocnemius tendon

Figure 17.1.13

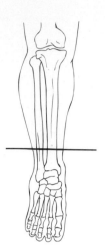

1. Tibialis anterior is predominantly tendinous here.

2. Peroneus longus tendon lies lateral to peroneus brevis tendon.

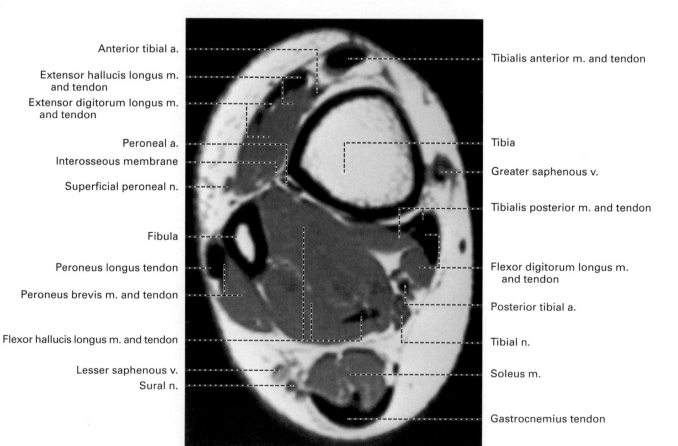

Anterior tibial a.

Extensor hallucis longus m. and tendon

Extensor digitorum longus m. and tendon

Peroneal a.

Interosseous membrane

Superficial peroneal n.

Fibula

Peroneus longus tendon

Peroneus brevis m. and tendon

Flexor hallucis longus m. and tendon

Lesser saphenous v.
Sural n.

Tibialis anterior m. and tendon

Tibia

Greater saphenous v.

Tibialis posterior m. and tendon

Flexor digitorum longus m. and tendon

Posterior tibial a.

Tibial n.

Soleus m.

Gastrocnemius tendon

1. Tibialis posterior and flexor digitorum longus are predominantly tendinous while flexor hallucis longus remains largely muscular.

2. This image is near the inferior edge of the interosseous membrane with the peroneal vessels continuing to reside posterior to it.

3. The long extensors of the foot are tendinous except for extensor digitorum longus, which still has some muscular component as its tendons develop.

Figure 17.1.14

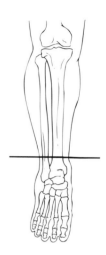

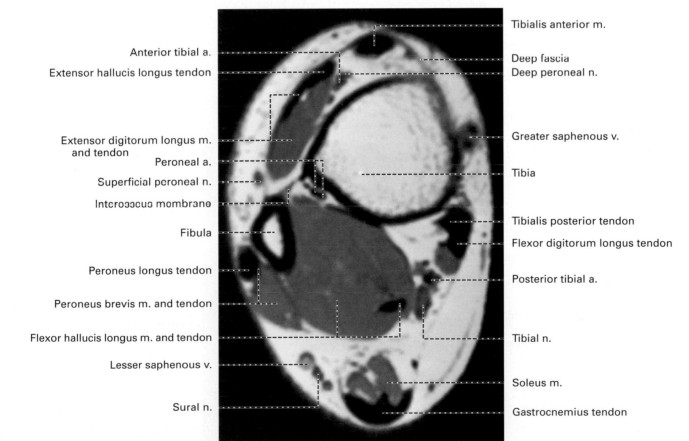

Anterior tibial a.
Extensor hallucis longus tendon

Extensor digitorum longus m. and tendon
Peroneal a.
Superficial peroneal n.
Interosseous membrane
Fibula

Peroneus longus tendon

Peroneus brevis m. and tendon

Flexor hallucis longus m. and tendon

Lesser saphenous v.

Sural n.

Tibialis anterior m.

Deep fascia
Deep peroneal n.

Greater saphenous v.

Tibia

Tibialis posterior tendon
Flexor digitorum longus tendon

Posterior tibial a.

Tibial n.

Soleus m.

Gastrocnemius tendon

Figure 17.1.15

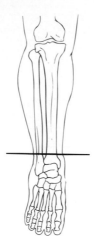

1. Peroneus tertius is now identifiable. This muscle is the inferior part of extensor digitorum longus. It differentiates when extensor digitorum longus tendon becomes identifiably separate from the residual extensor digitorum longus muscle. Peroneus tertius develops its own tendon distinct from extensor digitorum longus tendon.

2. Soleus has become completely tendinous; joining with the tendon of gastrocnemius it forms the prominent calcaneal (Achilles) tendon.

3. Flexor hallucis longus is the only residual muscle in the posterior compartment at this level. It has a prominent tendon medially but its muscular component continues to the inferior edge of the posterior tibia.

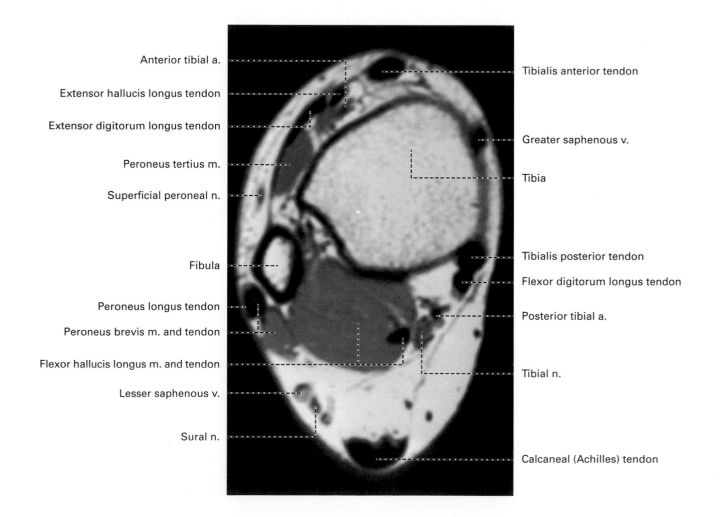

1. The anterior and posterior tubercles of the tibia form the margins of the tibial concavity for the fibula.

2. Tibialis posterior tendon lies posterior to the developing medial malleolus within the malleolar sulcus.

3. Note the relation of important structures in the posterior compartment. The order of these structures posterior to the medial malleolus is tibialis posterior tendon, flexor digitorum longus tendon, posterior tibial vessels, tibial nerve, and flexor hallucis longus. The mnemonic for this arrangement is Tom, Dick, and nervous Harry (*T*om: *t*ibialis posterior; *D*ick: flexor *d*igitorum longus; nervous: neurovascular bundle; and *H*arry: flexor *h*allucis longus).

Figure 17.1.16

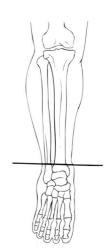

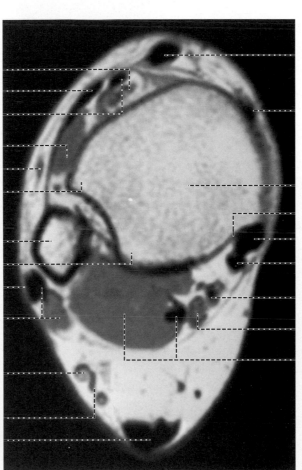

Anterior tibial a.
Extensor digitorum longus tendon
Extensor hallucis longus tendon

Peroneus tertius m.
Superficial peroneal n.
Tibia, anterior tubercle

Fibula
Tibia, posterior tubercle
Peroneus longus tendon

Peroneus brevis m. and tendon

Lesser saphenous v.

Sural n.
Calcaneal (Achilles) tendon

Tibialis anterior tendon

Greater saphenous v.

Tibia
Malleolar sulcus
Tibialis posterior tendon
Flexor digitorum longus tendon

Posterior tibial a.

Tibial n.

Flexor hallucis longus m. and tendon

Figure 17.2.1

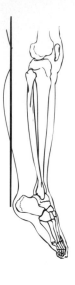

1. The medial and lateral heads of gastrocnemius are separated by a median raphe.

2. The lesser saphenous vein courses adjacent to this medial raphe until it migrates laterally and inferiorly.

3. The sural nerve is adjacent and slightly deep to the lesser saphenous vein.

4. The calcaneal (Achilles) tendon is seen as the tendinous continuation of the soleus and gastrocnemius muscles.

5. The bulk of gastrocnemius is on the medial side of the calf.

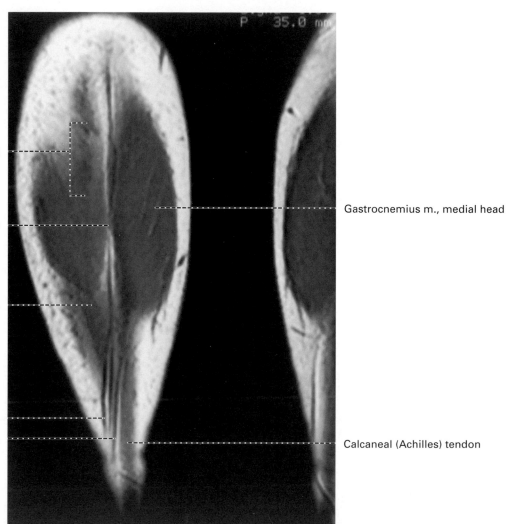

Gastrocnemius m., lateral head

Median raphe

Soleus m.

Lesser saphenous v.

Sural n.

Gastrocnemius m., medial head

Calcaneal (Achilles) tendon

1. Til
   mu

2. Th
   the

3. Ev
   not

4. Be
   me
   str
   do

Ir

Extens

Exter

1. Note that there is a tendinous division between the lateral head of gastroc-nemius and soleus. A similar division is seen radially.

2. The lesser saphenous vein seen distally is lateral to the calcaneal (Achilles) tendon.

Figure 17.2.2

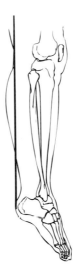

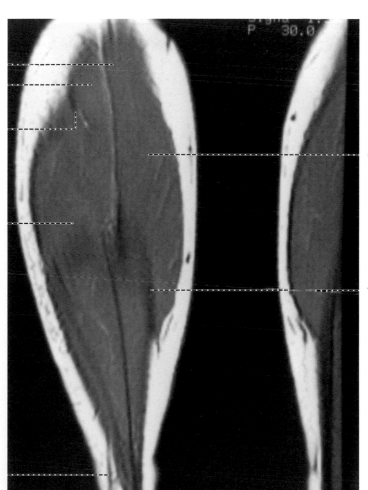

Lesser saphenous v.

Gastrocnemius m., lateral head

Tendinous division between gastrocnemius m., lateral head, and soleus m.

Gastrocnemius m., medial head

Soleus m.

Tendinous division between gastrocnemius m., medial head, and soleus m.

Lesser saphenous v.

Calcaneal (Achilles) tendon

Figure 17.2.13

1. The only muscles demonstrated in this section are those in the proximal anterior compartment. These include extensor hallucis longus, extensor digitorum longus, tibialis anterior, and the long extensors (dorsiflexors) of the foot. Note that these muscles are lateral to the tibia.

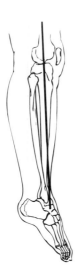

F

E

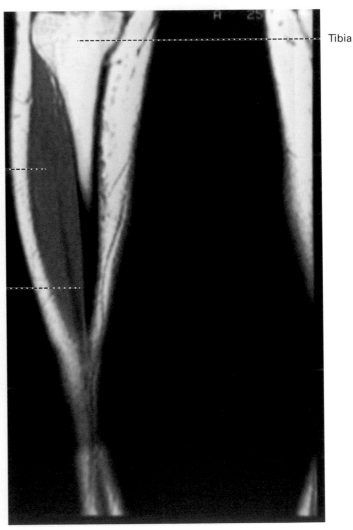

Tibia

Extensor digitorum longus and extensor hallucis longus mm.

Tibialis anterior m.

1. This is the most anterior section of the leg. It demonstrates the subcutaneous anteromedial aspect of the tibia and the extensor digitorum longus and hallucis longus muscles.

Figure 17.2.14

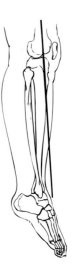

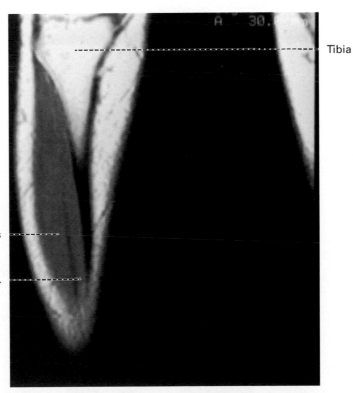

Tibia

Extensor digitorum longus
and extensor hallucis longus
mm.

Tibialis anterior m.

Figure 17.3.1

1. The greater saphenous vein, part of the superficial venous system of the lower limb, is adjacent to the anterior border of gastrocnemius (medial head).

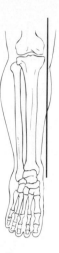

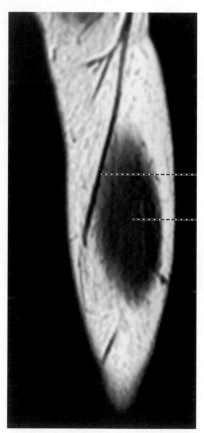

Greater saphenous v.

Gastrocnemius m., medial head

1. The junction between gastrocnemius (medial head) and soleus is well defined medially.

2. As the greater saphenous vein courses distally it is adjacent to the antero-medial border of soleus.

3. Tibialis posterior tendon is identifiable distally just superior and posterior to the medial malleolus.

4. Immediately posterior to tibialis posterior tendon is the tendon of flexor digitorum longus.

Figure 17.3.2

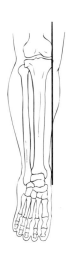

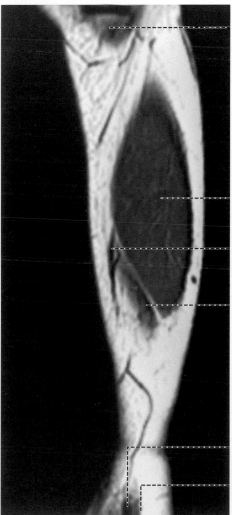

Medial tibial condyle

Gastrocnemius m., medial head

Greater saphenous v.

Soleus m.

Tibialis posterior tendon

Flexor digitorum longus tendon

Figure 17.3.3

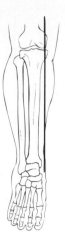

1. Parts of the pes anserinus (goose's foot) complex are seen superiorly, including semitendinosus.

2. Semimembranosus tendon inserts on the posterior medial tibial condyle.

3. The proximal and distal tibia are included in this image.

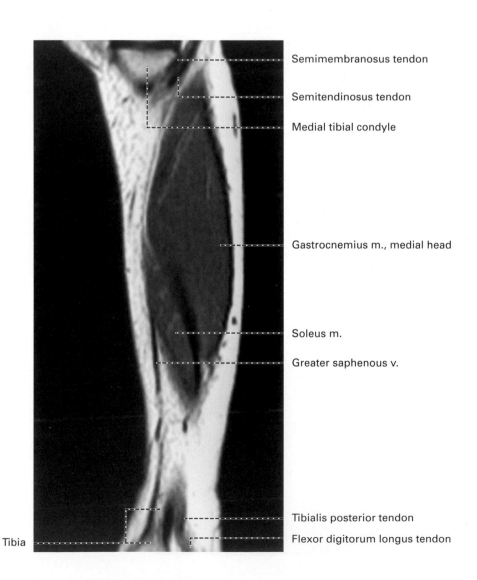

Semimembranosus tendon

Semitendinosus tendon

Medial tibial condyle

Gastrocnemius m., medial head

Soleus m.

Greater saphenous v.

Tibia

Tibialis posterior tendon

Flexor digitorum longus tendon

1. Flexor hallucis longus muscle is now seen in the midcalf region.

2. The medial edge of the calcaneal (Achilles) tendon is imaged posteriorly.

Figure 17.3.4

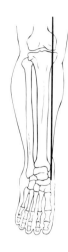

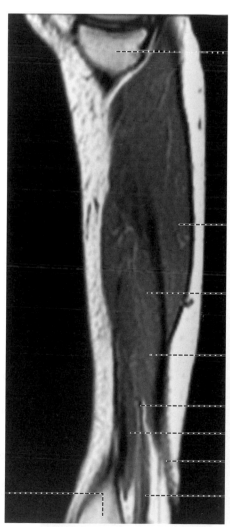

Tibia

Gastrocnemius m., medial head

Soleus m.

Flexor hallucis longus m.

Posterior tibial a. and tibial n.

Tibialis posterior m.

Calcaneal (Achilles) tendon

Tibia

Flexor digitorum longus tendon

Figure 17.3.15

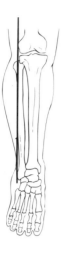

1. The fibular collateral ligament attaches to the proximal fibula. It is more medial than the tendon of biceps femoris. These structures may be indistinguishable at their fibular attachment.

2. The deep peroneal nerve is well visualized because of its accompanying fat. It is distal to its division from the common peroneal nerve, which occurs at the fibular neck.

3. Peroneus longus and brevis are the two muscles in the lateral compartment.

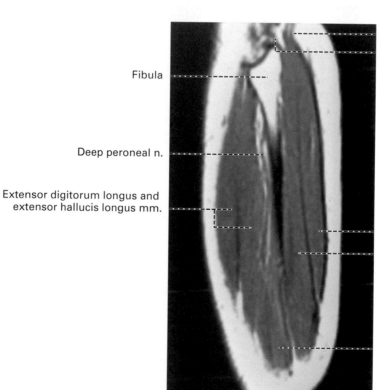

1. Biceps femoris tendon and fibular collateral ligament appear nearly conjoint as they attach to the proximal fibula.

2. The common peroneal nerve is coursing around the fibular neck. It will subsequently divide into its deep and superficial branches.

Figure 17.3.16

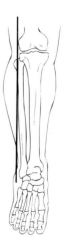

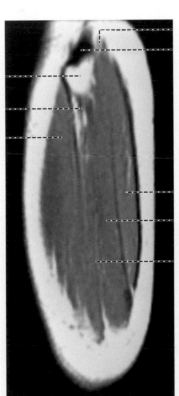

Common peroneal n.

Conjoint biceps femoris tendon and fibular collateral lig.

Fibula

Common peroneal n.

Extensor digitorum longus and extensor hallucis longus mm.

Gastrocnemius m.

Soleus m.

Peroneus longus and brevis mm.

Figure 17.3.17

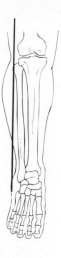

1. The common peroneal nerve is seen just proximal to its division into superficial and deep branches. The deep peroneal nerve courses inferiorly, adjacent to the anterior tibial artery not seen in this image.

2. Peroneus longus is posterolateral to peroneus brevis.

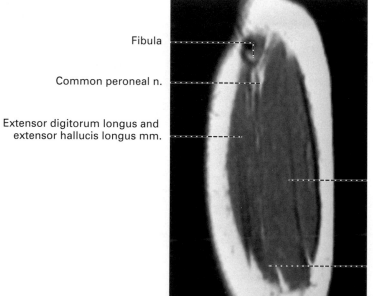

Fibula

Common peroneal n.

Extensor digitorum longus and
extensor hallucis longus mm.

Gastrocnemius m.

Peroneus longus and brevis mm.

1. The lateralmost portion of the common peroneal nerve is identified in this lateral image plane.

Figure 17.3.18

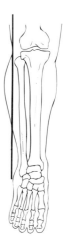

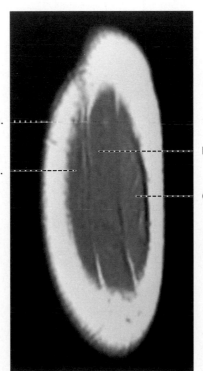

Common peroneal n.

Extensor digitorum longus and extensor hallucis longus mm.

Peroneus longus m.

Gastrocnemius m., lateral head

Chapter 18

ANKLE

Figure 18.1.2

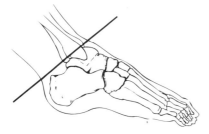

1. The posterior tubercle of the tibia forms the lateral margin of what is referred to clinically and radiographically as the posterior malleolus.

2. Note that muscle fibers of peroneus brevis extend inferiorly to the level of the tibiotalar joint.

3. The extensor retinaculum is well defined anteriorly and serves to keep the extensor tendons from bowing in the concavity of the ankle anteriorly. Note that tibialis anterior tendon lies anterior to this retinaculum.

4. The greater saphenous vein lies along the extensor retinaculum near the anteromedial surface of the tibia. The lesser saphenous vein is posterolateral in the soft tissues between the calcaneal (Achilles) and the peroneal tendons.

5. This portion of the tibia, superior to the tibiotalar joint, is known as the plafond, a French word meaning ceiling or roof.

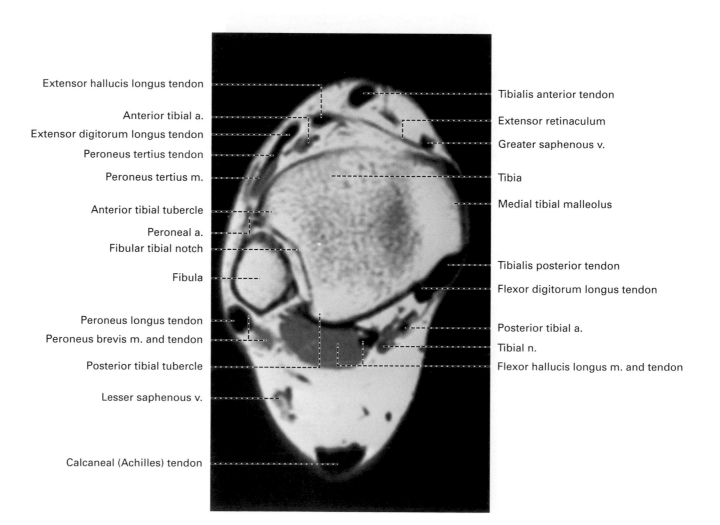

1. This image is at the level of the tibiotalar joint.

2. The posterior malleolus is loosely defined as that portion of the posterior tibia extending inferior to the highest portion of the tibiotalar joint. At this level, the medial and lateral malleoli are also seen.

3. The anterior and posterior inferior tibiofibular ligaments are both demonstrated. They are important structures for maintaining the integrity of the ankle mortice; they attach to the anterior and posterior tubercles of the tibia.

4. Note that flexor hallucis longus has formed a prominent tendon by this level, but it still has some muscle fibers.

5. Peroneus tertius tendon is now identifiably separate from the rest of the tendons of extensor digitorum longus.

6. The greater saphenous vein lies anterior to the medial malleolus.

Figure 18.1.3

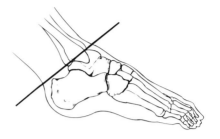

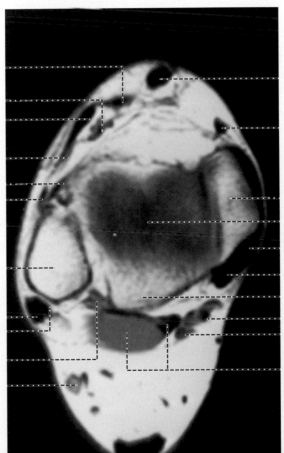

Extensor hallucis longus tendon

Anterior tibial a.

Extensor digitorum longus tendon

Peroneus tertius tendon

Anterior inferior tibiofibular lig.

Peroneal a.

Lateral malleolus

Peroneus longus tendon
Peroneus brevis tendon

Posterior inferior tibiofibular lig.

Lesser saphenous v.

Calcaneal (Achilles) tendon

Tibialis anterior tendon

Greater saphenous v.

Medial tibial malleolus

Tibiotalar joint

Tibialis posterior tendon

Flexor digitorum longus tendon

Posterior tibial malleolus

Posterior tibial a.

Tibial n.

Flexor hallucis longus m. and tendon

Figure 18.1.4

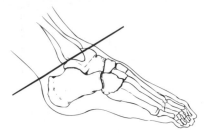

1. The trochlea of the talus is also referred to as the dome of the talus.

2. The deltoid ligament arises from the anteromedial aspect of the medial malleolus.

3. The structures posterior to the medial malleolus include posterior tibialis tendon, flexor digitorum longus tendon, neurovascular structures (posterior tibial artery and tibial nerve), and flexor hallucis longus tendon. These are referred to mnemonically as Tom, Dick, and nervous Harry.

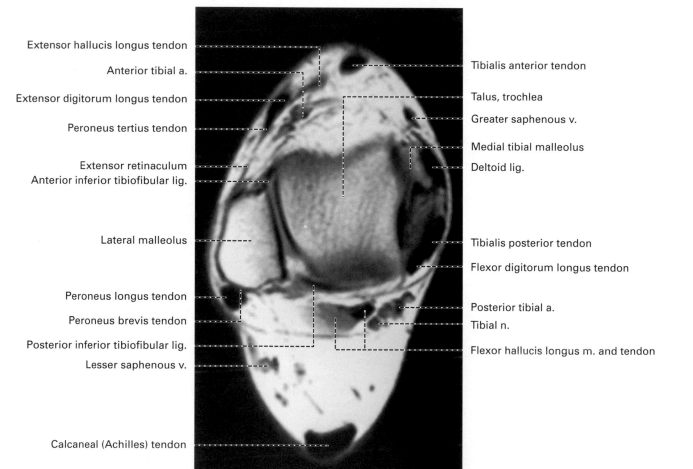

Extensor hallucis longus tendon
Anterior tibial a.
Extensor digitorum longus tendon
Peroneus tertius tendon
Extensor retinaculum
Anterior inferior tibiofibular lig.
Lateral malleolus
Peroneus longus tendon
Peroneus brevis tendon
Posterior inferior tibiofibular lig.
Lesser saphenous v.
Calcaneal (Achilles) tendon

Tibialis anterior tendon
Talus, trochlea
Greater saphenous v.
Medial tibial malleolus
Deltoid lig.
Tibialis posterior tendon
Flexor digitorum longus tendon
Posterior tibial a.
Tibial n.
Flexor hallucis longus m. and tendon

1. The lateral aspect of the extensor retinaculum is demonstrated as it attaches to the lateral malleolus. Part of the lateral or peroneal retinaculum is visible, as is the fascia of flexor hallucis longus.

2. The prominent posterior talofibular ligament extends from the posterior surface of the fibula to the posterior process of the talus. It is one of the three major lateral stabilizing ligaments, the other two being the anterior talofibular ligament and the calcaneofibular ligament.

3. The anterior talofibular ligament is seen at its proximal fibular attachment site.

4. The deltoid ligament has superficial and deep components. The superficial deltoid ligament has anterior (tibionavicular), middle (tibiocalcaneal), and posterior (posterior tibiotalar) parts. The deep deltoid ligament has only the anterior tibiotalar portion.

5. Note that the tendon of tibialis posterior courses along the superficial surface of the deltoid ligament.

Figure 18.1.5

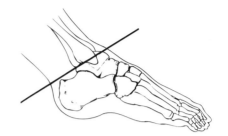

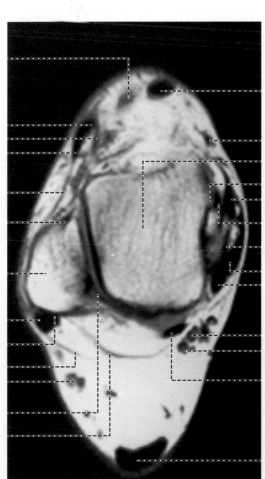

Extensor hallucis longus tendon

Extensor digitorum longus tendon
Anterior tibial a.
Peroneus tertius tendon

Extensor retinaculum

Anterior inferior tibiofibular lig.

Lateral malleolus

Peroneus longus tendon

Peroneus brevis tendon

Peroneal retinaculum
Lesser saphenous v.

Posterior talofibular lig.

Flexor hallucis longus m., fascia

Tibialis anterior tendon

Greater saphenous v.

Talus, trochlea

Talus, medial tubercle
Tibionavicular and tibiocalcaneal parts
of deltoid lig.
Anterior tibiotalar part of deep deltoid
lig.
Posterior tibiotalar part of superficial
deltoid lig.
Tibialis posterior tendon
Flexor digitorum longus tendon

Posterior tibial a.

Tibial n.

Flexor hallucis longus tendon

Calcaneal (Achilles) tendon

Figure 18.1.6

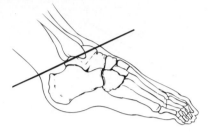

1. In this image, the anterior tibial artery has become the dorsalis pedis artery as it moves more superficially and courses along the dorsum of the foot.

2. Note the posterior process of the talus. An ununited posterior process is known as the os trigonum.

3. Flexor hallucis longus courses in a sulcus known as the posterior sulcus of the talus. It is bounded by the medial and lateral tubercles of the talus. The lateral tubercle is also known as the posterior process of the talus.

4. The calcaneofibular ligament attaches to the fibula adjacent to the fibular attachment of the fascia of flexor hallucis longus.

5. The superficial and deep components of the deltoid ligament are again noted. Tibialis posterior tendon continues along the surface of the deltoid ligament.

Extensor hallucis longus tendon

Extensor digitorum longus tendon

Dorsalis pedis a.
Peroneus tertius tendon

Inferior extensor retinaculum

Anterior talofibular lig.

Calcaneofibular lig.

Lateral malleolus

Peroneus longus tendon

Peroneus brevis tendon

Lesser saphenous v.

Flexor hallucis longus m., fascia

Talus, posterior process

Tibialis anterior tendon

Greater saphenous v.

Talus, body

Anterior tibiotalar part of deep deltoid lig.
Tibionavicular and tibiocalcaneal parts of deltoid lig.

Posterior tibiotalar part of deltoid lig.

Tibialis posterior tendon

Flexor digitorum longus tendon

Talus, posterior sulcus

Posterior tibial a.
Tibial n.

Flexor hallucis longus tendon

Calcaneal (Achilles) tendon

1. Several retinacula are demonstrated in this image. These include the flexor retinaculum (about the tendons of the posterior compartment muscles), the peroneal retinaculum (about the tendons of the same name), and the inferior extensor retinaculum.

2. The anterior talofibular ligament is prominent enough to be seen easily in the axial plane.

3. The calcaneofibular ligament courses obliquely and therefore is only partially seen in several images. It runs along the deep surface of the peroneal tendons.

4. The superior portion of the tarsal sinus is visible in this image. This sinus divides the talus into its posterior talocalcaneal articulation and its medial and anterior talocalcaneal articulations. It contains the strong interosseous talocalcaneal ligament.

Figure 18.1.7

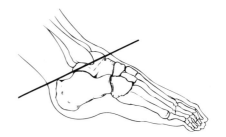

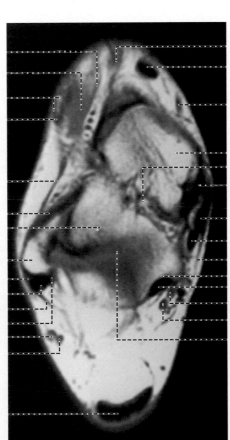

Dorsalis pedis m.
Extensor digitorum brevis m.
Extensor digitorum brevis tendons
Peroneus tertius tendon

Inferior extensor retinaculum

Anterior talofibular lig.
Talus, posterior part of body

Lateral malleolus

Peroneus longus tendon
Peroneus brevis tendon
Peroneal retinaculum
Calcaneofibular lig.
Lesser saphenous v.
Sural n.

Calcaneal (Achilles) tendon

Extensor hallucis longus tendon
Tibialis anterior tendon

Greater saphenous v.

Talus, anterior part of body
Tarsal sinus
Deltoid lig.

Tibialis posterior tendon

Flexor digitorum longus tendon
Flexor retinaculum
Talus, posterior sulcus
Flexor hallucis longus tendon
Posterior tibial a.
Tibial n.

Posterior talocalcaneal joint

Figure 18.1.8

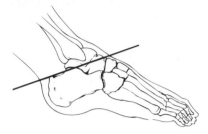

1. Extensor digitorum brevis, the short intrinsic extensor of the toes, arises anteriorly from the proximal superior surface of the calcaneus and from the inferior extensor retinaculum, deep to the tendons of the long extensors of the toes.

2. The lateral talocalcaneal ligament courses nearly parallel but deeper to the calcaneofibular ligament.

3. The medial talocalcaneal ligament courses from the medial tubercle of the talus (medial margin of the posterior sulcus of the talus, in which runs the tendon of flexor hallucis longus) to the sustentaculum tali. Therefore, it lies just anterior to flexor hallucis longus tendon.

4. Note that there is now a separate retinaculum for the tendon of flexor hallucis longus.

5. The talonavicular joint is visible. Its capsular fibers blend with the tibionavicular fibers of the deltoid ligament. This is the most anterior extent of the deltoid ligament; that is, it courses around the talar head to reach the talonavicular capsule.

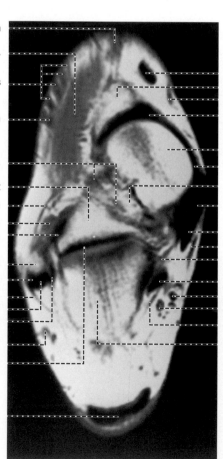

Extensor hallucis longus tendon
Extensor digitorum brevis m.
Extensor digitorum longus tendons
Peroneus tertius tendon
Interosseous talocalcaneal lig.
Talus, posterior part
Inferior extensor retinaculum
Lateral talocalcaneal lig.
Anterior talofibular lig.
Lateral malleolus
Peroneus longus tendon
Peroneal retinaculum
Peroneus brevis tendon
Calcaneofibular lig.
Lesser saphenous v.
Posterior talocalcaneal joint
Calcaneal (Achilles) tendon

Tibialis anterior tendon
Navicular
Greater saphenous v.
Talonavicular capsule and fibers of tibionavicular part of deltoid lig.
Talus, head
Deltoid lig., tibionavicular part
Tarsal sinus
Tibialis posterior tendon
Flexor digitorum longus tendon
Flexor retinaculum
Medial talocalcaneal lig.
Flexor hallucis longus tendon
Posterior tibial a.
Tibial n.
Retinaculum to flexor hallucis longus tendon
Calcaneus

1   At this level, the axial images of the ankle look similar to longitudinal images of the foot.

2. This image is at the level of the sustentaculum tali of the calcaneus. This is an important landmark. Posterior to it runs the tendon of flexor hallucis longus. Attaching to the sustentaculum tali from above are the medial talocalcaneal ligament and the tibiocalcaneal contribution of the deltoid ligament.

3. The tendons of flexor digitorum longus and tibialis posterior are located anteromedial to the sustentaculum tali.

4. Extending anteriorly from the sustentaculum tali is the plantar calcaneonavicular (or "spring") ligament.

5. Note that the orientation of the oblique tarsal sinus is nearly orthogonal to the plane of the posterior talocalcaneal joint.

Figure 18.1.9

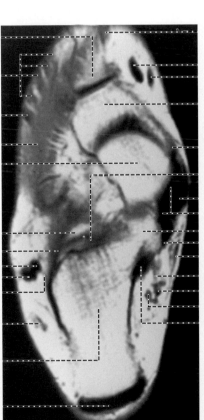

Middle cuneiform bone	Extensor hallucis longus tendon
Extensor digitorum longus tendons	Tibialis anterior tendon Greater saphenous v.
Peroneus tertius tendon	Navicular
Extensor digitorum brevis m.	Talocalcaneonavicular capsule
Talus, head	Posterior talocalcaneal joint
	Tibialis posterior tendon Plantar calcaneonavicular ("spring") lig.
Talus, posterior facet	Sustentaculum tali Flexor digitorum longus tendon
Lateral talocalcaneal lig.	Flexor retinaculum
Peroneus brevis tendon Peroneus longus tendon	Retinaculum to flexor hallucis longus tendon Posterior tibial a.
Calcaneofibular lig.	Tibial n.
Lesser saphenous v.	Flexor hallucis longus tendon
Calcaneus	
Calcaneal (Achilles) tendon	

Figure 18.1.10

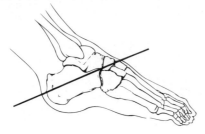

1. The plantar calcaneonavicular ("spring") ligament is broad and thick; it attaches to the plantar surface of the navicular. It not only stabilizes the relationship of navicular to calcaneus, but supports the head of the talus as it courses plantar to that bone.

2. Note that tibialis posterior tendon is medial to the plantar calcaneonavicular ligament while the tendons of flexor digitorum longus and flexor hallucis longus course along its lateral border.

3. Two more short intrinsic muscles arise at this level, quadratus plantae and abductor hallucis.

4. The three cuneiforms can be seen at this level. Note that all three articulate with the navicular.

5. The calcaneofibular ligament is seen attaching to the calcaneal tubercle laterally. Its contiguity with the deep surface of the peroneal tendons persists.

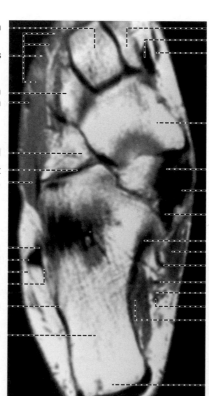

Left labels:
- Middle cuneiform
- Extensor digitorum longus tendons
- Lateral cuneiform
- Peroneus tertius tendon
- Cuboid
- Calcaneocuboid joint
- Extensor digitorum brevis m.
- Peroneus brevis tendon
- Peroneus longus tendon
- Peroneal retinaculum
- Calcaneofibular lig.
- Calcaneal tubercle
- Calcaneus
- Calcaneal (Achilles) tendon

Right labels:
- Medial cuneiform
- Tibialis anterior tendon
- Greater saphenous v.
- Navicular
- Plantar calcaneonavicular lig.
- Tibialis posterior tendon
- Flexor digitorum longus tendon
- Flexor hallucis longus tendon
- Abductor hallucis m.
- Medial plantar a.
- Medial plantar n.
- Lateral plantar a.
- Lateral plantar n.
- Quadratus plantae m.
- Calcaneal tuberosity

1. This section is at the level of the insertion of the tibialis posterior tendons. Note that this subject has an accessory ossicle in the substance of the tibialis posterior tendon known as the os tibiale externum.

2. This subject also demonstrates a well-defined separate lateral slip of the plantar calcaneonavicular ("spring") ligament.

3. The calcaneonavicular portion of the bifurcate ligament is well demonstrated here, but the accompanying calcaneocuboid component is less well visualized.

4. Some of the more inferior fibers of the calcaneofibular ligament are seen as they insert on the prominent calcaneal tubercle laterally.

5. Fibers from the tibialis anterior tendon are seen inserting on the medial plantar aspect of the medial cuneiform. Other fibers of the tibialis anterior continue to the base of the first metatarsal.

Figure 18.1.11

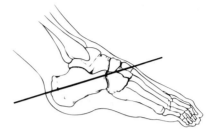

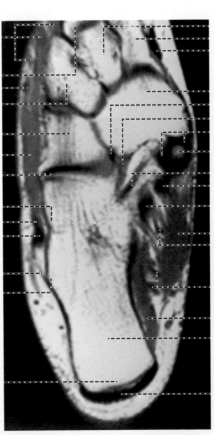

Extensor digitorum longus tendons

Second metatarsal, base
Peroneus tertius tendon
Lateral cuneiform

Cuboid

Extensor digitorum brevis m.

Calcaneocuboid joint

Peroneal trochlea
Peroneus brevis tendon
Peroneus longus tendon

Calcaneofibular lig.

Calcaneal tubercle

Calcaneal tuberosity

Middle cuneiform
Medial cuneiform
Tibialis anterior tendon

Navicular
Bifurcate lig., calcaneocuboid part
Bifurcate lig., calcaneonavicular part
Tibialis posterior tendon, broad insertion

Os tibiale externum

Lateral plantar calcaneonavicular lig.
Flexor digitorum longus tendon

Flexor hallucis longus tendon

Abductor hallucis m.
Medial plantar nn. and vessels

Lateral plantar nn. and vessels

Quadratus plantae m.

Calcaneus

Calcaneal (Achilles) tendon

Figure 18.1.12

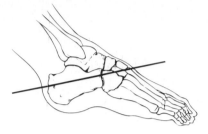

1. On the plantar surface of the navicular is a continuation of the fibers of the tendon of tibialis posterior. These fibers insert on the three cuneiform bones, the cuboid, and metatarsals two, three, and four.

2. Inferiorly note the medial tuberosity of the navicular. This prominence forms the insertion of the majority of the tibialis posterior tendon.

3. At this level, the peroneal tendons start to diverge, with peroneus brevis coursing toward the base of the fifth metatarsal and peroneus longus running along the deep plantar surface of the midfoot.

4. The medial cuneiform has a complex shape and is the largest of the three cuneiforms.

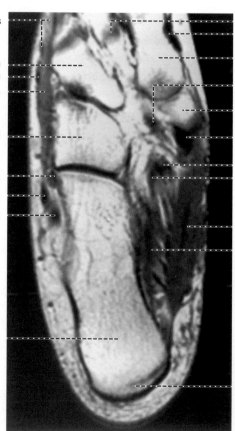

Extensor digitorum longus tendons

Lateral cuneiform
Peroneus tertius tendon
Extensor digitorum brevis m.

Cuboid

Lateral calcaneocuboid lig.

Peroneus brevis tendon

Peroneus longus tendon

Calcaneus

Middle cuneiform, plantar cortex
Tibialis anterior tendon

Medial cuneiform

Tibialis posterior tendon extension to cuneiforms
Navicular tuberosity

Tibialis posterior tendon

Flexor digitorum longus tendon
Flexor hallucis longus tendon

Abductor hallucis m.

Quadratus plantae m.

Calcaneal tuberosity

1. Abductor digiti minimi arises predominantly from the lateral process of the calcaneus. Some fibers come from the very distal part of the medial calcaneal process.

2. The fibers of the plantar calcaneocuboid ligament are visualized in this section. It is also known as the short plantar ligament.

3. This section is at the level of the decussation of flexor hallucis longus coursing medially and flexor digitorum longus continuing laterally.

Figure 18.1.13

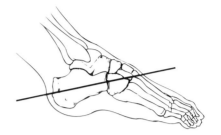

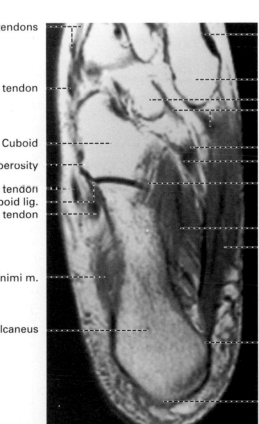

Extensor digitorum longus tendons

Peroneus tertius tendon

Cuboid

Cuboid tuberosity

Peroneus brevis tendon
Lateral calcaneocuboid lig.
Peroneus longus tendon

Abductor digiti minimi m.

Calcaneus

Tibialis anterior tendon

Medial cuneiform

Lateral cuneiform
Continuations of tibialis posterior tendon

Flexor digitorum longus tendon
Flexor hallucis longus tendon

Plantar calcaneocuboid (short plantar) lig.

Quadratus plantae m.

Abductor hallucis m.

Calcaneus, medial process

Calcaneal tuberosity

Figure 18.1.14

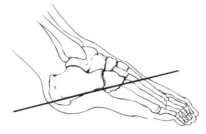

1. Flexor hallucis longus tendon is now on the medial aspect of flexor digitorum longus tendon.

2. The larger lateral plantar neurovascular structures are visible between fibers of quadratus plantae and abductor digiti minimi muscles. The medial plantar neurovascular structures lie initially between abductor hallucis and quadratus plantae, then between digitorum brevis and abductor flexor hallucis.

3. The medial and lateral processes of the calcaneal tuberosity are noted. These prominences serve as the origin for many of the short intrinsic muscles on the plantar surface of the foot.

4. Peroneus longus tendon is now in the peroneal groove of the cuboid.

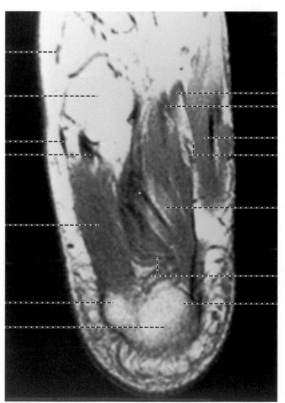

1. This section demonstrates the oblique course of peroneus longus tendon along the plantar surface of the cuboid. Its destination is the lateral aspects of the metatarsal and medial cuneiform. It runs deep to the intrinsic muscles of the plantar surface of the foot.

2. Flexor digitorum brevis is now visible. It is volume averaged with fibers of quadratus plantae.

3. The tendon of abductor hallucis is forming but will not insert until it reaches the base of the proximal phalanx of the great toe.

Figure 18.1.15

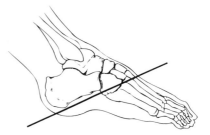

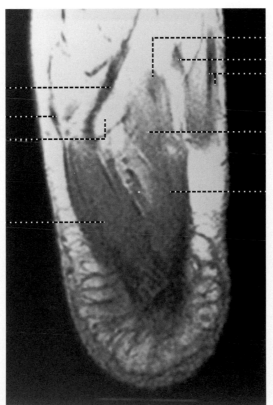

Peroneus longus tendon

Peroneus brevis tendon

Cuboid

Abductor digiti minimi m.

Flexor digitorum longus tendon

Flexor hallucis longus tendon
Abductor hallucis m. and tendon

Flexor digitorum brevis m.

Quadratus plantae m.

Figure 18.1.16

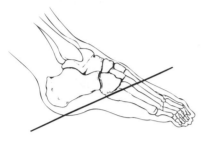

1. Peroneus brevis tendon inserts along the lateral aspect of the base of the fifth metatarsal.

2. The larger lateral plantar vessels extend between abductor digiti minimi and flexor digitorum brevis. They ultimately proceed distally in the foot to form the plantar arch after uniting with the deep plantar branch of the dorsalis pedis vessels.

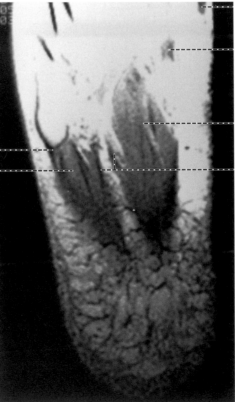

Abductor hallucis tendon

Flexor hallucis longus tendon

Flexor digitorum brevis m.

Peroneus brevis tendon

Abductor digiti minimi m.

Lateral plantar nn. and vessels

1. Note the prominent calcaneal (Achilles) tendon formed by contributions of soleus and gastrocnemius tendons. It represents the thickest, strongest tendon in the body. It attaches to the middle of the posterior surface of the calcaneus along the upper border of the calcaneal tuberosity.

2. A portion of the fat pad of the heel is demonstrated inferior to the calcaneus.

Figure 18.2.1

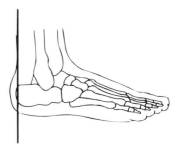

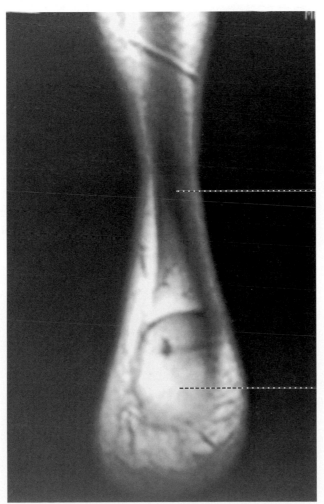

Calcaneal (Achilles) tendon

Calcaneus

Figure 18.2.2

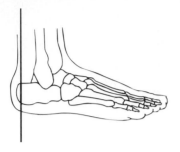

1. The insertion of soleus into the calcaneal (Achilles) tendon is noted in this image.

2. The sural nerve, with the more superficial lesser saphenous vein, is demonstrated in the lateral subcutaneous tissue. It is formed from branches of the tibial and peroneal nerves.

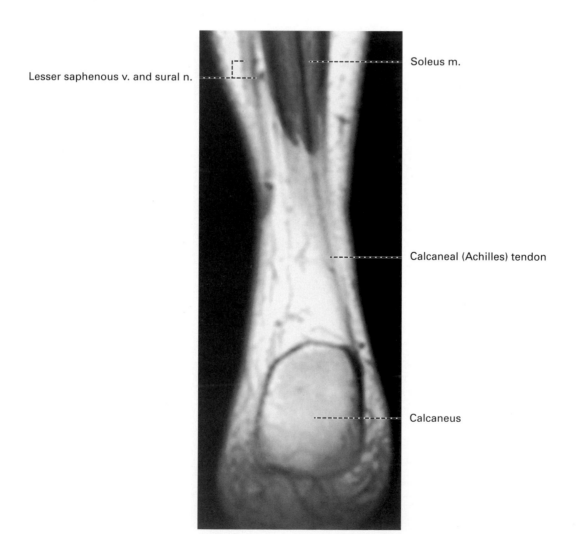

Lesser saphenous v. and sural n.

Soleus m.

Calcaneal (Achilles) tendon

Calcaneus

1. This section includes the posterior part of flexor hallucis longus. Of the deep posterior compartment muscles (tibialis posterior, flexor digitorum longus, and flexor hallucis longus), its muscle fibers extend most distally, nearly to the posterior talar sulcus.

2. The two saphenous veins are imaged in this section: the lesser saphenous vein laterally and the greater saphenous vein medially.

3. The inferior calcaneal surface serves as the origin of many of the short plantar muscles of the foot.

Figure 18.2.3

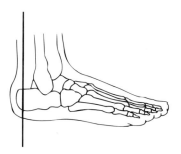

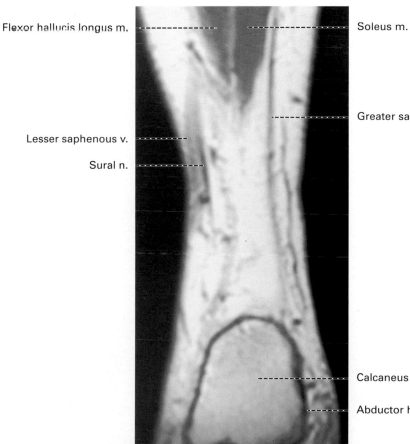

Flexor hallucis longus m.

Soleus m.

Greater saphenous v.

Lesser saphenous v.

Sural n.

Calcaneus

Abductor hallucis m.

Plantar aponeurosis

Figure 18.2.4

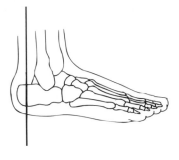

1. The lesser saphenous vein and the sural nerve remain closely paired as they descend. The sural nerve is also known as the lesser saphenous nerve.

2. The increased linear signal intensity between the lateral compartment muscles (peroneus longus and brevis) and flexor hallucis longus (posterior compartment muscle) represents the plane of the intermuscular septum.

3. The medial and lateral tubercles (processes) of the calcaneus serve as the origin of the first layer of intrinsic muscles of the sole of the foot (abductor hallucis, flexor digitorum brevis, and abductor digiti minimi).

4. Quadratus plantae, a muscle in the second layer of intrinsic muscles of the sole of the foot, has two heads, medial and lateral. The medial head is larger and more muscular and arises from the medial surface of the calcaneus.

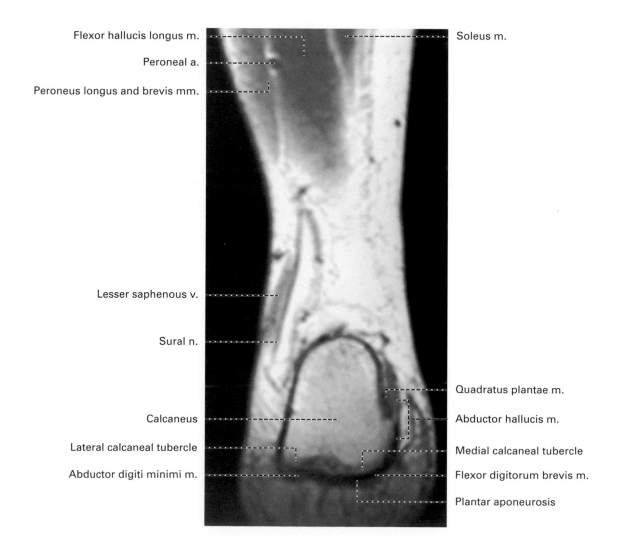

Flexor hallucis longus m.

Peroneal a.

Peroneus longus and brevis mm.

Lesser saphenous v.

Sural n.

Calcaneus

Lateral calcaneal tubercle

Abductor digiti minimi m.

Soleus m.

Quadratus plantae m.

Abductor hallucis m.

Medial calcaneal tubercle

Flexor digitorum brevis m.

Plantar aponeurosis

1. Flexor hallucis longus remains a broad muscle as it descends.

2. The peroneal vessels are noted as they penetrate the intermuscular septum between the posterior and lateral compartments.

3. The plantar aponeurosis is closely applied to the superficial surface of flexor digitorum brevis.

Figure 18.2.5

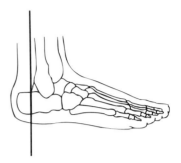

Flexor hallucis longus m.

Peroneus longus and brevis mm.

Peroneal a., perforating branches

Tibial n. and posterior tibial a.

Flexor hallucis longus m.

Quadratus plantae m.

Calcaneus

Abductor hallucis m.

Abductor digiti minimi m.

Flexor digitorum brevis m.

Plantar aponeurosis

Figure 18.2.6

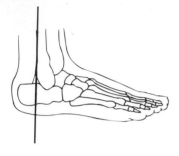

1. The calcaneal attachment of the calcaneofibular ligament is demonstrated. It is one of the ligaments that stabilizes the lateral ankle.

2. The tendons and muscle fibers of peroneus longus and peroneus brevis are posterolateral to the fibula.

3. Note the branches of the plantar vessels situated between quadratus plantae and abductor hallucis proximally and calcaneus and flexor digitorum brevis more distally.

4. Flexor digitorum longus tendon is medial to the neurovascular structures, which include the tibial nerve and the posterior tibial artery and veins.

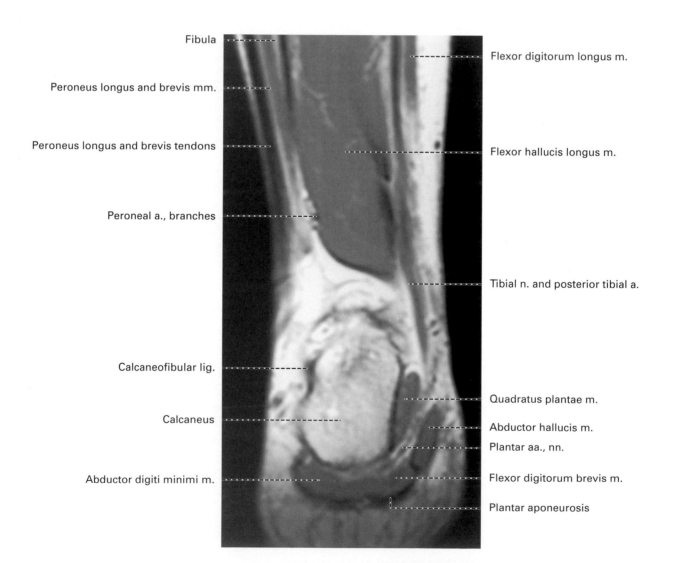

1. This image demonstrates the proximal tendon of flexor hallucis longus just lateral to the tibial nerve and posterior tibial vessels.

2. The posterior process of the talus is lateral to the tendon of flexor hallucis longus as it travels within the posterior sulcus of the talus.

3. The posterior malleolus of the tibia is demonstrated. Note that the muscle fibers of flexor hallucis longus extend to the inferior edge of this posterior tibial prominence.

4. The abductor of the little toe is prominent posterolaterally near its origin from the calcaneus. On the plantar aspect of the foot it mirrors the abductor hallucis.

Figure 18.2.7

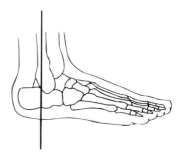

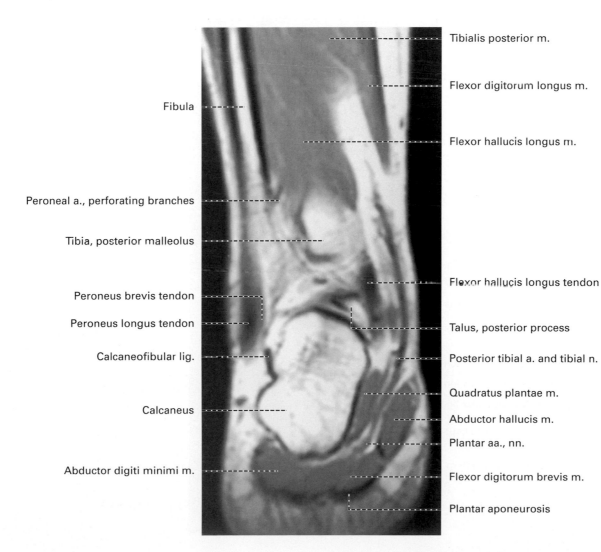

Figure 18.2.8

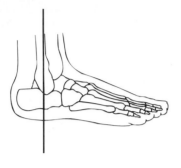

1. The calcaneofibular ligament is deep to the peroneal tendons. It attaches to the apex of the lateral malleolus.

2. Shown is a portion of the posterior talofibular ligament, a nearly horizontal course. This ligament is longer and thicker than the anterior talofibular ligament; it attaches to the posterior process of the talus.

3. The posterior inferior tibiofibular ligament has a more superior location and more oblique course than the posterior talofibular ligament.

4. At this level, the tendon of peroneus longus is lateral to that of peroneus brevis.

5. Flexor hallucis longus passes inferior to the medial surface of the talus just medial to the posterior subtalar joint.

6. The two most medial tendons, posterior to the medial malleolus, are the tendons of tibialis posterior and flexor digitorum longus. In the coronal plane, at this level, it is difficult to distinguish them.

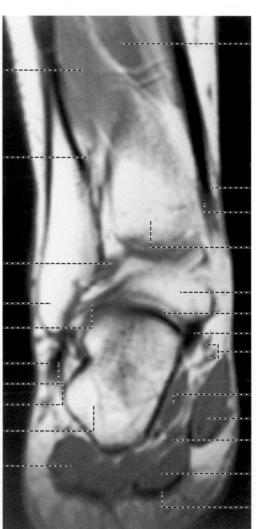

Flexor hallucis longus m.

Peroneal a., perforating branches

Posterior inferior tibiofibular lig.

Fibula, lateral malleolus

Posterior talofibular lig.

Peroneus longus tendon

Peroneus brevis tendon

Calcaneofibular lig.

Calcaneus

Abductor digiti minimi m.

Tibialis posterior m.

Flexor digitorum longus tendon

Tibialis posterior tendon

Tibia

Talus

Posterior talocalcaneal joint

Flexor hallucis longus tendon

Medial plantar a., n.

Quadratus plantae m.

Abductor hallucis m.

Lateral plantar a., n.

Flexor digitorum brevis m.

Plantar aponeurosis

Figure 18.2.9

1. The lateral malleolus is more inferior and posterior than the medial malleolus.

2. A portion of the fibular attachment of the calcaneofibular ligament can be identified in this section.

3. Flexor hallucis longus tendon is contiguous with the medial surface of the calcaneus, adjacent to the posterior subtalar joint and posterior to sustentaculum tali, under which it will subsequently course.

4. The tarsal sinus is an oblique canal that houses the interosseous talocalcaneal ligament.

5. Portions of the deltoid ligament are imaged deep to the tendons of flexor digitorum longus and tibialis posterior.

6. The lateral plantar vessels and nerve course lateral to the abductor digiti minimi.

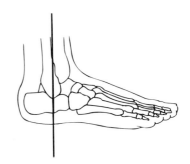

Extensor digitorum longus m.

Peroneal a.

Lateral malleolus

Anterior talofibular lig.

Peroneus brevis tendon

Peroneus longus tendon

Tarsal sinus

Calcaneus

Abductor digiti minimi m.

Greater saphenous v.

Tibia

Tibialis posterior tendon

Flexor digitorum longus tendon

Deltoid lig., superficial, posterior part

Talus

Flexor hallucis longus tendon

Medial plantar a., n.

Abductor hallucis m.

Quadratus plantae m.

Lateral plantar a., n.

Flexor digitorum brevis m.

Plantar aponeurosis

Figure 18.2.10

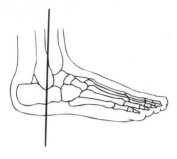

1. Sustentaculum tali is a medial extension of the calcaneus. It contributes to the middle subtalar joint.

2. Flexor hallucis longus tendon passes inferior to the sustentaculum tali.

3. The anterior talofibular ligament is nearly perpendicular to this plane. It travels in a nearly true axial plane to insert along the anterior neck of the talus.

4. The deltoid ligament, the deep portions of which descend from the medial malleolus to the sustentaculum tali, blends imperceptibly with the tendinous fibers of the tibialis posterior and flexor digitorum longus.

5. The greater saphenous vein is superficial. It courses superior and posterior to the medial malleolus. This location, and the ease of its stabilization against the underlying tibia, makes it a frequently used vein for emergency "cut-down" access.

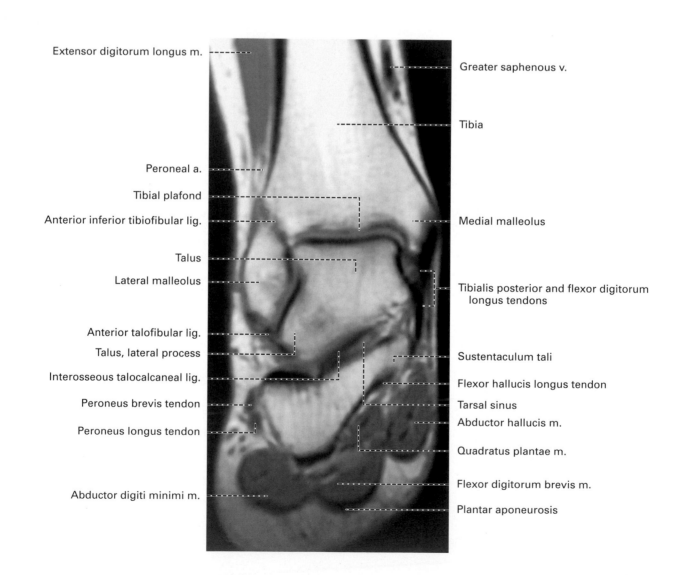

Extensor digitorum longus m.

Greater saphenous v.

Tibia

Peroneal a.

Tibial plafond

Anterior inferior tibiofibular lig.

Medial malleolus

Talus

Lateral malleolus

Tibialis posterior and flexor digitorum longus tendons

Anterior talofibular lig.

Talus, lateral process

Sustentaculum tali

Interosseous talocalcaneal lig.

Flexor hallucis longus tendon

Peroneus brevis tendon

Tarsal sinus

Peroneus longus tendon

Abductor hallucis m.

Quadratus plantae m.

Flexor digitorum brevis m.

Abductor digiti minimi m.

Plantar aponeurosis

1. The oblique anterior inferior tibiofibular ligament is noted as it attaches to the anterior tibial tubercle.

2. Flexor hallucis longus tendon remains lateral to the tendon of flexor digitorum longus. Distally, these tendons cross near the junction of the hindfoot and midfoot (talonavicular joint).

3. The medial malleolus is more anterior and superior than the lateral malleolus. Thus the "mortice" joint at the talocrural junction is oblique in relation to the coronal plane.

4. The tibial horizontal portion of the tibiotalar joint is known as the plafond, which in French means ceiling or roof.

5. Note that no muscles are associated with the anteromedial surface of the tibia.

Figure 18.2.11

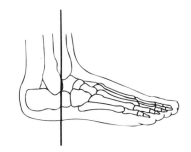

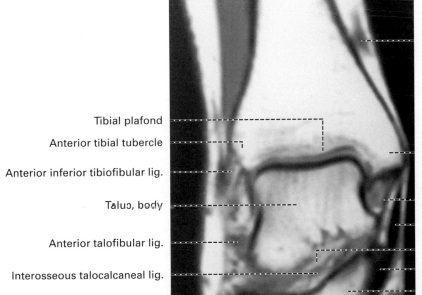

Extensor digitorum longus m.

Tibial plafond
Anterior tibial tubercle
Anterior inferior tibiofibular lig.
Talus, body
Anterior talofibular lig.
Interosseous talocalcaneal lig.

Peroneus brevis tendon
Peroneus longus tendon

Abductor digiti minimi m.

Tibia

Greater saphenous v.

Medial malleolus

Deltoid lig., deep part
Tibialis posterior tendon
Tarsal sinus
Flexor digitorum longus tendon
Sustentaculum tali
Flexor hallucis longus tendon

Abductor hallucis m
Quadratus plantae m.

Flexor digitorum brevis m.

Plantar aponeurosis

Figure 18.2.12

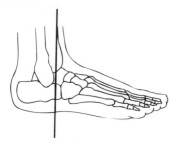

1. The anterior part of the tarsal sinus is seen in this section. The prominent interosseous talocalcaneal ligament is identified.

2. Note the origin of extensor digitorum brevis from the lateral surface of the calcaneus.

3. Peroneus longus is beginning its oblique course under the hindfoot and midfoot, deep to the intrinsic muscles of the foot. It is passing into a groove in the distal calcaneus prior to crossing the calcaneocuboid joint.

4. The calcaneonavicular ligament is seen arising from the sustentaculum tali.

5. This section demonstrates the deep (anterior tibiotalar part) and superficial (tibiocalcaneal part) components of the deltoid ligament.

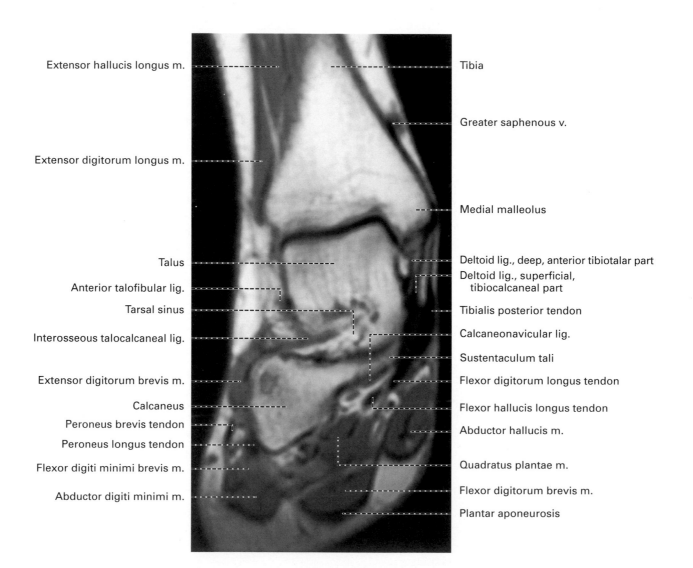

Extensor hallucis longus m.

Extensor digitorum longus m.

Talus

Anterior talofibular lig.

Tarsal sinus

Interosseous talocalcaneal lig.

Extensor digitorum brevis m.

Calcaneus

Peroneus brevis tendon

Peroneus longus tendon

Flexor digiti minimi brevis m.

Abductor digiti minimi m.

Tibia

Greater saphenous v.

Medial malleolus

Deltoid lig., deep, anterior tibiotalar part

Deltoid lig., superficial, tibiocalcaneal part

Tibialis posterior tendon

Calcaneonavicular lig.

Sustentaculum tali

Flexor digitorum longus tendon

Flexor hallucis longus tendon

Abductor hallucis m.

Quadratus plantae m.

Flexor digitorum brevis m.

Plantar aponeurosis

1. Calcaneocuboid ligament is seen in cross section in this image.

2. Peroneus longus tendon courses obliquely at the level of the calcaneocuboid joint.

3. A small slip of peroneus tertius tendon is noted. This muscle is an extension of extensor digitorum longus. It inserts on the dorsal surface of the base of the fifth metatarsal bone.

4. Note the calcaneonavicular ligament coursing immediately inferior to this portion of the talus. This ligament is important in supporting the talar head, thus preserving the longitudinal arch of the foot.

Figure 18.2.13

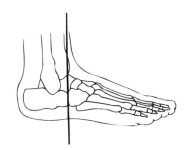

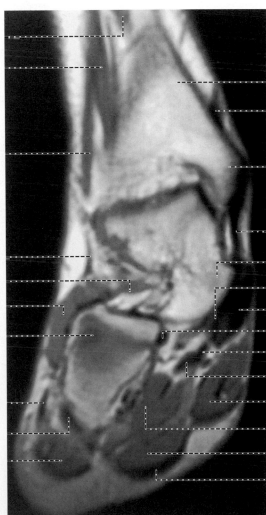

Tibialis anterior tendon

Extensor hallucis longus m. and tendon

Extensor digitorum longus tendon

Peroneus tertius tendon

Interosseous talocalcaneal lig.

Extensor digitorum brevis m.

Calcaneocuboid joint

Peroneus brevis tendon

Peroneus longus tendon

Flexor and abductor digiti minimi mm.

Tibia

Greater saphenous v.

Medial malleolus

Deltoid lig., anterior tibiotalar part

Talus, head and neck

Calcaneonavicular lig.

Tibialis posterior tendon

Calcaneocuboid lig.

Flexor digitorum longus tendon

Flexor hallucis longus tendon

Abductor hallucis m.

Quadratus plantae m.

Flexor digitorum brevis m.

Plantar aponeurosis

Figure 18.2.14

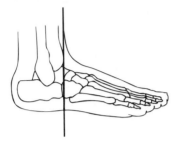

1. This image demonstrates the distal attachment of the anterior talofibular ligament.

2. This subject has an os tibiale externum, a sesamoid bone in the distal tendon fibers of tibialis posterior.

3. The calcaneonavicular ligament is larger near its attachment to the navicular.

4. Peroneus longus is seen within the cuboid sulcus.

5. Peroneus brevis tendon inserts on the dorsolateral surface of the base of the fifth metatarsal.

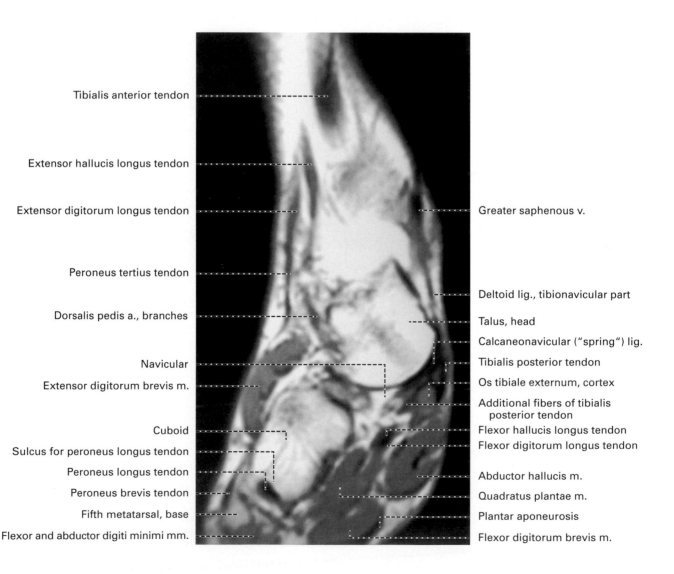

Tibialis anterior tendon

Extensor hallucis longus tendon

Extensor digitorum longus tendon

Greater saphenous v.

Peroneus tertius tendon

Deltoid lig., tibionavicular part

Dorsalis pedis a., branches

Talus, head

Calcaneonavicular ("spring") lig.

Navicular

Tibialis posterior tendon

Extensor digitorum brevis m.

Os tibiale externum, cortex

Additional fibers of tibialis posterior tendon

Cuboid

Flexor hallucis longus tendon

Flexor digitorum longus tendon

Sulcus for peroneus longus tendon

Peroneus longus tendon

Abductor hallucis m.

Peroneus brevis tendon

Quadratus plantae m.

Fifth metatarsal, base

Plantar aponeurosis

Flexor and abductor digiti minimi mm.

Flexor digitorum brevis m.

1. The dorsalis pedis and the deep peroneal nerve are located anteriorly between the tendons of extensor hallucis longus and extensor digitorum longus. Also note that this neurovascular group courses medial to extensor digitorum brevis and lateral to the talonavicular joint.

2. Tibialis posterior tendon inserts on the navicular tuberosity. There are a few fibers of tibialis posterior that extend distally to the cuneiforms. These fibers can be seen along the deep surface of the navicular tuberosity.

3. The tibionavicular portion of the broad deltoid ligament is demonstrated in this section.

Figure 18.2.15

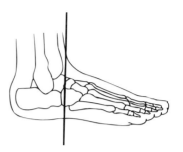

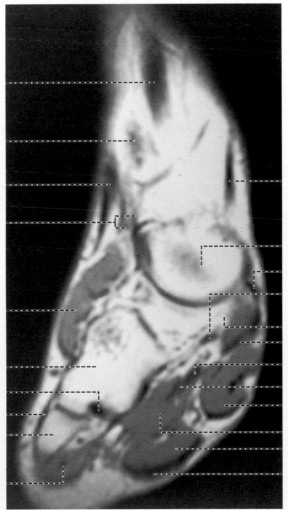

Tibialis anterior tendon

Extensor hallucis longus tendon

Extensor digitorum longus tendon

Dorsalis pedis vessels and deep peroneal n.

Extensor digitorum brevis m.

Cuboid

Peroneus longus tendon

Peroneus brevis tendon

Fifth metatarsal, base

Flexor and abductor digiti minimi mm.

Greater saphenous v.

Talus, head

Deltoid lig., tibionavicular attachment

Additional fibers of tibialis posterior tendon

Navicular tuberosity
Tibialis posterior tendon

Flexor hallucis longus tendon

Flexor digitorum longus tendon
Abductor hallucis m.

Quadratus plantae m.
Flexor digitorum brevis m.

Plantar aponeurosis

Figure 18.2.16

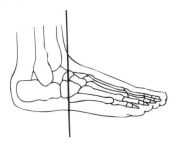

1. Peroneus longus tendon is in the sulcus at the medial margin of the cuboid.

2. The tibialis posterior tendon, which extends from the navicular to the cuneiforms, is seen as a prominent structure on the inferior surface of the navicular bone.

3. The dorsalis pedis vessels remain medial to the talonavicular joint.

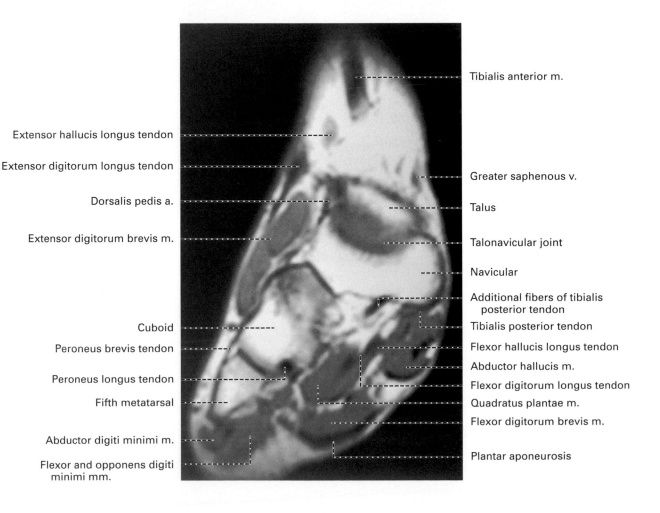

1. This image is at the level of the articulations of the cuboid and navicular with the cuneiforms.

2. Peroneus longus tendon is deep to the middle cuneiform.

3. Tibialis posterior is inserting onto the plantar surface of the middle cuneiform.

Figure 18.2.17

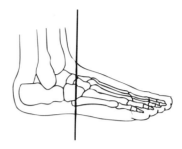

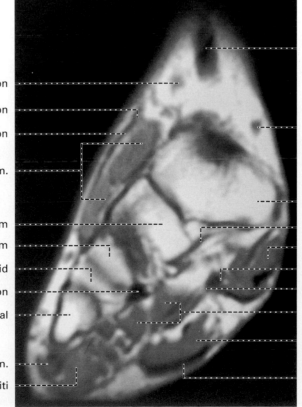

Extensor hallucis longus tendon
Extensor digitorum longus tendon
Peroneus tertius tendon
Extensor digitorum brevis m.
Middle cuneiform
Lateral cuneiform
Cuboid
Peroneus longus tendon
Fifth metatarsal
Abductor digiti minimi m.
Flexor and opponens digiti minimi mm.

Tibialis anterior m.
Greater saphenous v.
Navicular
Tibialis posterior tendon, fibers
Abductor hallucis m.
Flexor hallucis longus tendon
Flexor digitorum longus tendon
Quadratus plantae m.
Flexor digitorum brevis m.
Plantar aponeurosis

Figure 18.3.1

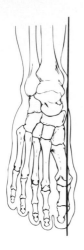

1. This medial section shows the abductor hallucis muscle and tendon.

2. Note flexor hallucis brevis inferior to the first metatarsal.

3. The great saphenous vein forms and ascends on the medial side of the foot.

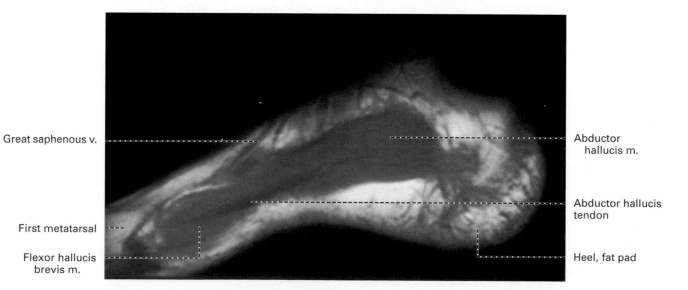

Great saphenous v.

Abductor hallucis m.

Abductor hallucis tendon

First metatarsal

Flexor hallucis brevis m.

Heel, fat pad

1. The tibialis posterior tendon is seen coursing anteriorly and inferiorly to insert on the plantar surface of the navicular tuberosity and cuneiforms.

2. The flexor digitorum longus tendon descends posterior to the tibialis posterior tendon.

3. The tibialis anterior tendon is partially outlined at its insertion onto the plantar surface of the medial cuneiform and base of the first metatarsal.

4. Flexor digitorum brevis is seen at its origin from the calcaneal tuberosity.

Figure 18.3.2

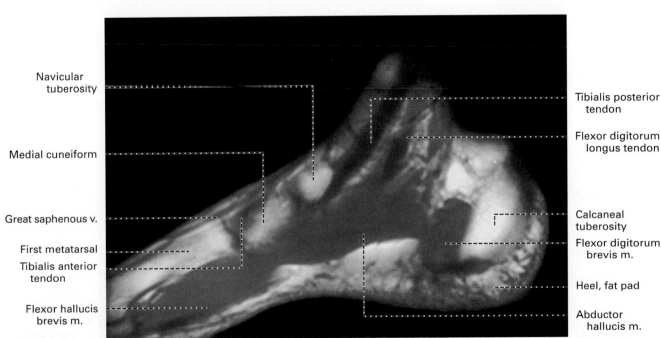

Navicular tuberosity

Medial cuneiform

Great saphenous v.

First metatarsal

Tibialis anterior tendon

Flexor hallucis brevis m.

Tibialis posterior tendon

Flexor digitorum longus tendon

Calcaneal tuberosity

Flexor digitorum brevis m.

Heel, fat pad

Abductor hallucis m.

Figure 18.3.3

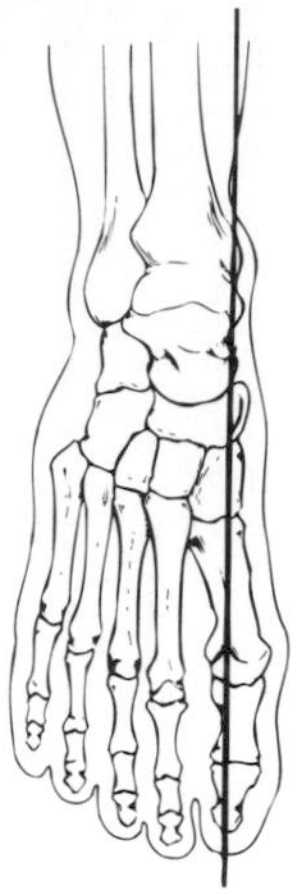

1. The long flexor tendons are located posterior to the medial malleolus and are arranged from anterior to posterior in the following order: (1) tibialis posterior tendon, (2) flexor digitorum longus tendon, and (3) flexor hallucis longus tendon.

2. The flexor hallucis longus tendon courses inferior to the sustentaculum tali.

3. Distally the flexor hallucis longus tendon is seen surrounded by flexor hallucis brevis (medial and lateral heads).

4. Note the branches of the plantar artery and nerve crossing flexor hallucis longus as they enter the foot.

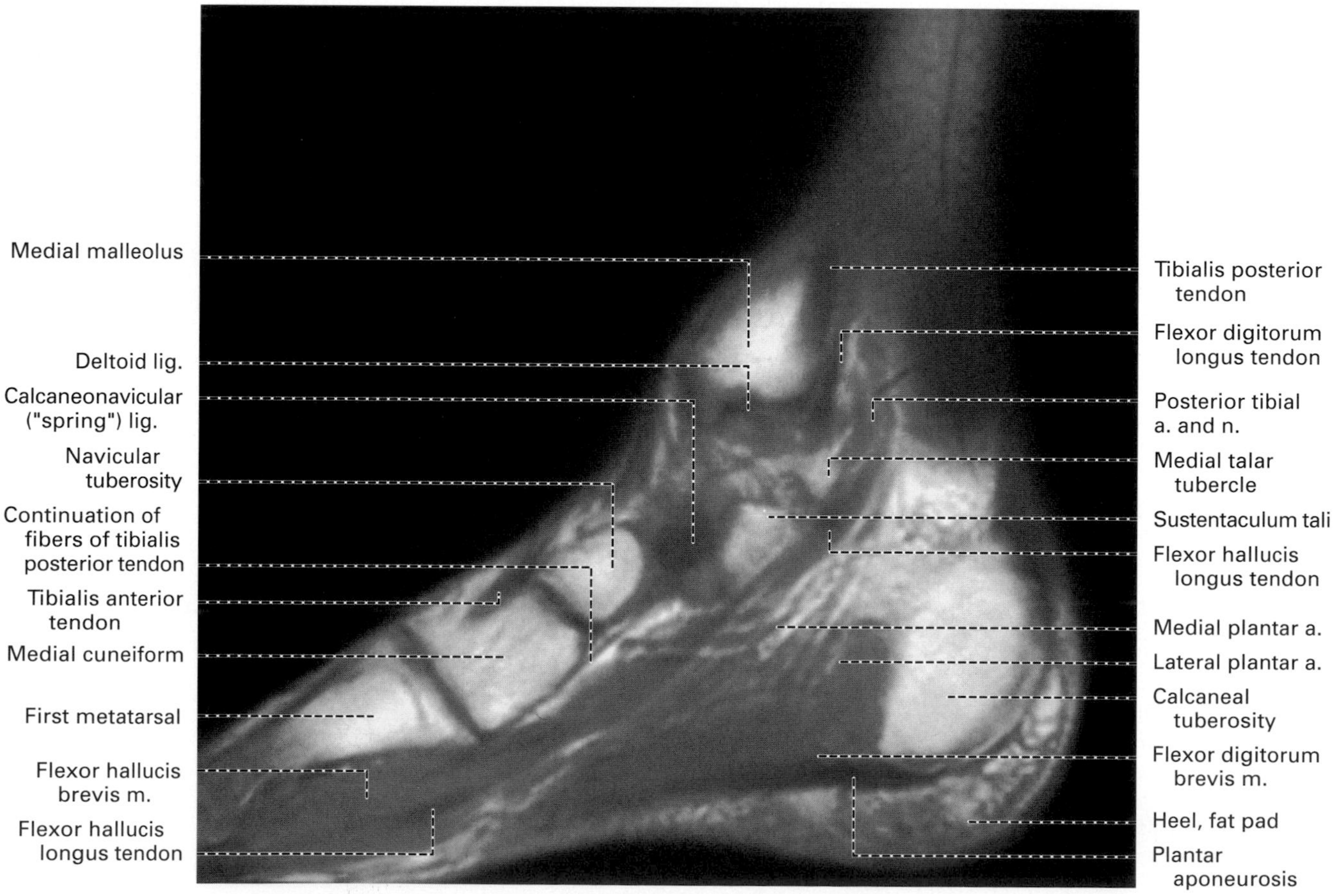
Medial malleolus
Deltoid lig.
Calcaneonavicular ("spring") lig.
Navicular tuberosity
Continuation of fibers of tibialis posterior tendon
Tibialis anterior tendon
Medial cuneiform
First metatarsal
Flexor hallucis brevis m.
Flexor hallucis longus tendon
Tibialis posterior tendon
Flexor digitorum longus tendon
Posterior tibial a. and n.
Medial talar tubercle
Sustentaculum tali
Flexor hallucis longus tendon
Medial plantar a.
Lateral plantar a.
Calcaneal tuberosity
Flexor digitorum brevis m.
Heel, fat pad
Plantar aponeurosis

1. The calcaneal (Achilles) tendon is partially demonstrated in this section.

2. The flexor digitorum brevis and quadratus plantae are closely related and difficult to separate.

3. The course of flexor hallucis longus in the midfoot is well demonstrated.

4. The thick muscle lateral to the first metatarsal is the oblique head of the adductor hallucis.

Figure 18.3.4

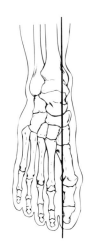

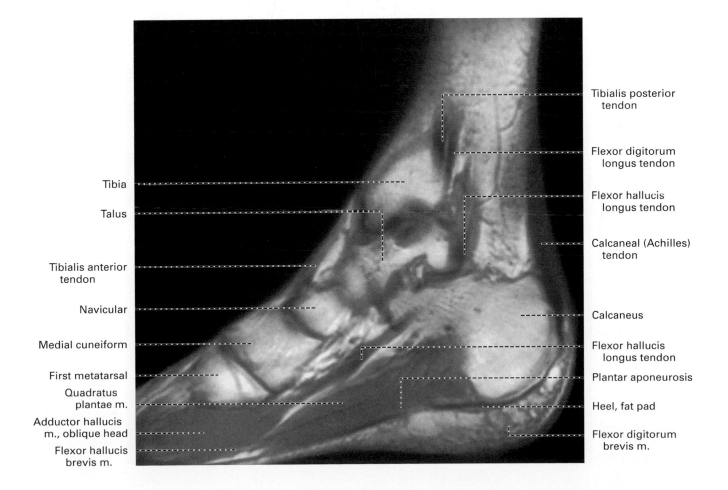

Tibialis posterior tendon

Flexor digitorum longus tendon

Flexor hallucis longus tendon

Calcaneal (Achilles) tendon

Calcaneus

Flexor hallucis longus tendon

Plantar aponeurosis

Heel, fat pad

Flexor digitorum brevis m.

Tibia

Talus

Tibialis anterior tendon

Navicular

Medial cuneiform

First metatarsal

Quadratus plantae m.

Adductor hallucis m., oblique head

Flexor hallucis brevis m.

Figure 18.3.5

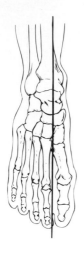

1. The calcaneal (Achilles) tendon is outlined in its entirety.

2. All three long flexor tendons are seen posterior to the distal tibia.

3. The posterior (lateral) and middle (medial) subtalar joints are demonstrated in this section.

4. Note the tibialis anterior tendon coursing obliquely anterior to the talus.

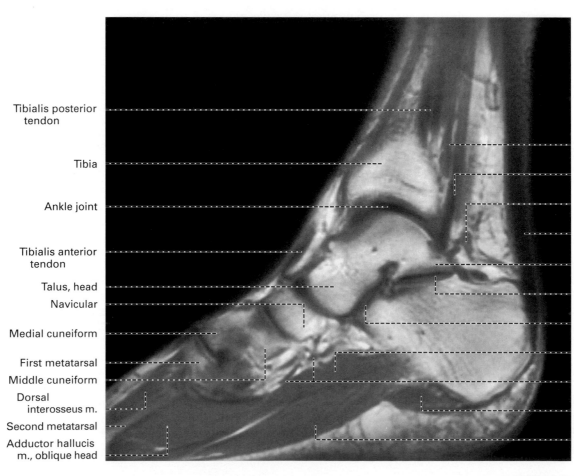

Tibialis posterior tendon

Tibia

Ankle joint

Tibialis anterior tendon

Talus, head

Navicular

Medial cuneiform

First metatarsal

Middle cuneiform

Dorsal interosseus m.

Second metatarsal

Adductor hallucis m., oblique head

Flexor digitorum longus tendon

Flexor hallucis longus tendon

Communicating a. from peroneal a.

Calcaneal (Achilles) tendon

Lateral talar tubercle

Posterior subtalar joint

Medial (middle) subtalar joint

Quadratus plantae m.

Medial plantar a., branches

Abductor digiti minimi m.

Flexor digitorum brevis m.

1. Note the position of the long flexor muscles posterior to the distal tibia.

2. The tarsal sinus is seen separating the posterior (lateral) and middle (medial) subtalar joints.

3. The soleus muscle is situated between the long flexor muscles and the calcaneal (Achilles) tendon.

4. Peroneus longus courses deep in the foot toward its insertion at the plantar aspect of the medial cuneiform and base of the first metatarsal.

5. Note the rich vascular network deep in the arch of the foot between quadratus plantae and the tarsal bones.

Figure 18.3.6

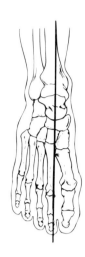

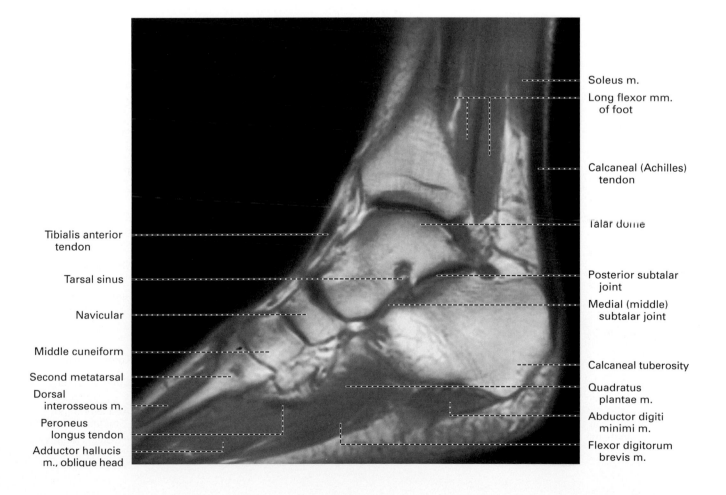

Soleus m.

Long flexor mm. of foot

Calcaneal (Achilles) tendon

Talar dome

Posterior subtalar joint

Medial (middle) subtalar joint

Calcaneal tuberosity

Quadratus plantae m.

Abductor digiti minimi m.

Flexor digitorum brevis m.

Tibialis anterior tendon

Tarsal sinus

Navicular

Middle cuneiform

Second metatarsal

Dorsal interosseous m.

Peroneus longus tendon

Adductor hallucis m., oblique head

Figure 18.3.7

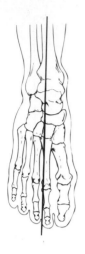

1. As the sections move laterally, the cuboid and abductor digiti minimi muscles can be seen.

2. Note the peroneus longus tendon as it exits the cuboid sulcus and proceeds medially.

3. The os trigonum represents an ununited posterior process of the talus (lateral tubercle) and is the talar attachment site for the posterior talofibular ligament.

4. Note the superficial position of the tibialis anterior tendon, which can normally be palpated under the skin.

5. The small anterior subtalar joint is depicted in this section. In some individuals, this joint is incorporated with the middle (medial) subtalar joint.

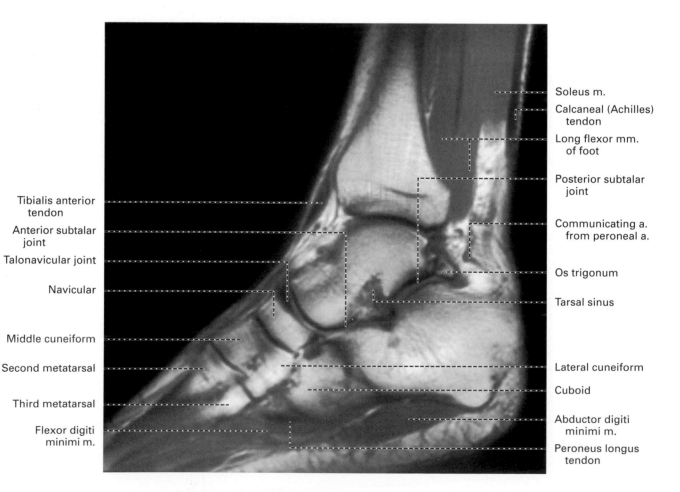

1. The anterior and posterior subtalar joints are demonstrated in this section.

2. The peroneus longus tendon is seen within the cuboid sulcus.

3. Anterior to the ankle joint, extensor hallucis longus and tibialis anterior tendons are both outlined.

Figure 18.3.8

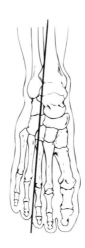

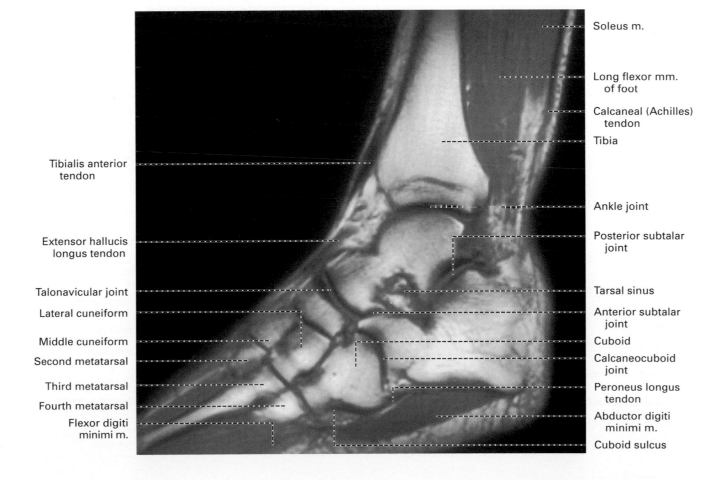

- Soleus m.
- Long flexor mm. of foot
- Calcaneal (Achilles) tendon
- Tibia
- Ankle joint
- Posterior subtalar joint
- Tarsal sinus
- Anterior subtalar joint
- Cuboid
- Calcaneocuboid joint
- Peroneus longus tendon
- Abductor digiti minimi m.
- Cuboid sulcus

Tibialis anterior tendon

Extensor hallucis longus tendon

Talonavicular joint

Lateral cuneiform

Middle cuneiform

Second metatarsal

Third metatarsal

Fourth metatarsal

Flexor digiti minimi m.

Figure 18.3.9

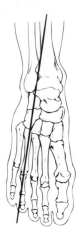

1. Flexor hallucis longus originates on the posteromedial surface of the fibula. Adjacent to it is peroneus brevis, which originates on the posterolateral surface of the fibula.

2. This section passes through the lateral process of the talus.

3. The peroneus longus tendon is seen within the cuboid sulcus.

4. Extensor digitorum brevis is seen on the dorsum of the foot.

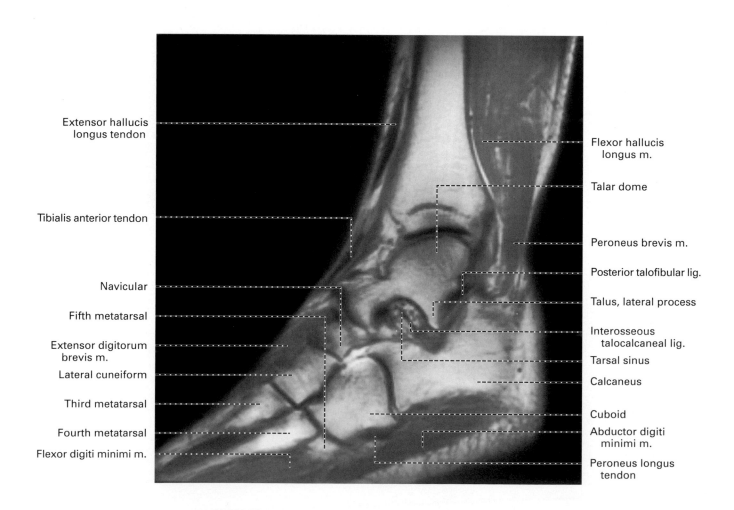

1. The peroneal tendons course posterior and inferior to the lateral malleolus.

2. In the midfoot, the peroneus longus tendon is seen entering the cuboid sulcus.

3. The interosseous talocalcaneal ligament is demonstrated connecting the two bones.

4. The muscles of the anterior compartment begin to appear in this section.

5. A portion of the bifurcate ligament is shown as it extends from the calcaneus to insert on the navicular.

Figure 18.3.10

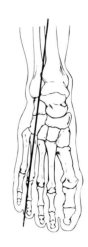

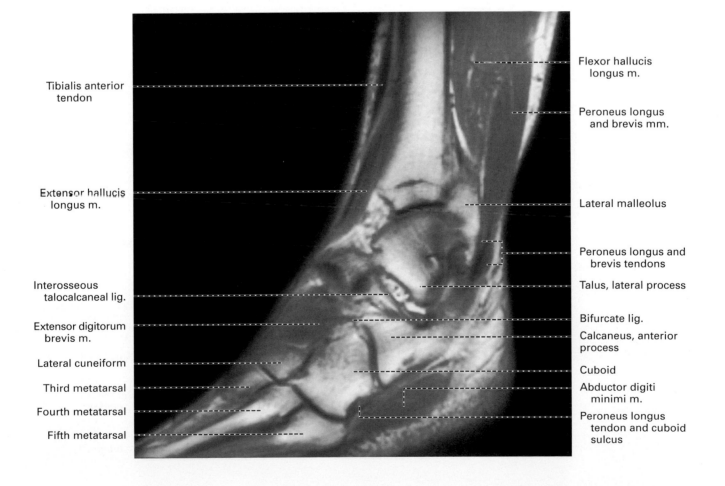

Tibialis anterior tendon

Extensor hallucis longus m.

Interosseous talocalcaneal lig.

Extensor digitorum brevis m.

Lateral cuneiform

Third metatarsal

Fourth metatarsal

Fifth metatarsal

Flexor hallucis longus m.

Peroneus longus and brevis mm.

Lateral malleolus

Peroneus longus and brevis tendons

Talus, lateral process

Bifurcate lig.

Calcaneus, anterior process

Cuboid

Abductor digiti minimi m.

Peroneus longus tendon and cuboid sulcus

Figure 18.3.11

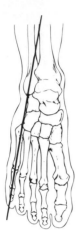

1. The peroneus longus and brevis muscles are closely related and difficult to separate.

2. The peroneus longus tendon courses posterior and inferior to the peroneus brevis tendon.

3. The peroneus longus tendon disappears from this section at the level of the calcaneus as it courses medially to enter the cuboid sulcus.

4. Peroneus brevis continues distally to insert onto the tuberosity of the fifth metatarsal.

5. Note the origin of the extensor digitorum brevis muscle from the anterior superior aspect of the calcaneus.

6. The long extensors of the foot are situated in the anterior compartment of the leg between the tibia and fibula.

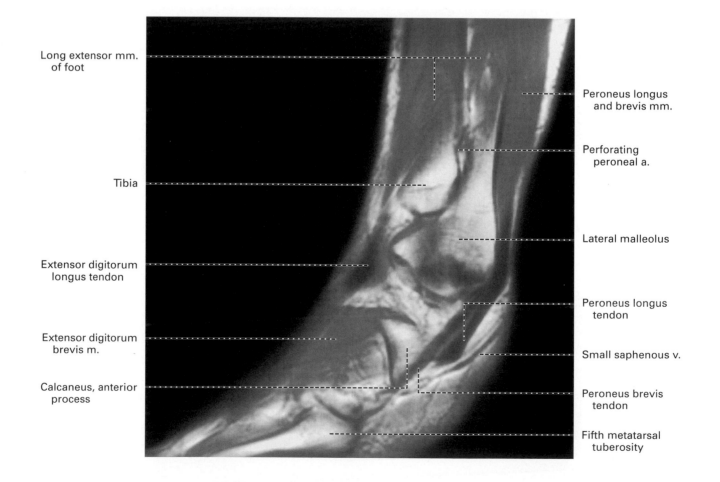

1. Note the relation of the peroneal muscles and tendons to the fibula and lateral malleolus.

2. The extensor digitorum longus tendon starts in the lower end of the anterior compartment, courses over the anterolateral aspect of the ankle, and divides into four smaller tendons on the dorsolateral aspect of the foot.

Figure 18.3.12

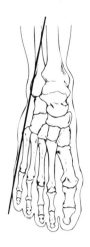

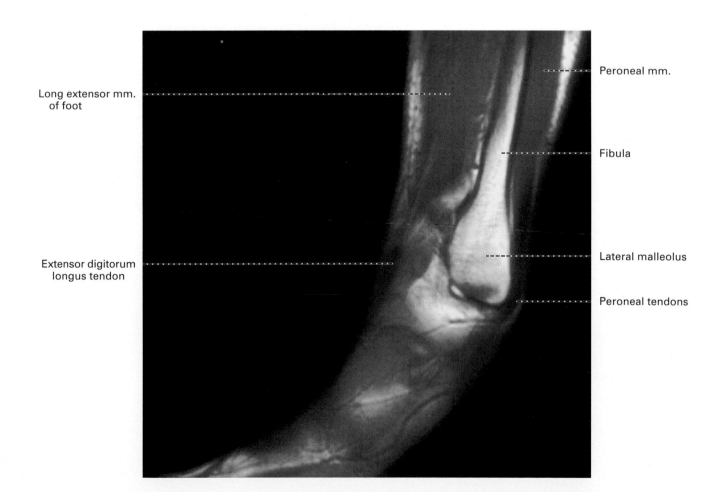

Long extensor mm. of foot

Extensor digitorum longus tendon

Peroneal mm.

Fibula

Lateral malleolus

Peroneal tendons

Chapter 19

FOOT

Table 19-1. Muscles of the Foot

Muscle	Origin	Insertion	Nerve Supply	Arterial Supply
Muscles of the dorsum				
Extensor digitorum brevis	Distal part of the lateral and superior surfaces of the calcaneus and the apex of the inferior extensor retinaculum	As the fiber bundles extend distally they become grouped into four bellies. Those fibers of the most medial and largest belly are known as extensor hallucis brevis. The tendon of this muscle inserts onto the base of the first metatarsal. The remaining fiber bundles are not so distinctly isolated as described for the great toe and their insertions are variable. The second toe inserts mainly onto the middle of the back of the base of the proximal phalanx and is often united with the tendon of the long extensor. The remaining three tendons are usually fused with the lateral margins of the corresponding tendons of the long extensor near the bases of the three middle phalanges and usually to the bases of the proximal phalanges of the corresponding toe.	Deep peroneal	Anterior tibial, dorsalis pedis
Muscles of the sole				
Flexor digitorum brevis	Medial process of the tuber calcanei, posterior third of the plantar aponeurosis, and the medial and lateral intermuscular septa	The tendons of the short (brevis) flexors pass superficial to those of the long flexor into the osteofibrous canals on the flexor surface of the digits. On the proximal phalanx of each toe the tendon of the short flexor divides and forms an opening through which the tendon of the long flexor passes. The tendons of the short flexor insert onto the base of the middle phalanx.	Surface near the medial edge of the muscle	Lateral plantar
Muscles attached to tendons of flexor digitorum longus				
Quadratus plantae (flexor accessorius)	Two heads, a small lateral and a large medial one. The lateral head arises from an elongated tendon from the lateral process of the tuberosity of the calcaneus, and from the lateral margin of the long plantar ligament. The medial head originates from the medial surface of the calcaneus in front of the tuberosity and from adjacent ligaments.	The two heads are separated at their origin by a short triangular space. The heads fuse to form a single belly but the fiber bundles of each head are separately inserted. From the lateral head the fibers insert into the lateral margin of the flexor tendon. The medial head inserts as an aponeurosis into the deep surface of the flexor tendon.	Lateral plantar nerve branch that passes obliquely across the superficial surface of the muscle parallel with the tendon of flexor digitorum longus	Lateral plantar

Continues

Table 19-1. *(Continued)*

Muscle	Origin	Insertion	Nerve Supply	Arterial Supply
Lumbricals	The three lateral lumbricals arise from the adjacent sides of the digital tendons of flexor digitorum longus. The first lumbrical arises on the medial margin of the second toe.	The fiber bundles of each muscle converge on both sides of a tendon that becomes free near the metatarsophalangeal joint and is inserted onto the medial side of the proximal phalanx of the appropriate toe. A tendinous expansion is inserted into the aponeurosis of the extensor muscle.	The three lateral lumbricals are usually supplied by branches of the deep ramus of the lateral plantar nerve. The medial lumbrical is supplied by the first common plantar digital branch of the medial plantar nerve. This nerve may supply the two more medial muscles, or the medial muscles may receive a double nerve supply.	Lateral plantar and plantar metatarsal
Intrinsic muscles of the great toe				
Abductor hallucis	Medial border of the medial process of the tuber calcanei, the deep surface of adjacent fascia, the flexor retinaculum, the septum between the muscle and the flexor digitorum brevis, the fibrous arch that extends on the deep surface of the muscle, and the long flexor tendons from the calcaneus to the navicular bone	Along with the tendon of the medial belly of flexor brevis onto the base of the proximal phalanx of the great toe. A tendinous expansion usually is joined to the extensor tendon.	Branch of medial plantar nerve	Medial plantar
Flexor hallucis brevis	Tendon attached to the first, second, and third cuneiform bones. The lateral fibers continue into the plantar calcaneocuboid ligament and the medial fibers into the expansion of the tendon of tibialis posterior.	The muscle has two bellies. The tendon of the medial belly passes obliquely, to be inserted into the tendon of abductor hallucis and, by a short tendon, into the medial part of the plantar surface of the base of the proximal phalanx. This tendon contains a sesamoid bone. The lateral belly joins the tendon of the oblique head of the abductor, and the two muscles insert, by a common tendon, which also contains a sesamoid bone, into the lateral part of the plantar surface of the base of the proximal phalanx.	Branch from the medial plantar or first plantar digital nerve. Rarely the lateral body may receive a branch from the lateral plantar nerve.	Medial plantar
Abductor hallucis (oblique head)	Tuberosity of the cuboid and the sheath of the tendon of peroneus longus, the plantar calcaneocuboid ligament, the third cuneiform, bases of the second and third metatarsals, and a fibrous arch that extends from the plantar calcaneocuboid ligament to the fascia on the interosseous muscles	By a flat tendon that is inserted in common with that of flexor brevis onto the lateral part of the plantar surface of the base of the proximal phalanx, and by a slip into the aponeurosis of the long extensor muscle on the back of the great toe	Branch of the deep ramus of the lateral plantar	Medial plantar

Continues

Table 19-1. *(Continued)*

Muscle	Origin	Insertion	Nerve Supply	Arterial Supply
Abductor hallucis (transverse head)	Joint capsules of the third, fourth, and fifth metatarsophalangeal joints and the deep transverse metatarsal ligaments	By a common tendon that splits and passes on each side of the tendon of the oblique head and is inserted into the sheath on the tendon of the long flexor of the great toe	Branch from the deep ramus of the lateral plantar	Medial plantar
Intrinsic muscles of the little toe				
Abductor digiti minimi	Lateral and medial processes of the tuber calcanei and the lateral and plantar surface of the body of the bone in front of these, the lateral intermuscular septum, the deep surface of the lateral plantar fascia, and the fibrous band extending from the calcaneus to the lateral side of the base of the fifth metatarsal bone	Onto the lateral surface of the proximal phalanx of the little toe and the metatarsophalangeal capsule. A slip may extend to the extensor tendon. The muscle usually glides over the tuberosity of the fifth metatarsal but may provide a second fasciculus that attaches to this bone (abductor osseus metatarsi quinti).	Lateral plantar	Posterior tibial
Flexor digiti minimi brevis	Sheath of peroneus longus, the tuberosity of the cuboid, and base of the fifth metatarsal	By short tendinous bands onto the base of the proximal phalanx of the little toe, the capsule of the corresponding joint, and the aponeurosis on the dorsal surface of the toe	Branch from superficial ramus of lateral plantar	Lateral plantar
Opponens digiti minimi	An inconstant muscle, it may arise from the sheath of peroneus longus and tuberosity of the cuboid by a thin tendon that passes over the tuberosity of the fifth metatarsal.	Onto the lateral surface of the fifth metatarsal	Branch from nerve to flexor brevis and the superficial ramus of lateral plantar	Plantar metatarsal
Interosseous muscles				
Interosseous, dorsal	Each of the three lateral dorsal interosseous muscles arise from the sides of the shaft and plantar surface of the bases of the metatarsal bones bounding the space in which each lies, from the fascia covering it dorsally, and from the fibrous prolongations from the long plantar ligament. The first (medial) has a similar origin except that its medial origin is by a tendinous slip from the peroneus longus tendon and occasionally by fiber bundles from the medial side of the proximal end of the first metatarsal.	The first and second interosseous muscles onto each side of the base of the proximal phalanx of the second toe; the third and fourth onto the lateral side of the bases of the proximal phalanges of the third and fourth toes. Each tendon adheres to the capsule of the adjacent joint.	Deep branch of the lateral plantar. The interosseous muscles of the fourth interspace are usually supplied by a branch from the superficial ramus of the lateral plantar.	Deep plantar
Interosseous, plantar	The plantar interosseous muscle arises from the proximal third of the medial plantar surface of the shaft, from the base of the metatarsal on which it lies, and from the fascial expansions of the long plantar ligament.	Onto a tubercle on the medial side of the base of the proximal phalanx of the digit to which it goes		Deep plantar

1. This section is toward the dorsum of the foot and shows the origin of the extensor digitorum brevis muscle from the anterolateral and superior aspect of the calcaneus.

2. Flexor hallucis longus and flexor digitorum longus tendons are seen as they course distally. At this level, which is superior to their crossing, the flexor hallucis longus tendon is lateral to the flexor digitorum tendon.

Figure 19.1.1

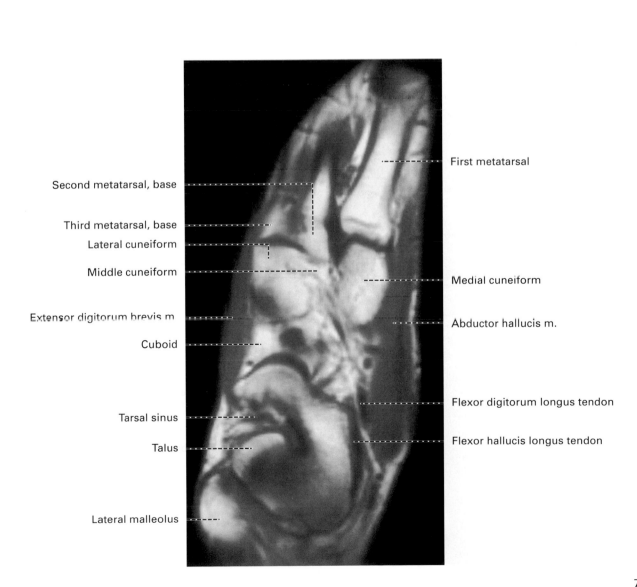

Second metatarsal, base

Third metatarsal, base

Lateral cuneiform

Middle cuneiform

Extensor digitorum brevis m

Cuboid

Tarsal sinus

Talus

Lateral malleolus

First metatarsal

Medial cuneiform

Abductor hallucis m.

Flexor digitorum longus tendon

Flexor hallucis longus tendon

Figure 19.1.6

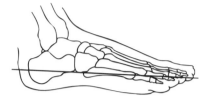

1. The flexor digitorum brevis muscle ends in the midfoot and divides into the short flexor tendons. The tendons of the short and long flexors are difficult to distinguish.

2. Flexor digitorum brevis is seen at its origin from the calcaneal tuberosity and in the midfoot immediately before it divides into its tendons.

3. Immediately medial to the origin of flexor digitorum brevis the medial head of quadratus plantae is demonstrated.

4. Flexor digiti minimi is seen medial to the fifth metatarsal.

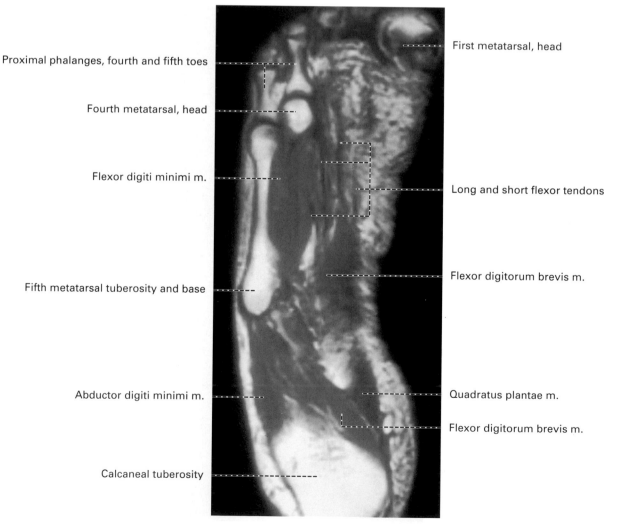

1. This section is through the fifth ray; the other rays are located superiorly.

2. Flexor digiti minimi, abductor digiti minimi, and flexor digitorum brevis muscles are partially demonstrated.

3. Both the longitudinal and transverse arches of the foot can be appreciated in this section.

Figure 19.1.7

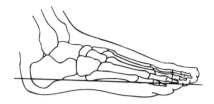

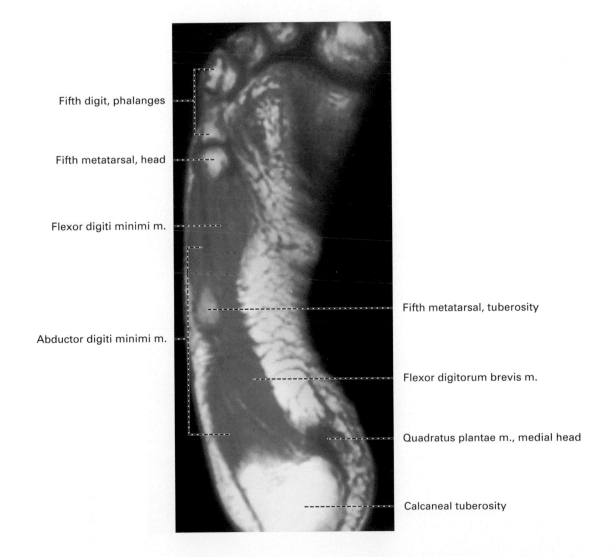

Fifth digit, phalanges

Fifth metatarsal, head

Flexor digiti minimi m.

Abductor digiti minimi m.

Fifth metatarsal, tuberosity

Flexor digitorum brevis m.

Quadratus plantae m., medial head

Calcaneal tuberosity

Figure 19.1.8

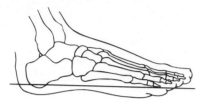

1. The lateral aspect of the foot is inferior to the medial aspect because of the presence of a transverse arch that is more pronounced at the midfoot.

2. Note the origin of abductor digiti minimi from the tuberosity of the calcaneus.

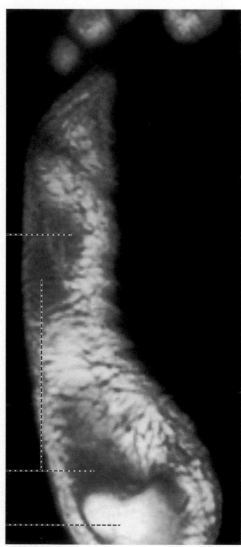

Flexor digiti minimi m.

Abductor digiti minimi m.

Calcaneal tuberosity

1. The deltoid ligament represents a collection of deep and superficial ligaments. The superficial ligaments include the tibionavicular, tibiocalcaneal, and posterior tibiotalar ligaments. A deep ligament, the anterior tibiotalar ligament, is seen as it attaches to the deep sulcus along the medial talar wall.

2. This is a helpful mnemonic for remembering the structures posterior to the medial malleolus: "Tom, Dick, and nervous Harry" (T, tibialis posterior tendon; D, flexor digitorum longus tendon; n, neurovascular branches of the tibial nerve and the posterior tibial artery, the medial and lateral plantar nerves and vessels; and H, flexor hallucis longus tendon.)

3. The tendons around the medial malleolus are superficial to the deltoid ligament and deep to the inferior flexor retinaculum.

4. Flexor hallucis longus lies in the posterior sulcus of the talus. This talar recess is bordered by a medial tubercle (receives the posterior tibiotalar ligament) and a lateral tubercle, also known as the posterior process, which receives fibers from the posterior talofibular ligament. The os trigonum is thought to represent an ununited lateral tubercle.

5. The superior peroneal retinaculum is demonstrated posterior to the lateral malleolus.

6. The sural nerve courses with the lesser saphenous vein.

Figure 19.2.1

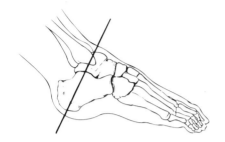

Extensor hallucis longus tendon

Extensor digitorum longus tendon
Peroneus tertius m.

Anterior tibiofibular lig.

Lateral malleolus

Talus

Posterior talofibular lig.

Peroneus longus and brevis tendons
Superior peroneal retinaculum
Calcaneofibular lig.

Lesser saphenous v.

Sural n.

Posterior talocalcaneal joint

Tibialis anterior tendon

Dorsalis pedis a.

Deep peroneal n.
Greater saphenous v.
Medial malleolus, tip

Deltoid lig. (superficial tibionavicular lig.)

Deltoid lig. (deep anterior tibiotalar lig.)

Flexor retinaculum

Deltoid lig. (superficial posterior tibiotalar lig.)

Tibialis posterior tendon

Flexor digitorum longus tendon

Talus, medial tubercle

Posterior sulcus

Medial and lateral plantar aa./nn., branches

Flexor hallucis longus tendon

Talus, lateral tubercle

Calcaneus

Calcaneal (Achilles) tendon insertion

Figure 19.2.2

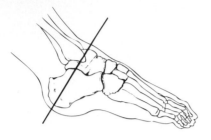

1. Abductor hallucis, one of the intrinsic muscles of the sole of the foot, arises from the medial surface of the body of the calcaneus and the medial process of the calcaneal tuberosity. It covers the entrance of the plantar nerves and vessels into the sole of the foot. It is at this level that the posterior tibial vessels become the medial and lateral plantar vessels and the tibial nerve becomes the medial and lateral plantar nerves.

2. Flexor hallucis longus tendon has its own retinaculum.

Extensor digitorum longus tendon

Peroneus tertius tendon

Talus

Posterior talocalcaneal joint

Lateral malleolus

Calcaneofibular lig.

Peroneus longus and brevis tendons

Superior peroneal retinaculum

Lesser saphenous v.

Sural n.

Tibialis anterior tendon

Extensor hallucis longus tendon

Greater saphenous v.
Dorsalis pedis a.
Deep peroneal n.
Deltoid lig. (anterior tibial lig.)

Flexor retinaculum
Deltoid lig., superficial fibers

Tibialis posterior tendon

Flexor digitorum longus tendon

Flexor retinaculum

Flexor hallucis longus tendon

Medial plantar a., n.

Lateral plantar a., n.

Retinaculum for flexor hallucis
longus tendon

Abductor hallucis m.

Calcaneus

1. The medial posterior and superior margin of the tarsal sinus can be seen in this section. It is formed by the paired opposing sulci of the talus and the calcaneus. It has an oblique course from posterosuperomedial to anteroinferolateral between the middle and posterior talocalcaneal articulations. It contains the interosseous talocalcaneal ligament.

2. The flexor retinaculum has a broad posterior extension attaching to the medial process of the calcaneus.

3. Peroneus longus (PL) tendon is usually posterior (P) and lateral (L) to peroneus brevis tendon (memory aid).

4. The calcaneofibular ligament is clearly demonstrated as it courses posteriorly, deep to the peroneal tendons.

Figure 19.2.3

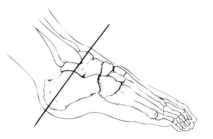

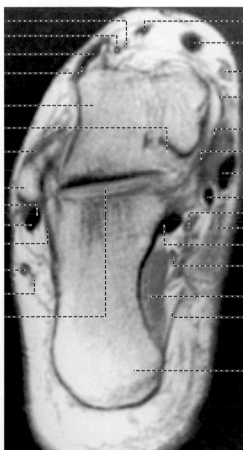

Dorsalis pedis a.	Extensor hallucis longus tendon
Deep peroneal n.	Tibialis anterior tendon
Extensor digitorum longus tendon	
Peroneus tertius tendon	Greater saphenous v.
	Flexor retinaculum
Talus	
Tarsal sinus	Superficial deltoid lig.
Anterior talofibular lig.	Deep deltoid lig.
	Tibialis posterior tendon
Lateral malleolus	Flexor digitorum longus tendon
Peroneus brevis tendon	Medial plantar n. and vessels
Peroneus longus tendon	Flexor retinaculum
Calcaneofibular lig.	Flexor hallucis longus tendon
Lesser saphenous v.	Lateral plantar n. and vessels
Sural n.	Abductor hallucis m.
Posterior talocalcaneal joint	Flexor retinaculum
	Calcaneus

Figure 19.2.8

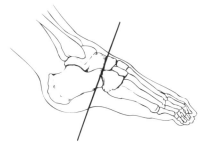

1. Flexor digitorum longus and flexor hallucis longus tendons are adjacent in this image. Further distally these tendons will cross to reach their destinations. This usually occurs at the level of the navicular.

2. The short calcaneocuboid component of the bifurcate ligament lies on the medial and dorsal aspect of that joint.

3. Extensor digitorum longus tendons are closely applied to extensor digitorum brevis muscle.

4. The long plantar ligament is seen in cross section deep to abductor digiti minimi and flexor digitorum brevis adjacent to the plantar medial surface of the calcaneus.

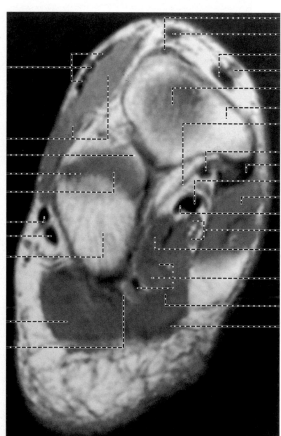

Extensor digitorum longus tendon

Extensor digitorum brevis m.
Cuboid
Calcaneocuboid joint
Calcaneocuboid lig. (part of bifurcate lig.)
Peroneus brevis tendon
Peroneus longus tendon
Calcaneus

Abductor digiti minimi m.
Long plantar lig.

Dorsal tibionavicular lig.
Extensor hallucis longus tendon
Tibialis anterior tendon
Greater saphenous v.
Talonavicular joint
Navicular tuberosity
Plantar calcaneonavicular ("spring") lig.
Additional slip of tibialis
Tibialis posterior tendon
Flexor digitorum longus tendon
Abductor hallucis m.
Flexor hallucis longus tendon
Medial plantar a., n.
Quadratus plantae m.

Lateral plantar a., n.

Flexor digitorum brevis m.
Plantar aponeurosis

1. Tibialis anterior tendon appears progressively more ovoid and flat as it approaches its insertion on the medial and plantar surfaces of the medial cuneiform and the base of the first metatarsal.

2. Multiple insertion slips of tibialis posterior tendon extend to the cuneiforms after the main portion of the tendon has inserted on the navicular tuberosity.

3. Flexor hallucis longus passes dorsal to flexor digitorum longus as they cross.

4. Abductor digiti minimi is the most prominent plantar muscle at this level.

5. The calcaneocuboid and cuboidonavicular joints are imaged at this level. The dorsal cuboidonavicular ligament is also demonstrated.

6. The strong plantar calcaneocuboid ligament is demonstrated in this section.

Figure 19.2.9

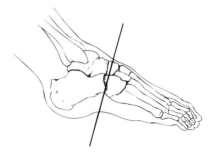

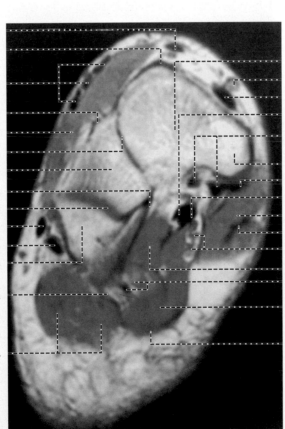

Extensor hallucis longus tendon
Dorsal talonavicular lig.

Extensor digitorum longus tendons

Dorsal cuboidonavicular lig.
Extensor digitorum brevis m.
Cuboidonavicular joint
Cuboid

Plantar calcaneocuboid lig.
Calcaneocuboid joint
Peroneus brevis tendon
Peroneus longus tendon
Calcaneus

Long plantar lig.

Abductor digiti minimi m.

Navicular
Greater saphenous v.
Tibialis anterior tendon
Flexor hallucis longus tendon
Additional slips of tibialis posterior tendon
Navicular tuberosity
Tibialis posterior tendon
Flexor digitorum longus tendon
Abductor hallucis m.
Abductor hallucis tendon
Medial plantar a., n.
Quadratus plantae m.
Lateral plantar a., n.
Flexor digitorum brevis m.

Plantar aponeurosis

Figure 19.2.10

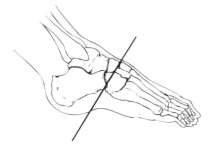

1. This section is at the level of the navicular-cuneiform joints. The navicular possesses three separate articular facets for the three cuneiform bones.

2. Observe that flexor hallucis longus crosses flexor digitorum longus on the dorsal surface of the latter.

3. Tibialis anterior tendon is now closely applied to the navicular as it forms the navicular-medial cuneiform joint. It will insert on the medial cuneiform and first metatarsal base.

4. Note the prominent slip of the tibialis posterior tendon continuing toward its insertion on the plantar surface of the lateral cuneiform. The distal plantar aspect of the navicular forms a groove or sulcus for this slip.

5. Slips of the plantar calcaneocuboid ligament are still observed. Fibers from the long plantar ligament are also identified.

6. Peroneus longus tendon begins its oblique course across the deep sole of the foot. It courses along the bony floor of the foot to insert along the lateral aspect of the medial cuneiform and base of the first metatarsal. This involves passage in a groove for peroneus longus, formed by the peroneal trochlea in the calcaneus, and through the peroneal sulcus of the cuboid. The distal portion of the long plantar ligament serves as the plantar retinaculum for the peroneus longus tendon.

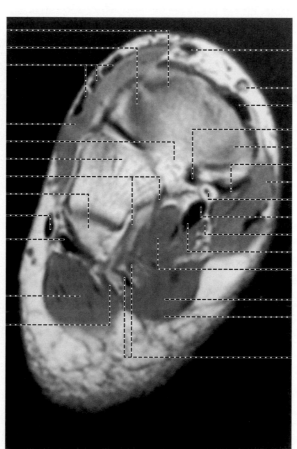

Navicular—middle cuneiform joint
Navicular—lateral cuneiform joint
Extensor digitorum longus tendons

Extensor digitorum brevis m.
Navicular
Cuboid
Plantar calcaneocuboid lig.
Calcaneus
Peroneus brevis tendon
Peroneus longus tendon

Abductor digiti minimi m.
Long plantar lig.

Extensor hallucis longus tendon

Greater saphenous v.
Tibialis anterior tendon

Tibialis posterior tendon, slip
Navicular—medial cuneiform joint
Tibialis posterior tendon
Abductor hallucis m.
Median plantar n., deep branch
Flexor hallucis longus tendon
Medial plantar a., n.
Flexor digitorum longus tendon
Quadratus plantae m.

Flexor digitorum brevis m.
Plantar aponeurosis

Lateral plantar a., n.

1. Since tibialis anterior tendon is initially along the dorsum of the midfoot it must migrate medially to reach the medial aspect of its insertion on the medial portion of the first metatarsal base and the medial cuneiform. Its insertion on the dorsomedial aspect of the medial cuneiform explains its dorsiflexing function of the foot at the talocrural joint.

2. The tendon of flexor digitorum longus is very closely applied to the quadratus plantae tendon on its dorsal surface.

3. The transverse arch of the midfoot (proximal transverse arch) occurs primarily at the cuneiforms. Note that the middle cuneiform appears and functions as a "keystone" of the arch.

Figure 19.2.11

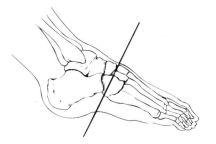

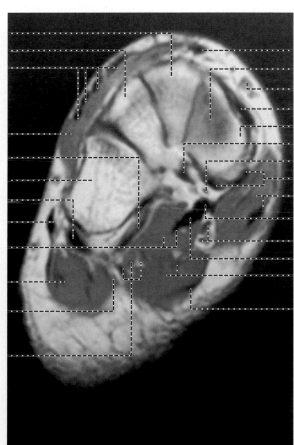

Middle cuneiform
Lateral cuneiform
Extensor digitorum longus tendons

Extensor digitorum brevis m.
Plantar calcaneocuboid lig.
Cuboid
Peroneus longus tendon
Peroneus brevis tendon
Quadratus plantae m. and tendon

Abductor digiti minimi m.

Long plantar lig.

Lateral plantar a., n.

Extensor hallucis longus tendon
Navicular—medial cuneiform joint
Greater saphenous v.
Tibialis anterior tendon
Medial cuneiform
Tibialis posterior tendon, slip
Median plantar n., deep branch
Tibialis posterior tendon
Abductor hallucis m. and tendon
Flexor hallucis longus tendon
Medial plantar a., n.
Flexor digitorum longus tendon
Flexor digitorum brevis m. and tendon
Plantar aponeurosis

Figure 19.2.12

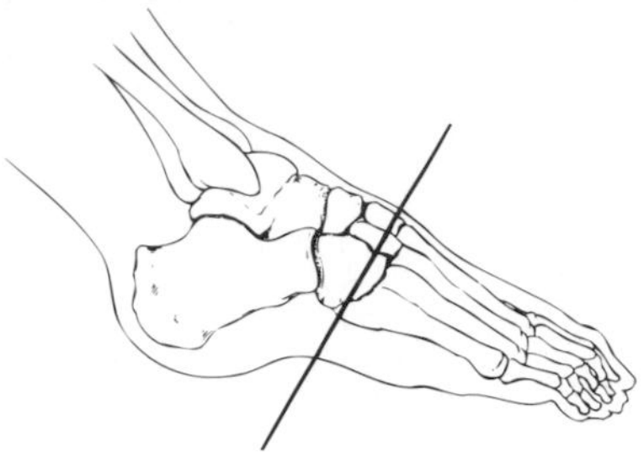

1. This section passes near the midfoot/forefoot junction.
2. Peroneus brevis inserts on the dorsolateral base of the fifth metatarsal.
3. Tibialis anterior tendon remains broad although a portion inserts on the medial cuneiform. The remainder will insert on the base of the first metatarsal.
4. Flexor hallucis brevis muscle and tendon are noted as they arise from continuations of slips of the tibialis posterior tendon.
5. Flexor digitorum longus tendon has divided into its digital tendons at this level.
6. Peroneus longus tendon courses obliquely along the plantar surface of the cuboid as it progresses medially and distally.
7. Some of the intercuneiform ligaments are demonstrated in this section. They and the intermetatarsal ligaments are important for maintaining the transverse arch of the foot.

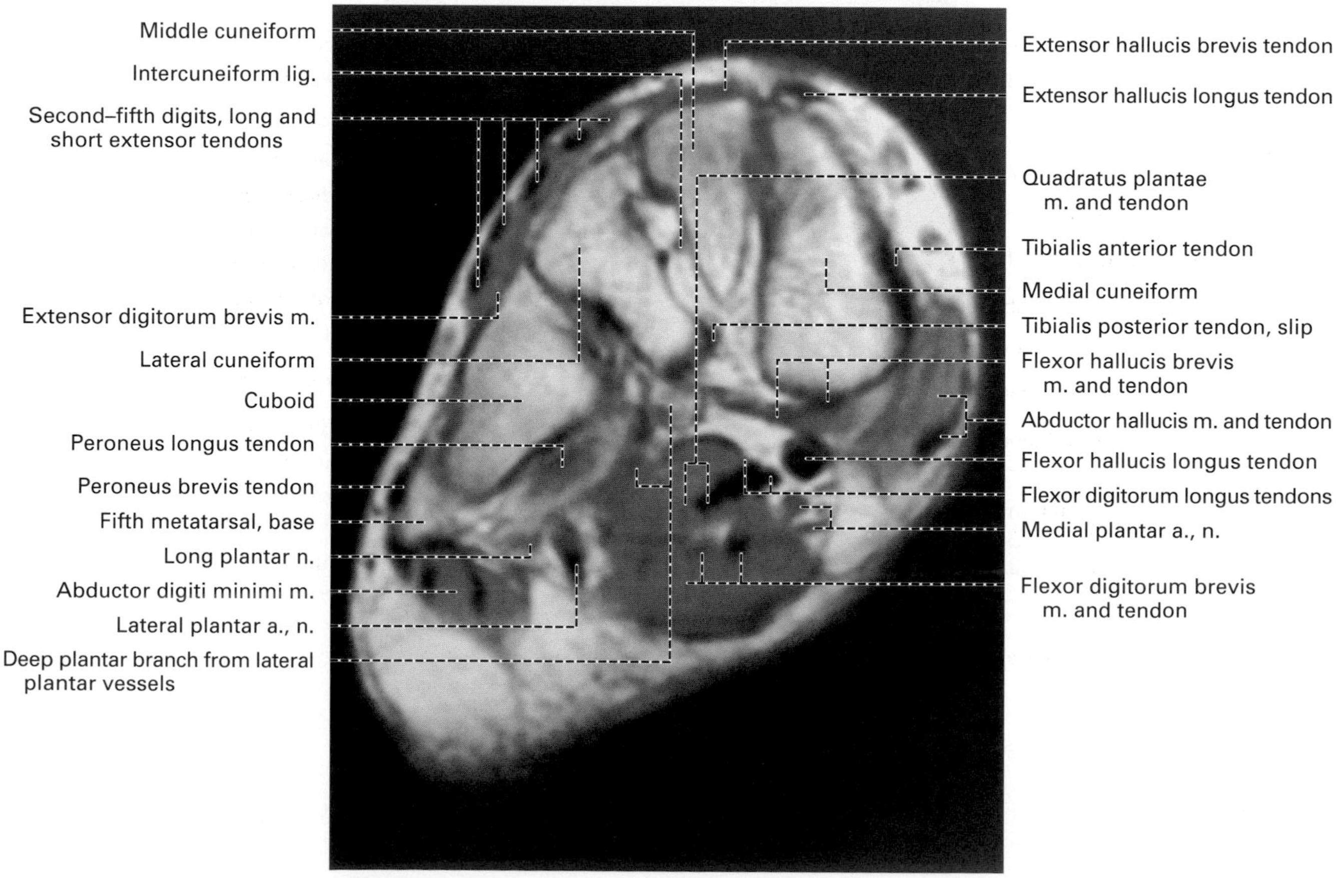
Middle cuneiform
Intercuneiform lig.
Second–fifth digits, long and short extensor tendons
Extensor digitorum brevis m.
Lateral cuneiform
Cuboid
Peroneus longus tendon
Peroneus brevis tendon
Fifth metatarsal, base
Long plantar n.
Abductor digiti minimi m.
Lateral plantar a., n.
Deep plantar branch from lateral plantar vessels
Extensor hallucis brevis tendon
Extensor hallucis longus tendon
Quadratus plantae m. and tendon
Tibialis anterior tendon
Medial cuneiform
Tibialis posterior tendon, slip
Flexor hallucis brevis m. and tendon
Abductor hallucis m. and tendon
Flexor hallucis longus tendon
Flexor digitorum longus tendons
Medial plantar a., n.
Flexor digitorum brevis m. and tendon

1. Adductor hallucis has two heads. The oblique head originates from the bases of the second through the fourth metatarsals and the sheath of the tendon of peroneus longus, as demonstrated here. The transverse head arises distally near the metatarsophalangeal joints.

2. The lateral plantar vessels are branching at this level.

3. Peroneus longus tendon is plantar to the cuboid, near the cuboid-fourth metatarsal joint, and is closely applied to the bone.

4. Flexor hallucis brevis is deep to flexor hallucis longus tendon. It develops a prominent muscle belly, which is "divided" into medial and lateral parts by the indentation caused by the tendon of flexor hallucis longus. These two "heads" continue distally and each develops its own tendons with separate sesamoids as is seen in more distal images.

5. The long plantar ligament is the longest of the ligaments of the tarsus. Its deep fibers attach to the cuboid while its more superficial portion extends to the metatarsal bases, forming a fibrous arch over the tendon of peroneus longus.

Figure 19.2.13

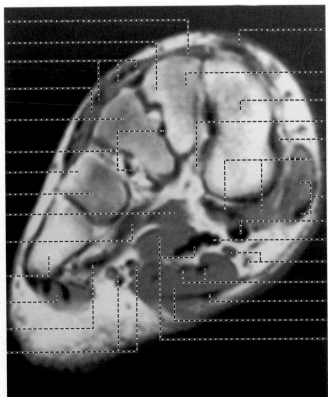

Extensor hallucis brevis tendon
Middle cuneiform
Digits, long and short extensor tendons
Extensor digitorum brevis m.
Third tarsometatarsal joint
Intercuneiform ligs.
Cuboid
Fourth tarsometatarsal joint
Adductor hallucis m., oblique head
Peroneus longus tendon
Fifth metatarsal, base
Abductor digiti minimi m.
Long plantar lig.
Branching lateral plantar aa., nn.

Extensor hallucis longus tendon
Second tarsometatarsal joint
Medial cuneiform
Deep plantar arch, branches
Tibialis anterior tendon
Flexor hallucis brevis m. and tendon
Abductor hallucis m. and tendon
Flexor hallucis longus tendon
Digits, long flexor tendons
Medial plantar a., n.
Digits, short flexor tendons
Plantar aponeurosis
Flexor digitorum brevis m.
Quadratus plantae m. and tendon

Figure 19.2.14

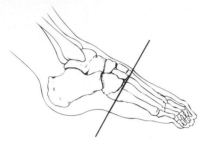

1. This section is at the first tarsometatarsal joint, which is the most distal of the tarsometatarsal joints.

2. Tibialis anterior tendon flattens and migrates to the posteromedial surface of the first metatarsal base. This explains how this muscle inverts and supinates the foot at the subtalar and midtarsal joints.

3. The medial migration of peroneus longus tendon is noted, now coursing on the plantar surfaces of the third and fourth metatarsal bases.

4. The short flexor of the little toe, flexor digiti minimi brevis, arises from the base of the fifth metatarsal as demonstrated here. At times some deep fibers of this muscle insert into the lateral part of the distal half of the fifth metatarsal; it is therefore termed opponens digiti minimi.

5. The long and short extensor tendons of the toe course together and are difficult to distinguish once they all become tendinous.

6. Flexor digitorum brevis remains muscular and plantar at this level, compared to flexor digitorum longus tendons.

7. The medial plantar nerves and vessels remain on the medial side of the long and short flexors of the toes and on the plantar side of the long and short flexors of the great toe.

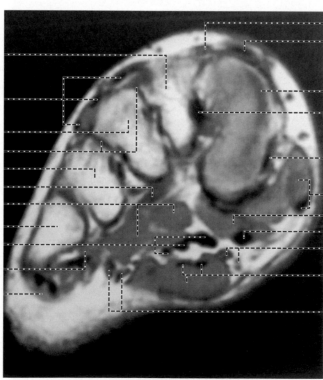

Second metatarsal, base

Second–fifth digits, long and short extensor tendons

Third metatarsal, base

Intermetatarsal joints

Fourth metatarsal, base

Peroneus longus tendon

Adductor hallucis m., oblique head

Fifth metatarsal, base

Digits, long flexor tendons

Flexor digiti minimi brevis m.

Abductor digiti minimi m.

Extensor hallucis brevis tendon

Extensor hallucis longus tendon

First tarsometatarsal joint

Intermetatarsal lig.

Tibialis anterior tendon

Abductor hallucis m. and tendon

Flexor hallucis brevis m.

Flexor hallucis longus tendon

Medial plantar a., n.

Flexor digitorum brevis m. and tendons

Lateral plantar a., n.

1. Note the insertion of peroneus longus tendon along the plantar base of the second metatarsal as well as the lateral surface of the first metatarsal base.

2. The lateral plantar nerves and vessels course lateral to the long and short flexor of the toes.

3. Adductor hallucis brevis (oblique head) becomes prominent in the plantar concavity of the forefoot.

Figure 19.2.15

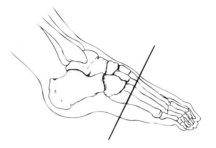

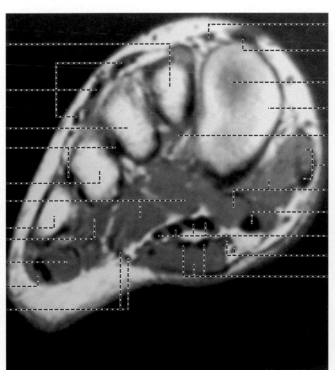

Second metatarsal

Second–fifth digits, long and short extensor tendons

Third metatarsal

Intermetatarsal ligs.

Fourth metatarsal

Adductor hallucis m., oblique head

Fifth metatarsal

Flexor digiti minimi brevis m.

Opponens digiti minimi m.

Abductor digiti minimi m.

Lateral plantar a., n.

Extensor hallucis brevis tendon

Extensor hallucis longus tendon

First tarsometatarsal joint

First metatarsal base

Peroneus longus tendon

Abductor hallucis m. and tendon

Flexor hallucis brevis m.

Flexor hallucis longus tendon

Flexor digitorum longus tendons

Medial plantar a., n.

Flexor digitorum brevis m. and tendons

Figure 19.2.16

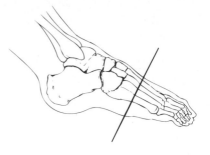

1. The first dorsal interosseous muscle is prominent at this level and is the largest of the four dorsal interossei.

2. Flexor hallucis brevis has become large at the level of the first metatarsal base. Its medial and lateral heads can be distinguished with the aid of the tendon of flexor hallucis longus on its plantar surface.

3. Abductor digiti minimi muscle is on the plantar and lateral surface of the fifth metatarsal.

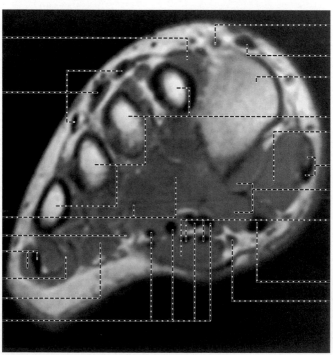

First dorsal interosseus m.

Second–fifth digits, long and short extensor tendons

Adductor hallucis m., oblique head

Lateral plantar a., n.

Abductor digiti minimi m. and tendon

Opponens digiti minimi m.

Flexor digiti minimi brevis m.

Flexor digitorum longus tendons

Extensor hallucis brevis tendon

Extensor hallucis longus tendon

First metatarsal, base

Second–fifth metatarsals

Flexor hallucis brevis m., medial head

Abductor hallucis m. and tendon

Flexor hallucis brevis m., lateral head

Flexor digitorum brevis m. and tendons

Flexor hallucis longus tendon

Medial plantar a., n.

1. This section is through the metatarsal shafts.

2. Coursing distally it is more difficult to distinguish flexor digiti minimi brevis from opponens digiti minimi.

3. All four dorsal interossei are identifiable. Each of these muscles is bipennate, with only one head arising from each adjacent metatarsal.

4. The three plantar interossei are also visible. They are unipennate and attach to the medial sides of the third, fourth, and fifth metatarsals. They function as adductors.

Figure 19.2.17

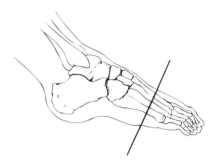

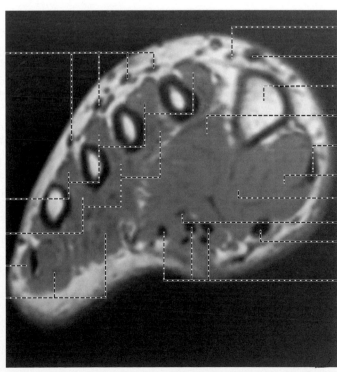

Long and short digital extensor tendons

Dorsal interosseous mm.

Plantar interosseous mm.

Abductor digiti minimi m. and tendon

Flexor and opponens digiti minimi mm.

Extensor hallucis brevis tendon

Extensor hallucis longus tendon

First metatarsal

Adductor hallucis m., oblique head

Abductor hallucis tendon

Flexor hallucis brevis m., medial head

Flexor hallucis brevis m., lateral head

Flexor digitorum longus tendons

Flexor hallucis longus tendon

Flexor digitorum brevis m. and tendons

Figure 19.2.18

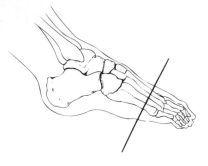

1. Near the distal metatarsals, proximal fibers from the transverse head of adductor hallucis are seen. They course medially to join the oblique head and insert on the proximal phalanx of the great toe.

2. The tendons of the long and short digital flexors blend at this level.

3. The proximal origin of the lumbricals arises from the medial aspect of the four digital tendons of flexor digitorum longus. As in the hand, their function is to flex the proximal phalanges at the metatarsophalangeal joints and extend the middle and distal phalanges at the interphalangeal joints.

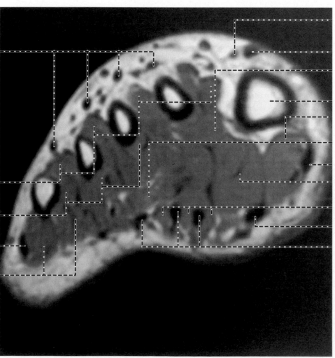

Extensor hallucis brevis tendon

Digits, long and short extensors

Extensor hallucis longus tendon

Adductor hallucis m., oblique head

First metatarsal

Flexor hallucis brevis m., medial head

Adductor hallucis m., transverse head

Abductor hallucis tendon

Dorsal interosseous mm.

Flexor hallucis brevis m., lateral head

Lumbrical mm.

Plantar interosseous mm.

Flexor hallucis longus tendon

Abductor digiti minimi tendon

Flexor digitorum brevis and longus tendons

Flexor and opponens digiti minimi mm.

1. The transverse head of adductor hallucis is apparent on this section. The two heads of this muscle join with each other and the lateral part of flexor hallucis brevis to insert along the base of the proximal phalanx of the great toe.

2. The short and long extensors of the digits are in the more superficial subcutaneous tissue as they progress distally over the metatarsophalangeal joints.

Figure 19.2.19

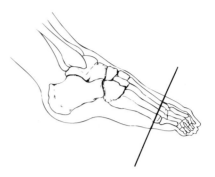

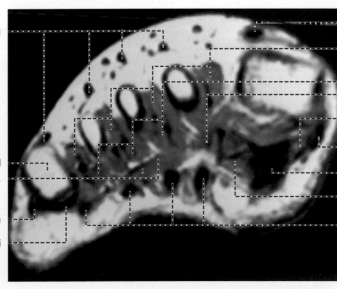

Digits, short and long extensor tendons

Fifth metatarsal, head

Adductor hallucis m., transverse head

Abductor digiti minimi tendon

Flexor and opponens digiti minimi tendons

Great toe, short and long extensor tendons

Dorsal interosseous mm.

Plantar interosseous mm.

Adductor hallucis m., oblique head

Flexor hallucis brevis m., medial head

Abductor hallucis tendon

Great toe, short and long flexor tendons

Flexor hallucis brevis m., lateral head

Digits, short and long flexor tendons

Figure 19.2.20

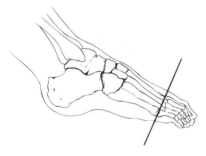

1. This section passes through the metatarsophalangeal joint of the little toe.

2. Note that the tendon of abductor hallucis blends with portions of the capsule of the metatarsophalangeal joint of the great toe.

3. The medial and lateral sesamoid bones of the tendons of the medial and lateral heads of flexor hallucis brevis are seen.

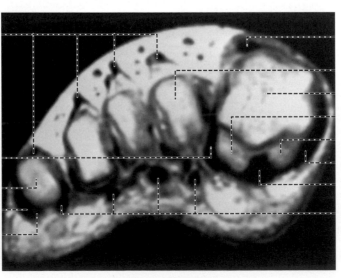

Digits, short and long extensor tendons

Adductor hallucis tendon

Fifth toe, metatarsophalangeal joint

Abductor digiti minimi tendon

Flexor and opponens digiti minimi tendons

Great toe, short and long extensor tendons

Second metatarsal, head

First metatarsal, head

Lateral sesamoid bone

Medial sesamoid bone

Abductor hallucis tendon

Flexor hallucis longus tendon

Digits, short and long flexor tendons

1. This section is at the level of the first through the fourth metatarsophalangeal joints and the proximal phalanx of the fifth toe.

2. Adductor hallucis tendon is adjacent to the tendon of the lateral head of flexor hallucis brevis.

3. Note the retinacula attaching the extensor tendons of capsules of the metatarsophalangeal joints.

Figure 19.2.21

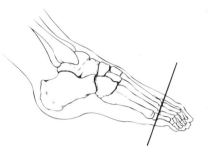

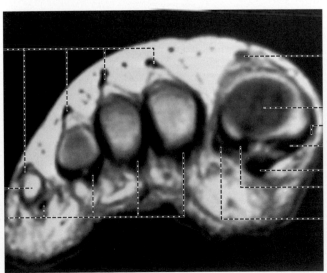

Digits, short and long extensor tendons

Great toe, extensor tendons

First metatarsophalangeal joint

Abductor hallucis tendon

Flexor hallucis brevis tendon, medial head

Flexor hallucis longus tendon

Flexor hallucis brevis tendon, lateral head

Fifth digit, proximal phalanx

Adductor hallucis tendon

Digits, short and long flexor tendons

Figure 19.2.22

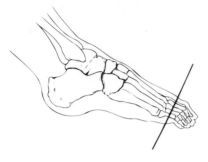

1. This level is near the insertion of abductor hallucis tendon and the medial head of flexor hallucis brevis onto the medial side of the base of the proximal phalanx of the great toe.

2. Similarly, adductor hallucis tendon (oblique and transverse heads) joins the lateral head of flexor hallucis brevis tendon and inserts onto the lateral side of the base of the proximal phalanx of the great toe.

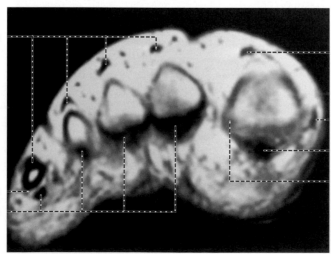

Digits, extensor tendons

Great toe, extensor tendons

Abductor hallucis tendon

Flexor hallucis longus tendon

Adductor hallucis tendons, insertion

Abductor digiti minimi tendon

Digits, flexor tendons

1. Abductor digiti minimi tendon inserts on the lateral aspect of the proximal phalanx of the little toe.

Figure 19.2.23

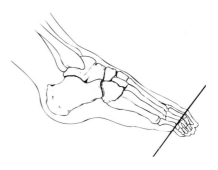

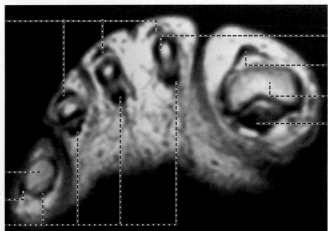

Second–fourth digits, extensor tendons

Second digit, proximal phalanx

Extensor hallucis longus tendon

Great toe, proximal phalanx

Flexor hallucis longus tendon

Middle phalanx of fifth digit, base

Abductor digiti minimi tendon, insertion

Second–fifth digits, flexor tendons

Figure 19.3.1

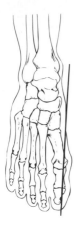

1. The abductor hallucis tendon is noted on this medial section. This tendon courses distally to insert at the base of the proximal phalanx of the great toe medially.

2. The flexor hallucis longus tendon is outlined at its insertion onto the base of the distal phalanx of the great toe.

3. The flexor hallucis longus tendon courses distally between the medial and lateral sesamoid bones.

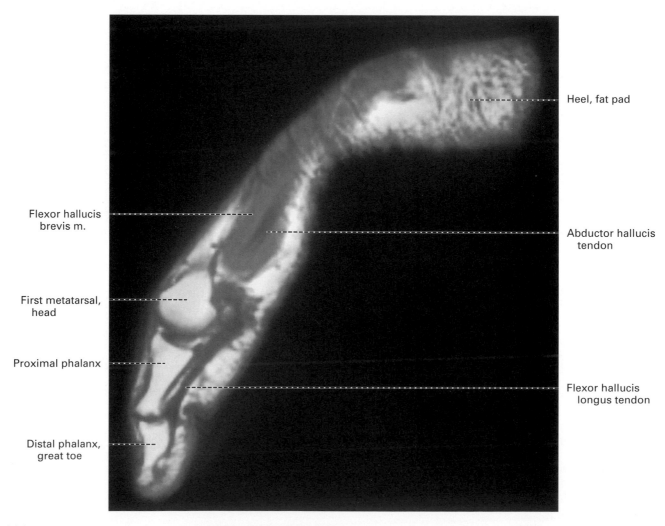

Flexor hallucis brevis m.

First metatarsal, head

Proximal phalanx

Distal phalanx, great toe

Heel, fat pad

Abductor hallucis tendon

Flexor hallucis longus tendon

1. This medial section shows the fleshy portions of the abductor hallucis and flexor hallucis brevis muscles.

2. The lateral sesamoid lies within the tendon of the lateral head of flexor hallucis brevis, which inserts onto the base of the proximal phalanx.

3. The tibialis anterior tendon is partially demonstrated in this section as it starts its insertion on the medial cuneiform and base of the first metatarsal.

Figure 19.3.2

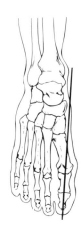

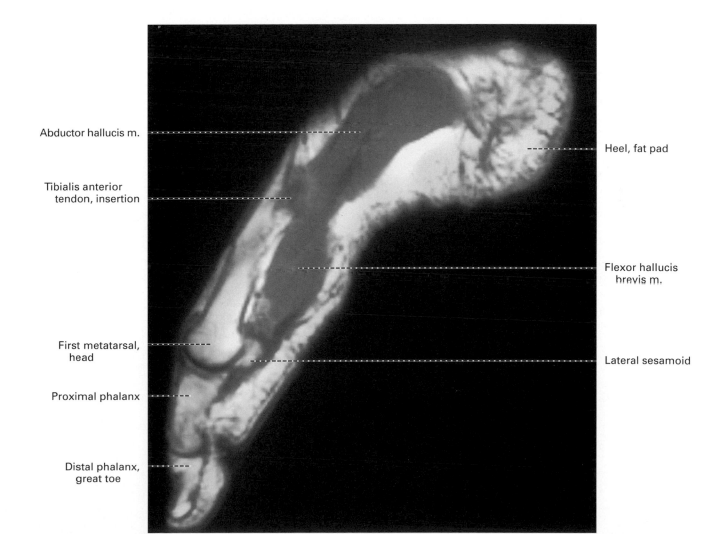

Abductor hallucis m.

Tibialis anterior tendon, insertion

First metatarsal, head

Proximal phalanx

Distal phalanx, great toe

Heel, fat pad

Flexor hallucis brevis m.

Lateral sesamoid

Figure 19.3.3

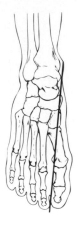

1. The tuberosity of the calcaneus is depicted. This serves as the origin of the plantar aponeurosis and the abductor hallucis, flexor digitorum brevis, quadratus plantae, and abductor digiti minimi muscles.

2. Note the insertion of the tibialis posterior tendon on the navicular and medial cuneiform.

3. The tibialis anterior tendon inserts on the medial cuneiform, and some fibers continue to insert on the base of the first metatarsal.

4. The belly of flexor hallucis brevis is also included in this section.

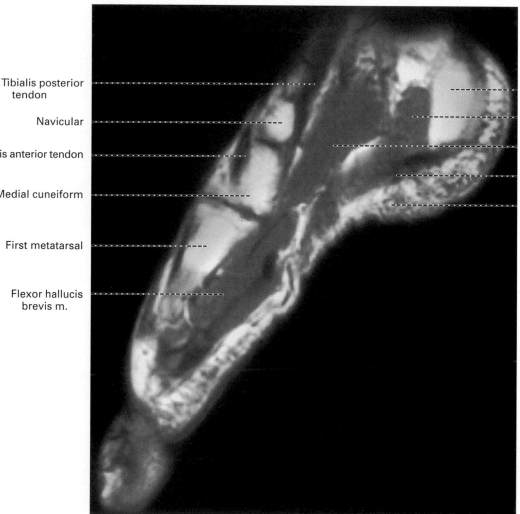

Tibialis posterior tendon

Navicular

Tibialis anterior tendon

Medial cuneiform

First metatarsal

Flexor hallucis brevis m.

Calcaneal tuberosity

Flexor digitorum brevis m.

Abductor hallucis m.

Plantar aponeurosis

Heel, fat pad

1. The course of the flexor hallucis longus tendon below the sustentaculum tali is demonstrated.

2. Note the close relation between flexor digitorum brevis and quadratus plantae muscles in the arch of the foot.

3. The adductor hallucis muscle is seen between the first and second metatarsals.

4. The distal portion of the flexor digitorum longus tendon is outlined as it courses to insert at the base of the distal phalanx of the second toe.

Figure 19.3.4

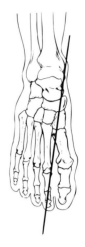

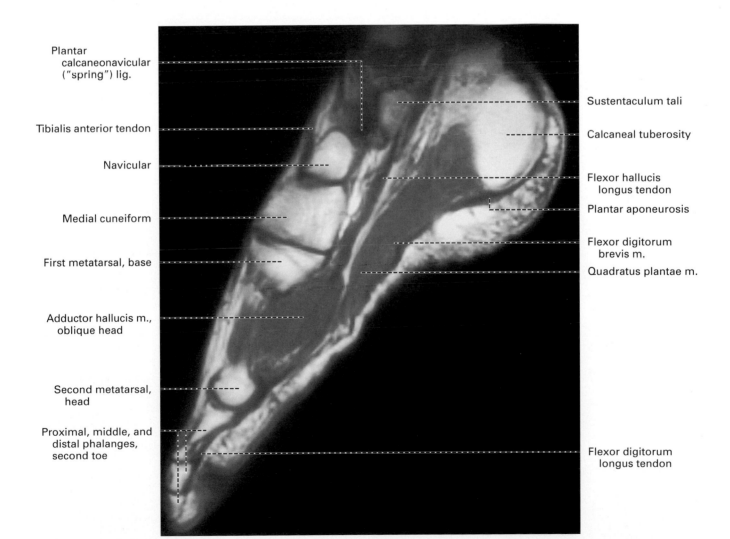

Plantar calcaneonavicular ("spring") lig.

Tibialis anterior tendon

Navicular

Medial cuneiform

First metatarsal, base

Adductor hallucis m., oblique head

Second metatarsal, head

Proximal, middle, and distal phalanges, second toe

Sustentaculum tali

Calcaneal tuberosity

Flexor hallucis longus tendon

Plantar aponeurosis

Flexor digitorum brevis m.

Quadratus plantae m.

Flexor digitorum longus tendon

Figure 19.3.5

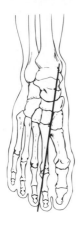

1. Note how the quadratus plantae muscle inserts on the tendon of the flexor digitorum longus.

2. In this section, abductor digiti minimi originates from the inferior aspect of the calcaneal tuberosity.

3. The calcaneal (Achilles) tendon inserts on the tuberosity of the calcaneus.

4. Note the belly of the first dorsal interosseous muscle with its origin from the second metatarsal. A portion of this muscle originates from the first metatarsal.

5. Tibialis anterior crosses over the head of the talus in this section.

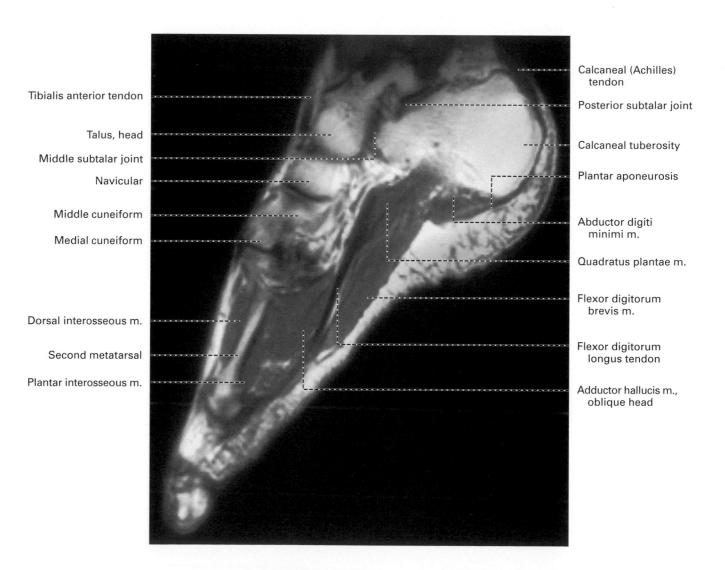

Tibialis anterior tendon

Talus, head
Middle subtalar joint
Navicular

Middle cuneiform

Medial cuneiform

Dorsal interosseous m.

Second metatarsal

Plantar interosseous m.

Calcaneal (Achilles) tendon
Posterior subtalar joint

Calcaneal tuberosity

Plantar aponeurosis

Abductor digiti minimi m.

Quadratus plantae m.

Flexor digitorum brevis m.

Flexor digitorum longus tendon

Adductor hallucis m., oblique head

Figure 19.3.6

1. The posterior (lateral) subtalar joint is included in this section.

2. The flexor digitorum brevis and quadratus plantae muscles are difficult to separate in this section.

3. The tarsal sinus and head of the talus are clearly delineated.

4. Note the relation of the tibialis anterior tendon to the head of the talus as this tendon courses inferior and medial to insert on the medial surface of the medial cuneiform and base of the first metatarsal.

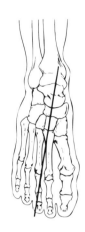

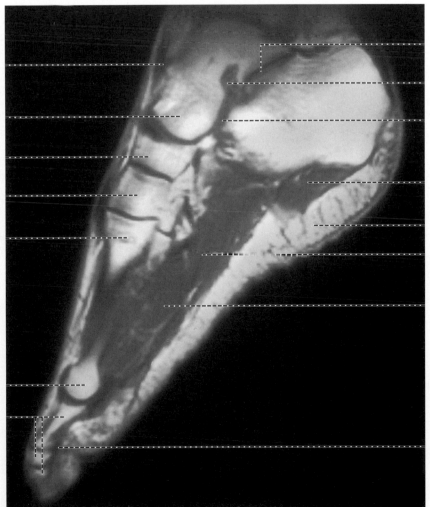

Tibialis anterior tendon

Talus, head

Navicular

Middle cuneiform

Second metatarsal, base

Third metatarsal, head

Proximal, middle, and distal phalanges, third toe

Posterior subtalar joint

Tarsal sinus

Middle subtalar joint

Abductor digiti minimi m.

Heel, fat pad

Flexor digitorum brevis and quadratus plantae mm.

Abductor hallucis m.

Flexor digitorum brevis tendon

Figure 19.3.7

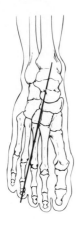

1. Both the posterior (lateral) and anterior subtalar joints are seen in this section.

2. Lumbrical and interosseous muscles can be identified.

3. Note the relation between the navicular and cuneiform bones.

4. The extensor hallucis longus tendon is seen on the dorsum of the foot.

5. The tendon of peroneus longus is seen entering the foot inferior to the cuboid.

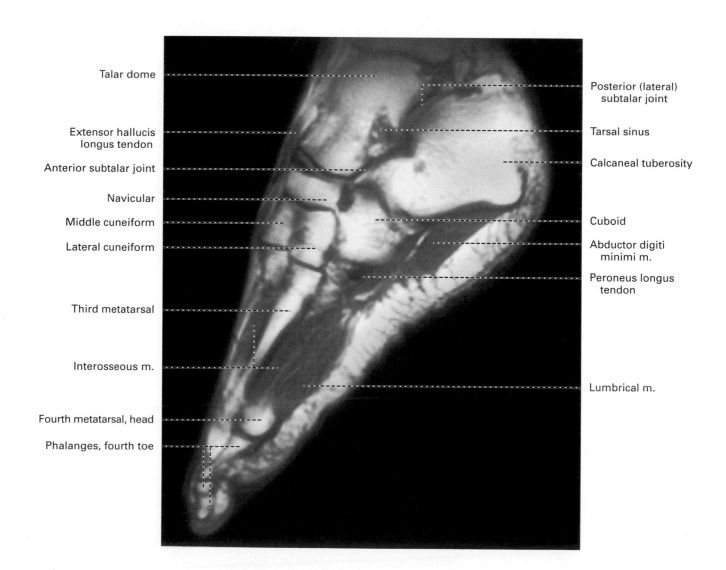

Talar dome

Extensor hallucis longus tendon

Anterior subtalar joint

Navicular

Middle cuneiform

Lateral cuneiform

Third metatarsal

Interosseous m.

Fourth metatarsal, head

Phalanges, fourth toe

Posterior (lateral) subtalar joint

Tarsal sinus

Calcaneal tuberosity

Cuboid

Abductor digiti minimi m.

Peroneus longus tendon

Lumbrical m.

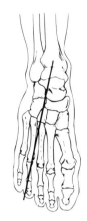

Figure 19.3.8

1. The lateral process of the talus and anterior process of the calcaneus are demonstrated.

2. The abductor digiti minimi and flexor digiti minimi muscles are noted over the lateral aspect of the foot.

3. Note the position of the cuboid between the calcaneus and fourth and fifth metatarsals.

4. The extensor hallucis longus tendon courses over the head of the talus.

5. The extensor digitorum brevis muscle is partially demonstrated.

6. The peroneus longus tendon is seen entering the cuboid sulcus.

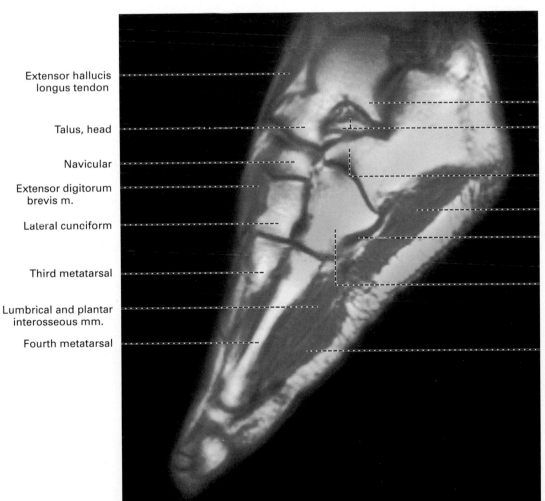

Figure 19.3.9

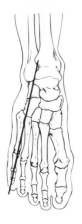

1. In this lateral section of the foot, the extensor digitorum longus tendon and extensor digitorum brevis muscle are well seen.

2. Abductor digiti minimi and flexor digiti minimi brevis muscles are situated over the lateral plantar aspect of the foot.

3. Peroneus longus is seen approaching the cuboid sulcus.

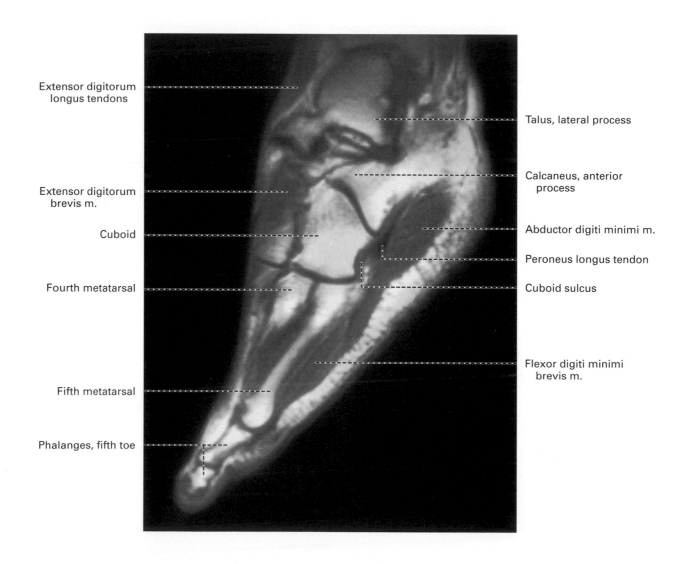

1. The peroneus longus and peroneus brevis tendons are outlined. The peroneus brevis tendon continues distally to insert onto the tuberosity of the fifth metatarsal. At the inferior lateral malleolus, the peroneus longus tendon lies posterior and lateral to the peroneus brevis tendon.

2. Flexor digiti minimi brevis lies on the plantar surface of the fifth metatarsal.

3. Note the origin of extensor digitorum brevis from the superior and lateral surface of the calcaneus (anterior process).

4. Extensor digitorum longus is demonstrated.

Figure 19.3.10

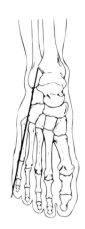

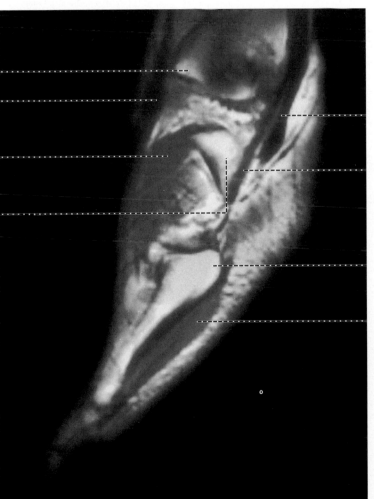

Talus, lateral process

Extensor digitorum longus tendon

Extensor digitorum brevis m.

Calcaneus, anterior process

Peroneus longus tendon

Peroneus brevis tendon

Fifth metatarsal, tuberosity

Flexor digiti minimi brevis m.

INDEX

Page numbers followed by t *indicate tables.*